SEASON OF BIRTH
ITS RELATION TO
HUMAN ABILITIES

SEASON OF BIRTH

ITS RELATION TO
HUMAN ABILITIES

ELLSWORTH
HUNTINGTON

YALE UNIVERSITY

Author of "Civilization and Climate,"
"Principles of Human Geography," *etc.*

New York
JOHN WILEY & SONS, INC.
LONDON: CHAPMAN & HALL, LIMITED
1938

PRINTED IN U. S. A.

PRESS OF
BRAUNWORTH & CO., INC.
BUILDERS OF BOOKS
BRIDGEPORT, CONN.

PREFACE

Two years ago, as part of a book entitled, *Civilization,* I planned to write a few pages on the effect of the seasons. Looking the matter up, I found some interesting suggestions as to birthdays of men of eminence, but nothing conclusive. Thinking to test the matter, I began gathering statistics. They proved so interesting that it seemed desirable to write an article about them. Further search made it clear that I had uncovered a great deposit of the richest kind of ore. Two years of work have made it possible to sink a trial shaft and make the preliminary assays which appear in the following pages. It is clear that further high-grade ore is available in large quantities for anyone who chooses to dig.

The first main result of the present study is what seems to be a convincing explanation of the highly puzzling fact that man has two different optima of temperature—physical and mental. Both appear to owe their origin to the selective effect of the climate in which the species *Homo sapiens* originated during the glacial period. The physical optimum apparently represents the season when conceptions were most likely to result in the birth of infants that were able to survive. The mental optimum represents the cooler season when births of this kind actually occurred.

The second main result takes the form of evidence which seems explicable only on the hypothesis that man inherits an extremely complex and delicate adjustment to climate and weather. This adjustment centers around four conditions. Two of these are the critical events of conception and birth. The third is the dangers to which the heat of summer exposes an infant. The fourth is the curious relation of low temperature not only to mental activity but also to the conception of persons who later display unusual intellectual

v

182265

ability. These relations dovetail together so perfectly that it seems as if they must play a great part not merely in our lives, but also in the scientific progress of the future.

This book is primarily a study of statistics. Nevertheless, statistical tables form only a minor item. Most of the statistics have been expressed in the form of diagrams which are much more important than the text. Diagrams have been used instead of tables because at a glance they bring out a great many relationships which even the most astute mathematician could not detect from the figures alone.

The amount of tabulation involved in the preparation of the diagrams has been enormous. It would never have been possible without the highly efficient and constructive assistance of Mr. Charles L. Ziegler who has been responsible for the greater part of the tabulation.

In addition to this I have been so fortunate as to have three most careful and interested secretarial assistants, Mrs. Jean Smith, Mrs. Ruth Mitchell, and Mrs. Greta Straton.

Another important line of assistance has come from a large number of institutions for the care of defectives and insane persons. The list of these is so long that it is placed in a separate appendix. Each of the persons and institutions there mentioned supplied data which in the aggregate represent hundreds of hours of work. And finally, Dr. D. L. Belding, Dr. Neil A. Dayton, Professor Stephen S. Visher, and Mr. Carl P. Tobey have voluntarily sent me statistical tables which they thought might be of use. To all of these kindly helpers I would express the hope that other people may treat them as well as they have treated me.

E. H.

New Haven, Conn.
June, 1937

CONTENTS

SEASON OF BIRTH
ITS RELATION TO HUMAN ABILITIES

Chapter I

SEASON OF BIRTH

The season at which people are born has far greater importance than is generally supposed. At certain seasons the number of babies is unusually large, and the proportion of girls is high. The children born at those times have a low death rate in infancy, and the survivors live to more than the average age. In addition, the births of persons who achieve distinction rise to high proportions. Such conditions indicate not only that reproduction is stimulated at certain seasons, but that the children then born are more vigorous than those born at other times. There is also a little hint that mentally defective children are born in unusual numbers at this same time. Such children, however, as well as those that are malformed show a more decided tendency toward birth at the time of year when evidences of vigor are least numerous. At the most favorable season, however, criminals and persons who suffer from insanity and tuberculosis, as well as those who achieve eminence, show an unusual number of births. This, too, is an evidence that reproduction is especially stimulated at certain seasons. It apparently means that the unstable or weak types of parents from whom such people are most likely to be born respond to the influence of the seasons more completely than do more stable or stronger types.

The season when these seemingly contradictory, but really harmonious, conditions occur among the most advanced nations is the late winter or early spring—February or March.

Its place in the calendar is apparently set by the fact that man is an animal. Like practically all animals he has a definite seasonal rhythm of reproduction. This rhythm appears to be an inheritance from a very ancient time, when relatively few children survived unless they were born at the best season. In our present sophisticated state children are born at all seasons, but on an average the ones born at the height of the old animal rhythm have an advantage over those born in its other phases. This book might be better if the author had been born in February instead of September.

The pioneer work of Lehmann and Pedersen (1907), and the fuller studies described by the author in *Civilization and Climate* (1915, 1924), indicated that the European races, at least, have two definite climatic optima, or sets of most favorable conditions. One optimum is physical, and its chief feature is an average temperature of 60° F. to 65° for day and night together. The other is mental and has been variously estimated as from 39° to 54°. In both cases humidity, variability of temperature, and other conditions such as sunlight play a part, but temperature is the dominant factor. Ever since these optima were discovered students have been greatly puzzled to know why a mean temperature of 60° to 65° F. rather than 70° to 75° or 50° to 55°, let us say, became established as the temperature at which man is best able to maintain a perfect balance between the production and loss of heat. Why should metabolism and the glandular functions proceed most perfectly at that particular temperature? A still more puzzling question has been: Why are there two optima of temperature? Why does not the brain function best at the same temperature as the other organs? This question has been so hard to answer that many people have totally rejected the idea of a mental optimum distinct from the physical optimum.

The most surprising feature of the study of births described in this book is that it seems to provide an answer to all these questions. Not till most of the facts had been collected and the book was more than half written did I realize that the conditions governing season of birth among our primitive ancestry apparently explain the mental as well as the physical optimum of temperature. Our bodies apparently function best at the temperature which prevailed in primitive times at the mating season, for children conceived at that season were best able to survive. This gives us a physical optimum. Our minds function best at the temperature which prevailed in primitive times at the normal season of birth. At that time, more than any other, the survival of the new generation depended upon the alertness of the parents. Thus a mental optimum became established at a temperature lower than the physical optimum. Such in brief are the main conclusions to which we are led by the facts set forth in this book.

It has long been known that the number of births varies from season to season, and that essentially the same variations repeat themselves from year to year. Sixty years ago an unnamed writer in a bulletin of the Department of Health in Michigan pointed out that this is presumably due to the weather or some other widely acting seasonal conditions, and not, as was often supposed, to the fact that marriages take place in great numbers in certain months. Since then we have gone a long way. Heape (1907) pointed out that in Cuba and elsewhere there is evidence of a distinct seasonal rhythm of births. Westermarck (1921) in his famous *History of Marriage* devotes an entire chapter to evidence of such a rhythm. He shows that it is especially strong among primitive people, and varies according to the climate. Ellis (1934) has amplified Westermarck's work. Many others have added bits of information here and there.

In 1912, Gini put the matter upon a sound statistical basis by publishing a large number of tables showing that the seasonal distribution of births varies greatly from country to country and even from one decade to another in the same country. He also discussed the interesting hypothesis that eminent people tend to be born in unusual numbers from January to March. He noted, to be sure, that a similar tendency is widely spread among ordinary people in many nations, but he thought that the tendency was especially strong among people of the highest eminence. He found, for example, that among minor lights, such as modern Italian senators, the tendency to be born in the late winter or early spring is not so strong as among more famous people. Therefore he concluded that there may be some connection between birth in cold weather and eminence.

Various other writers have followed Gini's lead. In 1925, Alleyne Ireland found that in a list of 2650 eminent persons selected by himself 382 were born in February in contrast to only 149 during June. He concluded, however, that during most of the year the seasonal course of births among men of genius is about the same as among the population as a whole. Since births in February represent conceptions in May, he thought that the excess of eminent births in February merely shows that "May, when all nature renews itself, is the natural breeding-month."

Kassel (1929) criticizes Ireland, but on the basis of a much smaller, although more carefully selected, list of eminent people he makes some rather sweeping suggestions. "For genius as a whole there are no favorite birth months, since the genius of the world seeks much the same month for the beginning of life as the ordinary population." He says, however, that the favorite month of birth for American and French genius is January; for German genius, December; for English, October; and for Italian, March. He even goes so far as to suggest that famous clergymen, poets, and scientists tend to be born in the half of the year from July onward, while philosophers, statesmen, and soldiers tend to be born in the other half. He recognizes, however, that, since his data pertain to only 431 persons all told, they cannot be very conclusive.

Pintner (1933) has thrown further light on this problem. When he uses the same data as Gini and Kassel, namely, a list of the world's most famous people, he finds, as they do, that eminent people show a strong tendency to be born in

January, February, or March.   He gets a similar result from the 1300 or more scientists who are starred in *American Men of Science* because their colleagues consider them leaders. Using all of the 9000 scientists in that book, however, he finds that, although the first quarter of the year has more than the average number of births, it does not have so many proportionally as does the early fall.   He found a similar seasonal distribution of births on tabulating 12,000 people in *Who's Who in America*.   Desiring to test the matter in another way, Pintner tabulated the intelligence quotients of thousands of school children in or near New York.   He found that on an average the children born in May and June, and also in September and October, have a slightly higher I.Q. than those born at other seasons.   Among the 17,000 children whom he investigated the average intelligence quotient was lowest among those born in January and February.   This is quite contrary to what one would expect from the seasonal distribution of the births of people of great eminence.   It is not contrary, however, to what we should expect when defective and inadequate groups as well as gifted groups are taken into account.

The study of the season of birth of defectives has hitherto led to equally contradictory conclusions.   Petersen (1934, 1935, 1936) presents data which seem to show that the births of physical defectives vary from season to season in about the same way as those of persons of unusual ability, the maximum of conceptions occurring in April, and of births in January. The conception of feeble-minded persons, he says (1935), follows quite an opposite course, with a minimum in April and a maximum in October.   He also concludes that the births of sufferers from schizophrenic insanity (dementia praecox) follow the same seasonal course as those of intellectual leaders.   Nevertheless, sufferers from manic-depressive insanity show a different seasonal distribution of births with a maximum of conceptions in midsummer.   Murphy (1936), from a comparison of defectives with their brothers and sisters, comes to the opposite conclusion—namely, that the season of birth has no relation to physical defects. Other investigators have also discussed the problem of the season of birth of defectives, but the statistical basis of all the studies except those of Gini and Pintner has been small.

Another phase of the problem is equally puzzling. The seasonal distribution of births varies not only from country to country, but also from decade to decade in the same country. In this respect births are like deaths, but there is one essential difference. In every country in the world, so far as I have been able to discover, the deaths fluctuate in harmony with the weather. Cold weather, especially if it is very dry, is always accompanied or soon followed by a rise in the death rate. Very hot weather, especially if it is humid, is accompanied by a similar but more sudden increase in deaths. Besson (1935) has shown that in Paris one can estimate the number of deaths with considerable accuracy merely from a knowledge of the weather. In the United States a weekly bulletin published by the Census Bureau gives a most illuminating curve showing the mortality in all cities of over 100,000 population. Spells of extremely hot or cold weather are invariably registered in the curve. In July, 1936, two weeks of unusual heat, especially in the central part of the country, sent the death rate skyrocketing to about 50 per cent above the normal. On the other hand, unusually warm weather in January, 1932, and again in January, 1934, took a bite out of the middle of the annual upward bulge in the mortality curve so that there were depressions in place of the usual peaks.

With births the case is somewhat different. In many countries they fluctuate in almost exactly the reverse fashion from deaths. Seasons of many deaths are seasons of few births; births increase as deaths diminish. Japan affords an extreme example of this, as I have shown in *Civilization and Climate* (1924). The population of that country is increasing with alarming rapidity. Nevertheless, during the summer the conceptions that lead to live births decline so much that in September, when they are at a minimum and deaths at a maximum, the conceptions are less numerous than the deaths. If such conditions prevailed permanently, the Japanese population would decline, instead of increasing by three quarters of a million or more per year. In many other countries, as I have shown elsewhere (1932, 1935), the conceptions and deaths follow opposite courses throughout the year. The work of Mills (1930, 1934) confirms the conclusion that such opposition is the rule in many countries. He lays special stress upon the small number of conceptions in hot weather, but cold weather also is associated with relatively lessened rates of reproduction.

In addition to all this, however, there are periods in most countries when the conceptions and deaths fail to fluctuate in opposite fashion. The deaths obediently follow the weather, except when there is some catastrophe such as famine or pestilence. The births, on the contrary, may follow the weather part of the year, but at other seasons they pursue their own course under the influence of conditions which apparently have little or nothing to do with climate.

The study described in this book examines millions of births in order to discover the reasons for their seasonal fluctuations and the degree to which the births at different seasons vary in quality. The first phase of the problem deals with factors which influence seasonal fluctuations in the number of births, regardless of the quality. One type of factors is purely cultural, and depends upon habits which have grown up in diverse parts of the world. Another type is climatic, and depends upon the weather. The season which happens to be the favorite for marriages is often cited as one of the most important cultural factors, but it has far less importance than is usually supposed. Religious fasts and festivals, on the contrary, have a pronounced effect upon the birth rate in some countries, and comparatively little in others. The demands of certain occupations upon people's energy may also play a part in causing the number of conceptions to vary from season to season. The greatest effect of all, so far as cultural factors are concerned, is produced by seasonal migrations whereby the men tend to be away from home during part of the year. The return home of the absentees in winter, especially at Christmas, is a persistent cause of a definite seasonal fluctuation in births. Yet in certain countries, and at certain epochs in other countries, the peak of births due to the midwinter holidays disappears entirely (Arctowski, 1935).

In this last respect the seasonal fluctuations arising from the weather are unlike those associated with cultural conditions. In hundreds of seasonal curves of births which were studied in preparing this book a peak of some sort is associated with the late winter or early spring, provided the winter is cool. The peak is sometimes smaller than peaks associated with certain cultural factors, but it is always present. Moreover, it always bears essentially the same relation to the weather, for it is the result of conceptions at the time when the weather is most nearly ideal. "In the spring a young man's fancy lightly turns to thoughts of love" for very good reasons. Man is an animal, as we constantly discover, and as we refuse with equal constancy to believe. Like all other higher animals, he has a definite seasonal rhythm of reproduction which makes it best for babies to be born in the late winter or early spring.

The facts set forth in later pages suggest that man acquired this fundamental animal rhythm because it favored the survival of the young. Let us adopt for the moment the widely accepted hypothesis that early man acquired his distinctive human characteristics in a climate that was warm, but not tropical. In such a climate the winter is short and cool, but not cold, and the summer fairly warm. Babies suffer relatively little from a moderately low temperature, but very greatly from high temperatures. Hence a primitive child born in March, let us say, has two advantages over a child born at other seasons, and especially over those born from June to September. First, its mother's ability to feed it will steadily increase for seven months or so in harmony with the growing demands of the child. The reason for this is that, except in recent decades and among the most advanced nations, the food supply during the winter has been poor in both quantity and quality, but begins to improve in the early spring. From that time onward the food becomes better until autumn, when grains, fruits, nuts, and fat animals are readily available. Thus by the time the March child of our early ancestors began to need much milk, its mother was beginning to be well fed. It had advantages like those which make it best for lambs to be born in April, and robins to be hatched in May. The green food, eggs, young animals, and probably the grubs and other insects of early spring, added vitamins to its milky diet, and the abundant food later in the season enabled its mother to feed it more and more bountifully in harmony with its growing needs. The same situation prevails among cows. During the eight months after their calves are born the cows whose calves arrive in February give more milk than do those whose calves are born at any other season (Huntington, 1933). Thus the February calf, like the February child, is unusually well fed.

The other main advantage of being born in February or March depends on the seasonal distribution of diseases. Before the advent of modern hygiene the death rate among infants had two peaks, one in winter, one in summer. In climates like that of New York the winter peak was of minor proportions. In climates with warm winters it practically disappeared, but in western Europe it was very prominent. The summer peak, which culminated in August or September, was truly appalling in regions such as much of the United States, where the summers are long and hot. It was due mainly to digestive disturbances, for children are born with a weak alimentary apparatus. The child born in February or March has the maximum chance of survival through the hot weather. Under normal, primitive conditions, it is still living on its mother's milk when the heat arrives, so that the great dangers from contaminated food are minimized. Moreover, it has lived long enough so that its digestive system is beginning to become stabilized and is by no means so easily disturbed as it was during the earliest months. Thus the child born at about the time when vegetation first begins to revive in the spring appears to have the best chance of survival. This may not be of much importance today with our modern methods of sanitation and diet, but it must have been of immense importance throughout most of man's long history. Therefore it is not surprising that in all middle latitudes thus far investigated we find evidence of at least a minor peak in the birth rate during the winter or early spring. Only in steadily warm regions, or in those in such high latitudes that the summers have no hot weather, do we find exceptions. The exceptions prove the rule, for they accentuate the importance of certain kinds of weather. So important is the fundamental annual rhythm of births that it is one of the main themes of the following pages.

This basic annual rhythm, which we may also call the physiological or animal rhythm, seems to offer an explanation of why the optimum temperature for health and efficiency varies so little from country to country, or race to race. People have the best health and greatest physical vigor when the mean temperature for day and night together averages from 60° to 70° F. (15.6°-21.2° C.). This seems to be equally true of races as diverse as the Finns of the far north and the Javanese close to the equator. Therefore it seems like a primitive trait acquired in the early stages of the existence of our species, and modified only a little by the diverse environments in which the various races of mankind have since lived. How slight the modification is may be judged from the fact that factory workers of west European descent in the northeastern United States work most effectively when the temperature averages 60° F., whereas the Cubans in the cigar factories of Florida work most rapidly at a mean temperature of 70° or less. Again, although the Javanese are a thoroughly equatorial people, they have the best health and greatest energy when they live at such an altitude that the temperature averages 70° or lower instead of 80°, as is the case where most of them live. In a general way we may say that a mean temperature of about 63° for day and night together is the optimum for physical well-being in man, and that the optimum rarely if ever falls below 60° or rises above 70° even among people who live in the coldest or hottest parts of the world. There may be exceptions, for the matter has not been studied among such people as the Eskimos of the far north and the Dinkas of the hot upper Nile in Sudan. There is, however, no question as to the small range of the optimum temperature among diverse races in contrast to the great range in the mean temperature of the regions where they live.

  This brings us to the interesting problem of why the human optimum happens to lie between the temperatures of 60° and 70° F. and why it varies so little from one climate to another. The usual answer is that the optimum temperature is the one at which there is the best balance between the cooling action of the air, and the warming action due to the combustion of food within our bodies. This is doubtless true, but for other animals which have essentially the same internal temperature as man the optimum external temperature appears to be quite different. We cannot quote chapter and verse for this, but it must be true because many animals thrive only in regions where the optimum human temperatures are never experienced. Polar bears, for example, never experience a mean monthly temperature much above 50° and their optimum may be lower. Tapirs and certain species of monkeys are unknown where even a single month has a temperature as low as 70°. Their optimum is probably more nearly 80°.

  Without further discussion, then, we may point out what seems to be the reason why the optimum temperature for human health occurs when the temperature for night and day together averages between 60° and 70° F. In preparing this book the seasonal distribution of births has been studied in more than 80 regions. In every one of these a major or minor maximum of births occurs when the mean temperature averages somewhere between 56° and 71° F. The median temperature at which this occurs is 62° F. In cool regions the rise toward this temperature appears to be especially effective in stimulating reproduction; but in hot regions the drop to 62° is more effective. This reproductive optimum is practically the same as the 63° which appears to be the average physical optimum on the basis of records of daily work and mortality. Such an agreement suggests that the optimum temperature for physical health was originally fixed by the selective action of the climate in which *Homo sapiens* became established as a distinct species. If parents were stimulated to reproduction by the temperature which happened to prevail 9 months before the most favorable season for the birth of children, their offspring would have the best chance to survive. Thus for generation after generation there presumably occurred a selection in favor of persons who inherited a tendency to have especially good health when the mean temperature rose to 60° or 70° in the spring.

The same hypothesis which best fits the physical optimum also fits the mental optimum. At the time of conception the best thing that parents can possibly do for their children is to be in perfect health. When a primitive child is born, however, the best thing the parents can do to insure its survival is to be as alert as possible. In other words, survival is best promoted if parents are physically at their best when their children are conceived and mentally at their best when the children are born. This, apparently, is the reason for two distinct optima of temperature. The discovery of the connection between reproduction and the two optima of temperature seems to me to be one of the chief features of this book.

If we are right about the optima, the human species presumably acquired its present physical adaptation to the weather under certain definite conditions of climate. These conditions appear to have been such that infants which were conceived when the temperature rose to 60° or 70° in the spring were born at the time most favorable for their survival. At that time the temperature averaged about 15° lower than at the time of conception. Hence the primitive parents whose physical vitality was especially stimulated by the higher temperature and whose mental activity was especially stimulated by the lower temperature were the ones whose progeny was most likely to survive. Their response to the weather became hereditary throughout the species by reason of natural selection. The final conclusion, then, is that on an average people feel most comfortable and vigorous with a noonday temperature of 70° or a little higher and a mean temperature of about 63° for day and night together because it is best that children should be born in the late winter or early spring. June has been rightly chosen as a favorite month for weddings. Nevertheless, our mental activity is greatest in the spring and fall when the temperature averages about 47° because that is the temperature at which it was best for our primitive ancestors to be *born*.

The differences between the children born at one season and another extend into many fields. A statistical study of the varying proportions of the two sexes at birth sounds like a dry subject. But statistics may be juicy. They seem, for example, to give the lie to the oft-repeated statement that girls possess more vitality than boys. According to the biologists all human being have 24 pairs of chromosomes. In 23 of these the members of each pair are alike, but among males the 24th pair consists of a so-called Y chromosome matched with an X chromosome, whereas in females both are of the X type. The relations of the X and Y chromosomes are such that the numbers of the two sexes in any large population should be equal at birth, unless some special circumstance favors one sex more than the other. Normally, however, about 105 boys are born for every 100 girls. Among stillbirths the proportion of males is often 125 for every 100 females, and among abortions at earlier stages of pregnancy it rises to 300 or 400. It is evident, then, that a great many potential females fail to materialize at all, or else perish very early. Some biologists explain the unequal numbers of the two sexes by assuming the existence of a special lethal form of certain genes which may occur in double doses in embryos that would otherwise become females, but is always neutralized by a stronger form in males. Hence a certain proportion of potential females never develop into embryos, and girls are less numerous than boys. Other biologists hold that the spermatozoa which contain X chromosomes and thus produce females are less vigorous than those having a Y chromosome, which produce males. Hence they have more difficulty in reaching the ova, and girls are correspondingly scarce.

Our investigations agree with this second explanation, but not with the first. They also indicate that when people are in the right physical condition the two kinds of spermatozoa are of nearly equal vigor. At the most favorable season of the year the two sexes are born more nearly in equal numbers than at any other season. Where the contrast in vigor from season to season is slight, as in Sweden, the contrast in the number of the two sexes is also slight. In Japan, on the contrary, where the contrast is great, girls may be as numerous as boys among children conceived in May or June at the end of the extremely delightful spring, but among those conceived in September at the end of the long, hot, humid season, there is an astonishing preponderance of boys. In view of all the available facts it seems probable that the numbers of the two sexes would be equal if the environmental conditions were perfect and if parents enjoyed perfect health.

If such perfect conditions should prevail, what difference would it make in the lives of the children? In the first place, they would presumably live long on an average. At any rate, among the people who are now born at the most favorable season the average duration of life is several years longer than among those born at the least favorable season. This is true even in comparatively good climates like that of the northern United States. It is probably true to a still greater degree in countries like Japan. There, however, we have not yet been able to test the matter, but we do know that, taking all the people together, regardless of when they were born, the average length of life is many years less in Japan than in England.

Length of life is of course dependent upon many factors beside the season at which one is born. Pearl (1934) has shown that long life is hereditary. People whose grandparents died at an average age above 80 years normally live about 10 years longer than those whose grandparents died at an average age of 50 or less. Mode of life also has a great influence upon how long people live. Workers in stone quarries where siliceous dust settles in the lungs die much earlier on an average than do farmers in the same neighborhood. Temperate clergymen are proverbially a very long-lived group in comparison with self-indulgent squires who eat, drink, and make merry to excess. Accidents, too, and such conditions as famines and pestilences shorten many lives. And the people in hot, humid climates die earlier than similar people in climates such as those of New Zealand, Belgium, and the state of Washington. But all this does not alter the fact that in the past, in New England for example, the people born in March, and attaining at least the age of 2 years, have lived on an average nearly 4 years longer than similar people born in July. Length of life depends upon the combined effect of many causes; the investigations here described show that season of birth must be added to the causes already known.

The data in this book support the idea that season of birth bears a close relation to genius and eminence. Unusually high ability is probably never the result of accidents. Accidents tend almost inevitably to injure rather than improve the delicate mechanism of the brain. Genius apparently arises from a fortunate combination of the genes within the chromosomes at the time of conception. In order to reach fruition it needs an environment sufficiently favorable to give the innate capacities full chance for expression. The facts set forth in this book indicate that the births of persons of unusual genius conform to the animal rhythm and to the temperature much more closely than do births in general. This is just what would be expected on the basis of what we have seen as to sex and length of life. The high percentage of girls and the long lives which are associated with birth at the most favorable season are indications of vigor. Unusual achievements are a similar indication. The fact that the births of persons of high distinction show more than the normal tendency to conform to the basic animal rhythm of the seasons merely shows that the weather helps the genes. One may surmise that people possessing an unusually favorable combination of genes are especially susceptible to outside influences. Hence even at the inception of life they are helped by the same seasonal conditions which increase the proportion of girls and increase the length of life. One may also surmise that throughout life people's health and mental vigor are influenced by the condition of the spermatozoa and ova at the time of conception. Perfect reproductive cells can be produced only when the health of the parents is perfect. An approach to such health is possible only under favorable conditions of many sorts, including mode of life, diet, and weather.

The births of people of uncommon ability show a tendency not only to follow the animal rhythm to an unusual degree, but to occur in weather somewhat cooler than that in which births are usually most numerous. This is especially interesting because studies which I have described in *Civilization and Climate* (1915, 1924) and later publications (1933) indicate that the optimum temperature for mental activity is lower than for physical. Low, but not excessively low, temperature has in some way become associated with mental activity. The scientific tendencies of the Swedes, and the philosophical tendencies of the Scotch, illustrate the matter. The innate quality of any given group and the accidental combinations of genes which produce genius are presumably the most important elements in the matter. Nevertheless, the fact that in our study of births we find a relationship between low temperature and intellectual activity may be highly significant. It leads us to suspect that cultural inventions which render people comfortable in cooler and more invigorating parts of the world have not only enabled civilization to move northwestward from ancient Egypt and Babylonia, but have thereby led to a higher level of mental activity among people as a whole. Not only have health and activity been promoted, but people have been born with greater vigor and with a higher percentage of potential leaders than would otherwise have been possible.

Turning now to defectives and weaklings of various kinds, we shall find in later chapters that the season of birth does not present so clear a picture among physical and mental defectives as among persons of eminence. There is some evidence that the inmates of homes for the feeble-minded tend to be conceived to an unusual degree in hot weather. This is what might be expected from the fact that persons of great achievement tend to be conceived in weather cooler than the physical optimum. It is not surprising that the facts in this respect are not clear. The defects which make people feeble-minded are partly innate and partly due to accidents or other environmental conditions which may occur at any time from conception onward. Even if the season of conception does have some relation to defects, its influence may not be evident among great numbers of defectives the majority of whom owe their defects to accidents having no connection with the seasons.

Criminals, insane persons, and sufferers from tuberculosis show a well-defined seasonal distribution of births which seems at first to contradict our conclusions as to men of genius. Among all these weaker types the basic animal rhythm of births is more strongly evident than among people in general. This agrees with Pintner's discovery that the intelligence quotient is low among people born in January and February. His data indicate that the number of births and the average intelligence quotient vary in opposite directions. A high average I.Q. accompanies a low birth rate. The new data given in this book show that when births are numerous not only is the average I.Q. low, but also the proportion of persons who will become criminals, or suffer from insanity, or tuberculosis, is high. The fact that this occurs at the season when the births of eminent leaders are most numerous furnishes strong, though unexpected, evidence as to the potency of the basic animal rhythm of reproduction. It apparently indicates that when the reproductive urge reaches its height in May or June two things occur. First, on an average the children who are then conceived are stronger and longer-lived than their brothers and sisters who are conceived at other seasons. This explains the high proportion of births of geniuses, or rather of persons whose innate ability finds expression in activities which lead to fame. True geniuses may be equally numerous at other seasons. Second, people who are emotionally or intellectually weak are especially likely to yield to the sexual stimulation which marks the chief season of reproduction. Such parents presumably are responsible for a large percentage of the persons who become criminals or suffer from insanity. Third, physically weak people who usually are not able to produce children may become parents under the stimulus of the primitive breeding season. Their children are probably especially susceptible to tuberculosis as well as to the influences which lead to crime and insanity. In this connection we shall find it especially interesting to note that outbreaks of insanity, as well as of suicide and sexual crimes, follow the seasonal rhythm of conceptions with extraordinary fidelity. Man, like the animals, is subject to a breeding season which is accompanied by heightened emotional instability. When effects like these are added to the well-known seasonal and regional variations in health, diet, and occupations, it becomes evident that weather and climate influence human welfare to an extraordinary degree.

This last point is so important that we may well devote the rest of this chapter to a brief statement of the chief ways

in which climate influences human conduct. These ways
may be divided into two great sections, namely, cultural, and
biological or physiological. There is no hard and fast line
between the two. At the extremes they are distinct, but in
the middle they overlap. Diet is partly a matter of climate
and partly of the cultural situation in any given region.
The fact that people use striped awnings in one region and
shutters in another is almost purely cultural, whereas the
sudden energy which one feels when a cool breeze arises after
a hot day is physiological with only the slightest cultural
element. Nevertheless, even in these cases culture and climate overlap. The use of awnings in contrast to shutters
may be determined by the amount of sunshine and the physiological discomfort which it produces. The degree of stimulus from the breeze may depend on the kind of clothing.
Between these two extremes such a matter as clothing depends almost equally upon cultural habits and biological
conditions as represented by human needs and the available
plants or animals in the given type of climate.

Each of the two great sections of climatic influences falls
into subdivisions. Cultural influences include those that are
economic, political, esthetic, and of other types, but for the
sake of brevity we shall confine ourselves to the economic
type. The physiological influences may be divided into four
types: dietetic, parasitic, energic, and genetic. These terms
will be defined later. They are arranged here in accordance
with the degree to which cultural conditions are intermixed
with those that are biological. Diet depends almost equally
on cultural habits and natural products as determined by
climate and other geographic factors. Genetic conditions,
such as the birth of men of genius, have little or no relation
to cultural conditions.

Everyone recognizes the economic relationships of climate.
The icecap of Antarctica, the center of the Sahara Desert, the
high, cold, level stony parts of the plateau of Tibet, and the
dense forests of the Amazon basin present environments in
which the chief differences are due to climate. It is beyond

the scope of human ingenuity to get a living and carry on the ordinary functions of life in the same way in all of them. They do not, to be sure, compel people to follow any particular occupations, or modes of life, or to use any special types of food, clothing, shelter, and transportation. But they do say categorically that all but a very few of the many possible methods of doing these things are doomed to failure. Moreover, they say with equal positiveness that the methods which succeed best in one of these environments are not the same as those which succeed best in the others. Thus the economic limitations of the various climatic environments exert a profound effect upon man's actions.

An economic effect of a different kind is produced by changes in the weather from one time to another. It would be the rankest folly for us to attempt to conduct ourselves in the same way in winter as in summer. Imagine the results of hours in the water and on the beach in bathing suits with the thermometer at zero Fahrenheit. Irregular changes in the weather likewise have a great effect upon our conduct because they alter our economic situation. Consider, for example, the Chinese floods which cause almost incredible famines and millions of deaths in China, or the droughts which cost America billions of dollars in taxes to be used for relief. In many regions, even in a progressive country such as the United States, the income of the average farmer is twice as great when the weather is good as in years when it is bad. Consider, too, the interruptions to transportation and the losses of property and life that arise from storm, flood, fog, frost, and snow. It would be easy to add indefinitely to the list of economic conditions which are influenced by climate and weather, and which thus lead to diverse types of human conduct.

We have said that the four types of climatic influences which are not economic are biologic. We may go farther and say that they all are important primarily because of their bearing on health. Modern investigations are making it clear that human health, efficiency, longevity, and mental activity are greatly modified by the proportions in which our diet contains carbohydrates, fats, proteins, acids, vitamins, and other ingredients. So powerful is this influence that ardent enthusiasts sometimes think that a good diet is the greatest of human needs. For our present purpose two points should be emphasized. The first is that the customary diet in any given region, as we have just seen, is partly due to the geographic environment—primarily the climate—and partly to cultural conditions. As civilization advances, the cultural element becomes steadily stronger. Hence the people who live in modern centers of culture often fail to appreciate the fact that until recently in all parts of the world, and even now among nine tenths of mankind, the main determinant of diet is the kind of crops which will yield the most food with the least labor. In other words, the diet depends mainly upon climate. Unfortunately the climates which are less favorable in other respects appear also to be those in which the normal diet is most poorly balanced and most likely to be deficient. Hence it is easy to confuse the effect of diet with that of the other conditions which we shall now consider.

The parasitic phase of climatic influences includes all diseases which are due to parasites or viruses, and which have a distinct regional distribution by reason of climate. Malaria, yellow fever, African sleeping sickness, yaws, pellagra, hookworm disease, and the more severe forms of dysentery are examples of diseases that are found mainly in the warmer portions of the earth because those are the regions most favorable to certain parasitic organisms and their carriers. Other diseases such as pneumonia, catarrh, rheumatism, and influenza are primarily associated with cooler climates. Moreover, in all climates where there is any marked contrast of seasons there is also a seasonal fluctuation in the types of disease. In the case of such diseases, just as in that of diet, the climatic influence becomes less evident as the stage of culture advances, and there is a corresponding modification of human conduct. The elimination of hookworm disease or malaria in warm regions produces a wonderful effect upon the amount and quality of people's work. The elimination of the digestive diseases of young children in summer in the most advanced regions has done away with an enormous drain on the community, not only physiologically and economically, but also emotionally. Nevertheless, in the world as a whole, the progress of knowledge and skill has made only a faint beginning in reducing the great differences in parasitic and other diseases which arise in response to differences in climate.

The term "energic," as applied to the next type of climatic effect, has probably puzzled many readers. I have used it to designate the direct effect of the weather upon our physical and mental energy. Regardless of whether people are well or ill, cultured or uncultured, active or inactive, a change in the weather produces a change in their physiological reactions. This manifests itself in feelings of lassitude or energy, in the amount of work done both physically and mentally, and in the accuracy with which we work and think. Among people who are in good health this direct effect of the weather has been measured in such activities as the work of factory operatives, and the carefully measured physical and mental reactions of individuals under controlled experimental conditions. The seasonal distribution of births as described in this book and in previous publications is likewise an evidence of variations in energy or health in direct response to the weather. A similar effect of the weather is also evident in such mental indices as the marks of students, the percentage of success in civil-service examinations, and the frequency of applications for the amendment of specifications for patents. Among people who are not in good health it is evident in the percentage of success among surgical operations, the degree of disturbance among sufferers from mental derangement, and above all in the fluctuations of the death rate which follow the weather with extraordinary fidelity not only from season to season, but even from day to day.

Back of all these direct responses to weather and climate lies the general process of metabolism within the human body. Sundstroem (1926), Balfour (1923), and others have shown how this acts in tropical as compared with temperate regions. Mills (1930) and Belding (1936) have found evidence of it in the activity of the reproductive glands. Petersen (1935, 1936) has published a series of remarkable curves showing how all sorts of physiological conditions vary constantly in harmony with the weather. These variations are evident in such conditions as the pulse rate, the rate of respiration, blood pressure, the amount of carbon dioxide expired from the lungs, and the relative proportions of calcium, phosphorus, and other elements in the blood. In January or February, according to Gachsen, the haemoglobin in the blood falls to a minimum, as does the number of red corpuscles, but the size of the corpuscles is at a maximum. At that same time, according to Linhard, people breathe most frequently and least deeply, their lungs are most poorly ventilated, and the tension of the CO_2 in them is at a maximum. In July and August the opposite is true. It seems clear that our physiological reactions, and hence our physical and mental states, are being constantly swayed back and forth—stimulated or depressed—by the daily, weekly, monthly, and seasonal swings of the weather. It seems probable that each type of climate has its own special grade of metabolic reactions, and its own level of activity.

The energic type of climatic influence is less affected by cultural conditions than is either the dietetic or the parasitic type. We do indeed warm and protect ourselves by means of clothes, houses, and fire. Nevertheless, the process of creating ideal air conditions has by no means gone so far as the similar process in respect to diet and parasitic diseases. Not even in hospitals have we any certainty that the ideal conditions of the atmosphere prevail, or that the fluctuations in temperature, humidity, sunshine, wind, and electrical potential which take place out-of-doors are prevented from producing an effect within doors. People who are in good health almost invariably go back and forth from indoors to outdoors. They also feel the outside influence by reason of the opening of doors and windows and the indraft of air which takes place even in the most tightly sealed of ordinary houses. Among the overwhelming majority of mankind the cultural modification of the physiological influence of the atmosphere is limited to the heating of houses and the prevention of drafts in ways which often do as much harm as good.

The present book adds still another to the types of physiological influence exerted by climate. I have called this type "genetic" because no other term seems right. The old definition of genetic, as given for example in Worcester's dictionary, is "relating to birth, generation, or origin." This is exactly the sense in which we here use the word. A newer meaning may be defined as "relating to the genes, or carriers of inheritance within the chromosomes." This however, is a very recent and highly specialized definition. Nevertheless, it applies to the type of climatic effect now under discussion, provided we make it clear that we do not imply that the effects of climate are passed on by inheritance. As to that we have no knowledge whatever. The facts set forth in this book, however, seem to make it clear that the weather at or shortly before the time of conception exerts an important effect upon the embryo, and that this effect continues throughout life. It is probable that the weather during pregnancy and at the time of birth also exercises an influence, but as to this the evidence is not clear. The one thing that stands out most clearly when all the facts set forth in this book are before us is that the human race inherits a highly sensitive mechanism which reacts to the weather. The reaction of parents at or before the time of conception has a direct and lasting effect upon the vigor of the embryo and of the resultant human being throughout the whole of life. Because this type of climatic influence acts without our knowing it, nothing has yet been done to change its course. Thus it stands in complete contrast to economic effects which are constantly altered as the result of man's inventive activity.

Perhaps we ought to reverse the order of the great types of climatic effects. First, most intimate, least known, and most enduring in its results, is the effect of the season of conception, which manifests itself in such traits as length of life and degree of mental activity. So intimately is this a part of our constitutional make-up that hitherto it has not been separated from traits which are due to biological inheritance. Second, from birth, or even from conception onward if we consider that the blood stream of the mother belongs also to the child, each individual is constantly subject to the direct action of the weather. His energy, both physical and mental, and his resistance to disease not only swing back and forth from day to day and season to season, but are raised or lowered to a definite level which harmonizes with the climate in which he lives. Third, the diseases which attack us vary in nature, severity, and geographical distribution according to differences in climate, as well as for other reasons. Still a fourth physiological effect is produced by our diet, which varies because of climate more than for any other cause. Thus we pass from the genetic effects of climate, which are purely biological in origin, to the energic, parasitic, and dietetic effects in which cultural conditions become more and more important. Only then do we come to the purely cultural phase which is here represented by economic influences of climate.

Through the action of these varied types of influence the cultural system of every part of the world has become more or less fully adapted to the kind of climate in which it happens to be found. It is no accident that certain parts of the world surpass others in standards of living, diet, health, transportation, the use of machinery, stability of government, education, and in a host of other respects. Those parts are the ones where diet, parasitic diseases, energy, and genetic strength are most favorably influenced by climate. Climatic advantages bring cultural advantages. Thus climate becomes by far the most important feature of man's natural environment. And the natural environment ranks with biological inheritance and cultural surroundings as one of the three all-inclusive factors which determine human behavior and make man what he is.

To some readers all this may suggest astrology. It may prompt some reviewer to entitle his review "Meteorological Magic," as was done by an able anthropologist in reviewing *Civilization and Climate* more than twenty years ago. The relation of this book to astrology, however, is like that of modern chemistry to alchemy. The old alchemists were wrong when they thought they could transmute lead into gold; they were right in thinking that one metal can be changed into another. Modern chemists all agree that radium, uranium, and thorium are distinct metals, and yet are stages in the breaking down of radium into lead. They also agree that theoretically other metals might be changed into gold, or the reverse, if only we knew how to make the necessary transfer of electrons. In the same way the old astrologers were quite wrong, and the modern ones are still more so, in thinking that there is value in a horoscope based on the positions of the planets at the time of birth. Nevertheless, the cold facts as to millions of births leave no doubt that on an average the people born in February and March differ decidedly from those born in June and July. In the middle latitudes of the northern hemisphere, as we shall soon see, they tend to be more numerous, more evenly divided as to sex, and longer-lived. By a curious quirk of fortune they also include a larger proportion not only of distinguished people, but also of unfortunates who become criminals or are afflicted with insanity or tuberculosis. Man is like the lower animals in having a definite seasonal rhythm of reproduction with a maximum of births in the late winter or spring.

CHAPTER II

THE BASIC ANIMAL RHYTHM: BELGIUM

Having sketched the chief conclusions of our investigation we must now turn to the detailed facts on which they are based. The data of this investigation include three main types. The first consists of official records of births in many countries, provinces, states, and cities. These include not only total births, both urban and rural, but also births in relation to such matters as legitimacy, stillbirth, occupations, religion, and race. As a rule, both early and late statistics have been used. Most of the data thus employed have been derived directly from official records. Another type of data is derived from dates of birth, and sometimes of death, as given in many encyclopedias, biographical dictionaries, books such as *Who's Who,* genealogical memoirs, and other reference books. Genealogical books dealing with individual families, by the way, contain a vast amount of valuable, accurate, and wholly unused data. A third kind of information has come from the records of schools, hospitals, insane asylums, prisons, and schools for the feeble-minded. The numerous institutions listed in Appendix A have assisted in supplying data of this sort. Their willingness to co-operate and the care with which they have assembled the necessary data deserve the most cordial thanks. Some data have also been taken from the published work of other investigators, especially Gini.

The data derived from these various sources are presented mainly in the form of seasonal curves rather than tables. The reason is that the curves, at a single glance, show a great number of features which even the most practised statistician cannot detect from the figures alone. As a rule, the month of birth is the basis on which the curves are drawn. It is generally indicated at the top of the diagram.

and the season of conception at the bottom. In some cases, however, the curves are arranged primarily according to month of conception, and the reader should carefully note which method is used. All curves of births, conceptions, and deaths are constructed in the same way unless otherwise indicated. In the curves for births, for example, the horizontal line marked 100 represents the average number of births per day for the year as a whole. Each month is represented by its average number of births per day, and this is always expressed as a percentage of the corresponding average for the year. When this method is used the difference in length among the months is eliminated. For example, if the births are as in Column B, the daily averages will be as in Column D, and the percentages for each month as in Column E.

A Period	B No. of Births	C No. of Days	D Births per Day	E Births per Day as Percentage of Yearly Average
Year.........	2192	365¼	6	100
January......	124	31	4	67
February.....	113	28¼ *	4	67
March.......	186	31	6	100
April........	240	30	8	133

*Allowing for leap year where necessary.

Thus all the curves are directly comparable with one another, no matter whether they are based on many persons or few. Where individual births have been tabulated the number is always stated. Where data for geographic regions are employed, the dates are given.

So complex a matter as the seasonal distribution of births is influenced by many diverse factors. One set of factors is purely climatic. The weather, in the broadest sense of the word, appears to have a direct effect upon people's physiological well-being, and thus upon the number of conceptions. The seasonal variations of another set of factors, including diet, shelter, and many occupations such as agriculture and fishing, also depend directly upon the weather, but in these cases the effect of the weather upon reproduction is indirect and may be greatly modified or even eliminated by human ingenuity. Still a third set of factors, such as religious observances and seasons of marriage, is largely cultural, but even in these cases the seasonal incidence of different kinds of customs usually depends indirectly upon the weather. There are, however, certain factors which are independent of the weather, but which in course of time may bring about pronounced changes in the seasons at which births occur. These include such conditions as industrialization and birth control, which change from decade to decade rather than from season to season.

In order to guide our thoughts in the following pages, a table of conditions which may influence season of birth is appended. It does not go into minor details, but includes all major factors so far as we are aware.

TABLE 1

Main Conditions Influencing Season of Birth

I. Factors which change with the seasons.
    A. Direct factors of climate or weather.
        1. Temperature.
        2. Humidity (including precipitation).
        3. Sunshine.
        4. Weather, in the sense of combinations of the three preceding factors, together with other factors such as wind. These combinations manifest themselves as alternations between storms and fair weather.

    B. Indirect factors which influence births mainly through physiological conditions.
        1. Diet.
        2. Clothing and shelter.
        3. Disease.
        4. Illegitimacy.
        5. Abortion, miscarriage, and stillbirths.

    C. Indirect factors which influence births mainly through cultural conditions.
        1. Religious observances, fasts, festivals, etc.
        2. Occupations.
        3. Seasonal migrations, vacations, etc.
        4. Season of marriage.

II. Factors which do not change with the seasons, but which may in the long
   run alter the seasonal distribution of births.
   1. Urbanization.
   2. Industrialization.
   3. Non-seasonal migration.
   4. Restriction of births.
   5. Decline or change in religious observances, old customs, etc.

Where so many factors are concerned it is often difficult
to discover how much is due to each.   The important thing
is to recognize that all the factors have some effect, and that

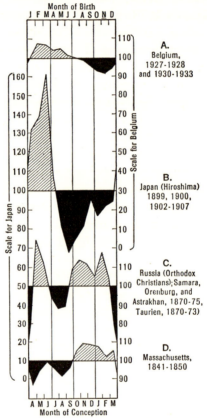

Fig. 1.—Seasonal Distribution of Births: Typical Curves.

they may combine in a great many ways.   In some cases the
seasonal curves appear to depend very closely upon the climate, whereas in others the climatic element is largely con-

cealed by a rather intricate combination of cultural conditions. Moreover, in a single area the cultural conditions may influence the seasonal distribution of births far more at one epoch than at another.

In order to gain a general view of the possible causes of seasonal variations in the birth rate, let us analyze the four highly diverse curves of Figure 1. These have been selected to illustrate extreme types of seasonal distribution of births. The Belgian curve (A) supplies an example of the highest statistical accuracy. It illustrates the conditions among people who have made a comparatively complete adjustment to modern methods of limitation of births, and have ceased to be greatly influenced by old religious customs, or by seasonal variations in occupations. Moreover, the Belgians are comparatively immobile—that is, there is very little seasonal migration among them. The net result is that the Belgian curve affords an excellent example of a seasonal distribution of births dependent almost entirely upon the weather.

The Japanese curve (B) is not so perfect statistically as the Belgian curve. Its main peak is not due to an excess of births, but to excessive zeal for knowledge as will be explained later. The curve is like that of the Belgians, however, in its freedom from any significant effect of religious restrictions, festivals, seasonal migrations, or even seasonal occupations, although this last is not quite certain. It appears to illustrate what happens when there is no limitation of births in a climate where the summer heat and humidity are very much greater than in Belgium. Thus we have two diverse curves both of which appear to owe their form largely to seasonal variations in the weather, but one of which contains a statistical error.

The other two curves in Figure 1 have been selected because they go to the opposite extreme. Both are influenced partly by faulty statistical methods and still more by cultural conditions. These two factors together alter the form of the curves so much that the influence of the weather is evident only part of the year. The old Russian curve (C in Figure

1) contains certain extreme statistical errors; it is based on a population which placed no limitation upon procreation except under the stress of religious compulsion, and in which the men practised a sort of seasonal migration; and it belongs to a climate characterized by extremely low temperature in winter. The curve for Massachusetts (*D*) nearly a century ago shows a mild, but persistent, type of statistical error; it represents people among whom migration produced unique effects; it does not appear to be much influenced by limitation of births; and it belongs to a climate which is almost if not quite as healthful as that of Belgium, but which is more extreme both in summer and winter. A comparison of these four curves will enable us to test every reasonable hypothesis as to the causes of seasonal fluctuations of births. It will disclose evidence of practically all the factors listed in Table 1 as changing from season to season, and it will show the fundamental climatic rhythm with all sorts of additions due to diverse conditions of culture.

In studying the Belgian curve of Figure 1 our problem is to examine all the factors which may reasonably be suspected of giving rise to a pronounced maximum of births in February and March and a minimum in October, November, and December. The minor minimum in April and the minor maximum in May are so small that we shall omit them. The two main features may be due to variations either in the number of conceptions from month to month, or in the abortions, miscarriages, and stillbirths which prevent the conceptions from giving rise to living births. At first we shall disregard this second alternative, and discuss the Belgian curve as if its form depended primarily upon the number of conceptions at different times of the year.

The curve looks as if its general form were due to an annual biological rhythm of reproduction. Such a rhythm may be inherent in the human species, or it may be due to the environment. A biological rhythm, independent of the environment, is by no means an impossibility. A monthly rhythm of this sort is characteristic of women. Even among them, however, the biological rhythm is subject to frequent environmental interruptions by such causes as over-exertion, drugs, disease, and climate. The menstrual periods of white women often become highly irregular in the tropics. Moreover, we are constantly finding new evidence that the reproductive rhythm of animals is set in motion by changes in the seasonal distribution of temperature, light, food, and other environmental conditions. With man the same seems to be true. An annual rhythm of reproduction is everywhere evident, but it varies from one climate or one social system to another. Hence the most probable hypothesis appears to be that the seasonal curve of births in Belgium represents an annual rhythm like that of animals and dependent either directly or indirectly upon climatic factors.

Before accepting this conclusion, let us first inquire whether there is any good reason for a seasonal rhythm such as that of Belgium in Figure 1. The answer, as we saw in the first chapter, appears to be affirmative. Even in man's present civilized state the rhythm of births, as seen in Belgium, appears to be such that children are born in greatest numbers at the season when they have the best chance of life. This will be fully explained in a later chapter. We shall see there that a highly complex and apparently hereditary mechanism gives young infants different degrees of sensitivity to the weather at different stages of their lives. This adaptation to the climatic environment presumably dates back to some primitive epoch. In the kind of climate where man acquired his most definite human characteristics the chief dangers of winter were probably already past by the end of February. The summer, with its much greater dangers from the digestive diseases which, till recently, killed so many children in warm weather, was so far away that the children had a good chance to become sturdy and resistant before it arrived. The season of abundant and healthful food was approaching, so that the mothers had a good prospect of being able to meet the increasing needs of the infants for milk. The young of many animals are born at about this time, or a little later, and the advantages are obvious.

In the previous chapter we saw that it is advantageous to calves to be born in cold weather. Figure 2 illustrates the matter. Its upper curve is based on the records of some 2000 cows for 17 years at the Walker-Gordon farms in New Jersey and Massachusetts. These cows receive the best food and care at all seasons. They are bred so that calves are born in approximately the same numbers each month of the year (Huntington, Williams, and Van Valkenburg, 1933). Figure 2 shows that the average daily yield of milk per cow is

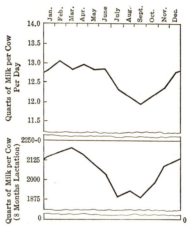

FIG. 2.—Milk Production on the Walker-Gordon Farms, 1916-1932.

large from February to June. As long as the temperature remains below approximately 60° F. (15.5° C.), the cows give abundant milk. When it rises higher, the yield of milk declines rapidly. Only when the temperature again falls below 60° F. does the amount increase once more. Moreover, Hays, Davidson, and others have shown that the total amount of butter fat in cow's milk, regardless of percentage, is low at high temperatures and high in cold weather. In other words, in the northeastern United States, calves are well fed by their mothers from December, and especially from February to June. They are poorly fed from July to November.

The records of a large number of cows investigated by J. A. Gowen lead to a similar conclusion. The lower curve of Figure 2 shows the average amount of milk given during the 8 months after parturition by cows whose calves were born at various seasons. The average calf born in March might have gotten from its mother about 2200 quarts of milk, whereas those born in July, August, and September had to be content with about 1900. March is about the time when calves are born in greatest numbers in a state of nature. Practically none are born in the summer and early autumn. It seems clear, then, that even when cows are kept under highly artificial and extremely favorable conditions at all seasons, they still show a pronounced seasonal rhythm in the production of milk. These cows are like modern people in that they are protected from the weather, receive abundant and nutritious food at all seasons, live in a climate different from that in which their species evolved, and produce young at all seasons. Nevertheless, their old reproductive rhythm is clearly evident in the fact that cows which produce calves at the optimum season give their young a much better start than do those whose calves are born out of season.

Rats supply a better illustration than cows. Their physiological responses to diet, disease, and weather are surprisingly like those of man. Figure 3 shows the seasonal distribution of birth among rats raised for many years by Dr. Helen D. King at the Wooster Institute in Philadelphia. It is based partly on data published in 1926 and partly on data communicated by Dr. King personally. The diagrams on the left are unsmoothed, and those on the right are smoothed.* They show the same systematic quality and the same kind of irregularities that we find in the corresponding

* The curves are smoothed by the formula $\dfrac{a + 2b + 2c}{4} = b'$. This merely means that in place of the actual data for any month we use the average of that month taken twice and of the preceding and following months taken once. Such smoothing can add nothing to the fluctuations of a curve. It merely smooths off the minor irregularities. When smoothed curves are mentioned anywhere in this book they have been smoothed by this formula.

curves for man. The most universal features are a maximum in April or May and a minimum in October or November. Curve *A* is the most important for our present purpose. It is based on rats that had been kept in captivity for 50 generations, which would correspond to 1500 years of civilization among mankind. They were well fed and well protected at all seasons, and were kept at room temperature. Under such

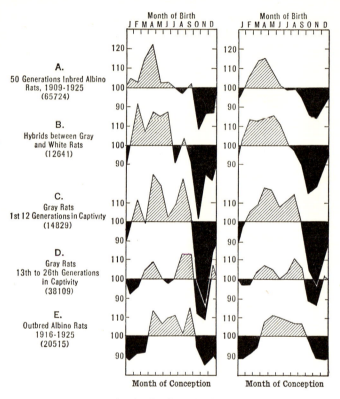

FIG. 3.—Seasonal Distribution of Births among Rats.

conditions they bred at all seasons. Nevertheless, in Curve *A,* for example, the birth rate, according to our index numbers, rose to 123 in April and fell to 78 in October. The most significant fact is that in their smoothed form Curves *B, E,* and especially *A,* although based on rats in Philadelphia, closely resemble the curve for modern men in Belgium. The amplitude, or swing from maximum to minimum, to be sure, is greater than in the Belgian curve, and the maximum does not come in quite the same month, but the general resemblance is obvious. Curves C and D are also similar, except for a peak in August, but exactly such a peak is one of the puzzling features of modern curves of birth in the United States. Similar curves for many other animals might be added.

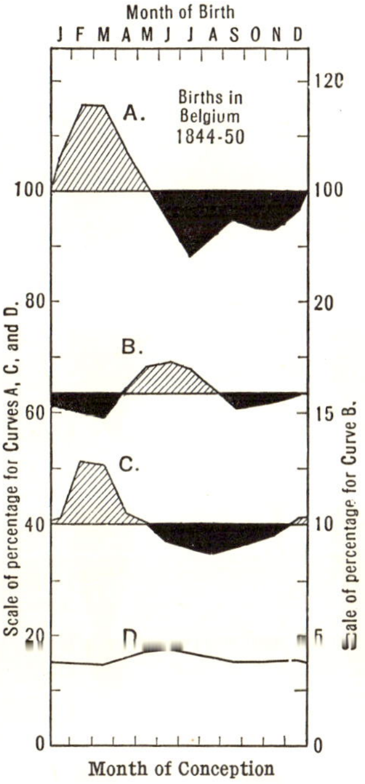

This gives great strength to the hypothesis that civilized man in Belgium, like the civilized cows in New Jersey and the civilized rats in Philadelphia, inherits an annual rhythm of reproduction. But what sets the rhythm in motion? How closely does it conform to modern conditions of climate? Does it show evidence of being an ancient adaptation to climate which still persists even though it may not be perfectly adapted to the climate of modern Belgium? A first step in answering these questions is to ascertain what differences there are in the chances of survival among Belgian children born at different seasons. In order to get data for this we have to go back almost a hundred years. Just why this is so, and how our results are obtained, are explained with greater detail in Chapter XIII. Here it must suffice to give the results.

FIG. 4.—Relation of Month of Birth to Survival During Infancy in Belgium, 1844-1850.

A century ago the seasonal distribution of both births and deaths in Belgium was approximately the same as now, although more extreme. Curve A in Figure 4 shows that births were at a maximum in February and March, declined to a minimum in July, and rose somewhat during the later part of the year. This brings the greatest number of births at the season when health is worst according to Curve *C,* whereas the minimum of births comes in July at practically the same time as the best health (August). On the other hand, Figure 4 shows that, although the seasonal differences are very slight, as appears in Curve *D,* the percentage of children who die during the first 2 years of life is lower among those born in February and March than among those born at any other season. This is more clearly evident in Curve *B,* which is the same as *D,* but on a four-fold greater scale. There we see that in general the chances of survival among Belgian infants were, and apparently still are, almost inversely proportional to the number of children born at any given season. When many children are born, only a small percentage of them die. In other words, the annual rhythm of births in Belgium is adjusted in such a way that it tends to increase the chances of survival, but the adjustment is not perfect. If all Belgian children had been born in February and March during the years here employed, the death rate per 1000 infants would have been reduced from 159.3 to 150.0. Six out of every 100 deaths of infants would have been avoided.

This looks as though the Belgians possessed an innate adjustment to climate of such a nature that conceptions tend to occur in largest numbers at the season which will cause births under the most favorable conditions. We shall later find a similar basic annual rhythm in many other places. Hence it seems probable that we are dealing with a universal human trait, acquired perhaps in the climate where our species originated, modified perhaps by experience in other climates. We assume that climate is the motivating factor because there is no other environmental agency by which a seasonal rhythm can be set in motion. Either the rhythm is an inherited trait which has no relation to environment, or it is set in motion by such factors as sunshine, temperature, and humidity which are climatic in nature. The facts set forth in later chapters seem to leave no alternative except the climatic explanation.

If the seasonal rhythm of births observed in Belgium is of climatic origin, we should expect some of the individual climatic factors to show special agreement with the seasonal distribution of conceptions. Let us see whether this is the

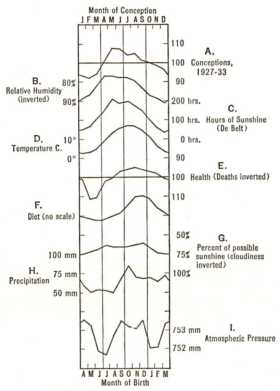

FIG. 5.—Possible Explanations of Seasonal Distribution of Births in Belgium.

case. A comparison of conceptions with the climatic factors is facilitated by setting the curve of births back 9 months to agree with the approximate time of conception. This is done in Curve *A* of Figure 5. The other curves in that diagram represent the main climatic elements, namely, relative humidity (inverted), hours of sunshine, temperature, percentage of possible sunshine (cloudiness inverted), precipitation, and atmospheric pressure. With these are curves for health and diet, the two main physiological conditions through which the weather may influence conceptions indirectly. Shelter and clothing might also be included, but their effects vary in almost perfect harmony with temperature and humidity, and hence cannot be separated from those factors. In Figure 5 diet is represented by an estimate of its approach to the ideal at different seasons. Health is represented by the inverted curve of deaths.

It is evident at a glance that atmospheric pressure (the lower curve) has no appreciable relation to conceptions. Precipitation is almost equally unrelated, for its two equal minima occur in February, when conceptions are at a minimum, and in May, when they are at a maximum. Cloudiness, which in its inverted form is equivalent to the percentage of possible sunshine, shows no more relation to conceptions than do atmospheric pressure and precipitation. This percentage, it should be noted, is quite different from the total hours of sunshine because it takes no account of the great variation in the length of the day from summer to winter.

Diet doubtless exerts a potent effect upon reproduction. Certain vitamins appear to be essential to the production of young. Nevertheless, the seasonal changes of diet in Belgium do not seem to be closely related to the seasonal changes in conceptions. The diet of the ordinary people in Belgium becomes of poor quality in winter, for then it consists far too largely of bread and potatoes with only a little meat, and no great supply of milk and eggs. The cabbages, root crops, apples, and other products of the garden and orchard which are abundant in the fall become more and more exhausted as the winter goes on. Thus in March or April the diet reaches its worst. The vast majority of Belgians cannot afford the winter fruits and vegetables which are now so common in America. If conceptions were largely influenced by seasonal changes in diet, one would expect their minimum to come in March or April rather than in February. In summer the discrepancy between diet and conceptions appears to be still greater. The first greens of the year—such things as dandelions—are eaten in April, but garden produce in sufficient quantities to form an important part of the diet of the ordinary people of both city and country is not available till June. Thereafter vegetables and fruits are eaten in greater and greater quantities until the optimum conditions are reached in the fall, presumably in September or October. The maximum number of conceptions, however, occurs in May. This does not preclude the possibility that diet may have an important effect upon reproduction, but it does show that the general form of the seasonal curve of births is quite different from what would be expected on the basis of diet.

Health in general seems to be more closely related to reproduction than does diet, but there are marked discrepancies. In winter, to be sure, the most deaths and the fewest conceptions occur at the same time, in February. Then, until May, the deaths diminish and the conceptions increase harmoniously. In June, however, the conceptions are scarcely as numerous as in May, and then they decline almost steadily. The deaths, on the contrary, decrease until August. In fact, among people at the reproductive ages, 21 to 45 years, the minimum of deaths, as will appear in Chapter XIII, is postponed until November. Thus the best conditions of health among parents lag 6 months behind the maximum of conceptions. It is doubtless true that relatively poor health due to the confinement, poor diet, exposure, and other unfavorable conditions of cold weather is largely responsible for the low conception rate in winter, but something else appears to determine the maximum of reproduction in the spring.

The three remaining curves of Figure 5 agree with that of conceptions more closely than do those thus far considered. The temperature reaches a minimum in January, which might well be connected with a minimum of conceptions as well as a maximum of deaths the following month. From February to May the temperature rises and the conceptions increase. About the end of May, however, when conceptions are close to their maximum, the temperature has risen only to 58° F. (14.5° C.). During July and August it rises to a maximum monthly average of 64°, but the conceptions decline. Thus births show about the same relationship to temperature, to diet, and to health except that the relationship to temperature is closest. There is, however, one important difference. It seems scarcely probable that conceptions are stimulated up to a certain point by improvements in diet and health, and thereafter are reduced in number by still further improvement. Of course, people may be over-nourished and grow fat, but that is another matter. On the other hand, we have abundant evidence that hot weather as well as cold reduces people's vitality, and leads to poor health and a high death rate. It is possible that the optimum temperature for reproduction may be as low as 58° F. in Belgium, although abundant statistical data and many laboratory experiments indicate that an average of about 63° for day and night together is more nearly the optimum for health among people of western European origin. Nevertheless, thousands of factory workers in the United States have been found to do their best work at a mean temperature of 59° for women and 60° for men (Huntington, 1915, 1924), and a temperature about like this may be the optimum for reproduction.

This would lead us to expect a second maximum of conceptions in September when the temperature again averages 58°. In Belgium we find only a very slight maximum, and this comes in August, but in other countries there is considerable evidence that after a warm but not unhealthful summer conceptions increase when cooler weather again brings the temperature not only down to the optimum, but to lower levels which are at first invigorating. In general, however, as will become clear in later pages, a rise of temperature to the optimum appears to be accompanied by increased reproduction more often than does a drop, even though the optimum is reached in both cases. Such a condition would produce the maximum number of births in the early spring when conditions are most favorable for the infants, but there would also be a minor maximum in the autumn which would result in births the next summer. We shall later find considerable evidence that this is the case. But we shall also find that, if the summer is of the right quality and there is no specially unfavorable season for births, a drop to the optimum temperature may be followed by the main maximum of births. In other words, modern conditions of abundant food and warm houses may in some places have modified the old climatic response. Nevertheless, in Belgium the temperature in summer may remain so close to the optimum that when it begins to drop there is no appreciable stimulation of reproduction. Another possibility is that when the amount of sunlight is increasing and the temperature is rising toward 62° the stimulating effect is much greater than when both light and heat are diminishing.

In Figure 5 the curve of total hours of sunshine (*C*), and the inverted curve of relative humidity (*B*), which we may call a curve of dryness, agree closely. This is natural, for they are expressions of almost the same thing. Their curves agree with that of conceptions to about the same degree as does the curve of temperature. In the spring the driest time is April and May, and the amount of sunshine is greatest in May, just when conceptions are at a maximum. In the winter, however, both dryness and sunshine are at a minimum in December, two months before the minimum of conceptions. Thus the season in which the temperature agrees most closely with the conceptions is the one when sunshine and dryness agree least closely.

The way in which the maxima of sunshine and of conceptions coincide in May may be significant. Numerous recent studies indicate that light has a pronounced effect in stimulating the reproductive glands of birds and other animals. Rowan (1931), for example, in *The Riddle of Migration* has presented some very interesting evidence tending to show that migration occurs among birds because changes in the amount of daylight tend to stimulate the reproductive glands and produce an urge which first sends birds to their breeding ground, and later leads to mating. Bissonnette (1936) gives a long list of animals in which sexual activity is stimulated by changes in the length of the day. For example, some aphids, some sheep and deer, and various other animals resemble our autumn plants, such as the chrysanthemum, which are stimulated to produce seeds by the short days of fall. Other animals, such as ferrets, field mice, hedgehogs, crows, canaries, poultry, and some other aphids, are stimulated to reproduction when the days become longer in the spring. In some animals, such as the hedgehogs and field mice, there is a sexual response to several factors, including light, temperature, and food. Moreover, in all animals that have been investigated thus far, improper food, and, especially, deficiencies in vitamins, fats, and salts (to quote Bissonnette), "may act as limiting factors which may prevent changes in sexual cycles [from occurring in response] to changes in length of day, or even suppress sexual cycles altogether."

Taking all the curves of Figure 5 into consideration, it appears that the number of conceptions varies more closely in harmony with the direct climatic factors of sunshine, relative humidity, and temperature than with indirect climatic effects such as seasonal variations in diet and health. Thus so far as we have yet gone the hypothesis of a direct climatic effect on reproduction fits the facts more closely than the hypothesis of an indirect climatic effect through diet and disease, or than the hypothesis of a biological rhythm independent of the environment. The direct climatic hypothesis involves the following possibilities, which may or may not prove tenable when we have investigated further: (1) The minimum of conceptions in winter may be due to low temperature, but it is impossible to say how large a part is played by concomitant conditions of diet, sunshine, humidity, housing, and clothing. (2) The maximum in May is subject to two possible explanations, both of which may work together: (a) Rising temperature may have a stimulating effect upon reproduction up to a mean of about 60°. At higher temperatures the effect may be reversed, but in Belgium the drop of temperature from the slightly higher level in summer to the supposed optimum may not be sufficient to stimulate reproduction once more. (*b*) Increasing sunlight and dryness may also have a stimulating effect until their optimum is reached. Then they may become harmful.

Another way to put the matter is that the seasonal quality of the Belgian curve of births is so clear that some sort of climatic hypothesis appears to be inevitable. About 15 per cent more children are born at the season of more numerous births than at the season when births are at a minimum. The season of most births is characterized by temperatures rising to a mean of about 60° F., and by the driest, sunniest weather of a country which is never very sunny or very dry. The gist of the hypothesis which thus emerges may be stated as three propositions: First, in Belgium this combination of weather, or else some factor in this combination, is especially stimulating to reproduction. Second, if births occur in harmony with the basic seasonal rhythm, that is, near its maximum, the chances of survival are greater than otherwise. Third, the relationship of weather and conceptions which leads to the most births in February and March is presumably inherited from some long past condition in which such a relationship was especially desirable. The obvious corollary is that the minimum birth rate occurs in October, November, and December because those were the least favorable months for survival at some past time, when the present climatic adaptations of the Belgians were acquired.

Before we accept this climatic hypothesis, or any other, we must inquire whether any cultural conditions can properly be invoked as more or less responsible for the seasonal variations of births in Belgium. The season of marriage may be a cultural condition of this sort. Because of Belgium's recent low birth rate of only about 17 each year per 1000 inhabitants, a large share of all births are the first births to the respective mothers. From 1927 to 1933, for example, almost

exactly 40 per cent of the total births were first births, provided we assume that 15 per cent of Belgian marriages were
childless, and that first births after more than 7 years of married life are negligible.   If marriages are exceptionally numerous at certain seasons in a population where first births
form so large a proportion of all births, we might reasonably
suppose that the number of conceptions soon after marriage

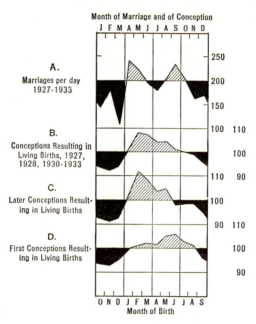

FIG. 6.—Relation of First and Later Conceptions to Date of Marriage in
Belgium.

forms an appreciable element in causing fluctuations in the
number of births from month to month.

Figure 6 shows to what extent this supposition is reliable.
Curves *A* and *B* make it possible to compare the number of
marriages month by month with the births 9 months later.
There is not much resemblance between the two curves.
The maximum of marriages (244 per day), to be sure, comes
in April, just a month before the maximum of conceptions.

This loses much of its significance, however, when we note that the preceding month, by reason of Lent, shows a minimum of marriages, only 109.

A more important consideration is that the percentage of first births arising from conceptions immediately after marriage is not so large as is generally supposed. Although no data on this point are available for Belgium, Gini (1930) gives a table for Italy which shows that in 1926 approximately 18 per cent of all first births occurred within 9 months

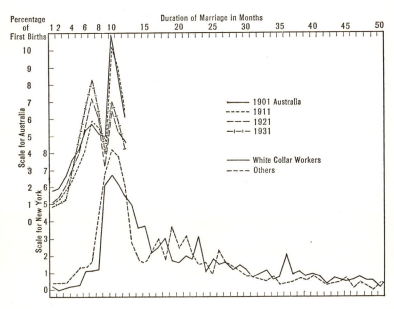

Fig. 7.—Relation of First Births to Date of Marriage. Upper four curves, Australia. Lower two, New York City.

of marriage, and 30 per cent more in the next 3 months. The Official Yearbook of the Commonwealth of Australia gives similar but more detailed figures, as appears in the upper part of Figure 7. There we see that 1 or 2 per cent of the first births occur during the first month after marriage. During succeeding months the percentage rises steadily. In 1901 it had reached nearly 6 per cent in the seventh month, and in later years had risen still higher at that time. In

1931 it was more than 8 per cent. This seems to mean that in Australia many marriages are contracted when girls first discover that they are pregnant because of extramarital sex relations. During the eighth and ninth months after marriage the percentage of first births falls once more, thus leaving a peak in the seventh month. The peak which would normally be expected among first births in the tenth month after marriage rose only to 11 per cent in the earlier days of Australia and has now fallen to 6 or 7.

American and Swiss, as well as Australian, data as to the number of first children born at various intervals after marriage are shown in Table 2A. The American data were collected in New York for the Milbank Memorial Fund, and have been most kindly placed at my disposal by Dr. Frank W. Notestein. They represent only 1762 births, but are especially valuable because they are divided into two occupational groups, and show the conditions long after the date

TABLE 2A

PERCENTAGE OF FIRST BIRTHS AT VARIOUS INTERVALS AFTER MARRIAGE

Duration of Marriage	New York, 1932		Switzerland, 1933		Australia			
	White Collar	Manual	Rural	Cities *	1911	1921	1931	1933
Months								
0–3	0.3	1.2	13.6	11.6	10.0	6.6	8.1	7.3
4–7	2.3	5.1	13.2	12.7	21.4	18.9	23.0	25.7
8	0.8	4.0	3.4	2.7	4.9	4.7	3.3	3.8
9–11	19.8	22.3	20.8	14.0	25.4	25.5	16.7	17.2
1 yr. or less	23.2	32.6	51.0	41.0	61.7	55.7	51.1	54.0
12–23	35.2	32.0	27.7	26.7	23.8	27.2	25.8	23.0
24–34	14.4	12.8	9.6	13.1	6.8	7.1	10.0	8.7
36–47	10.0	6.0	5.1	7.6	2.9	3.4	5.3	5.3
48–59	5.2	3.1	2.5	4.4	1.5	2.0	2.8	3.1
5 yrs. or more	12.0	13.5	4.1	7.2	3.3	4.6	5.0	5.9

*Over 10,000 population.

TABLE 2B

Estimated Normal Percentage of First Births Each Month During First Two Years After Marriage

Month	Per-centage	Month	Per-centage	Month	Per-centage
First	0.5	9th	8.5	17th	2.4
Second	0.5	10th	11.0	18th	2.2
Third	0.5	11th	10.0	19th	2.0
Fourth	0.7	12th	9.0	20th	1.9
Fifth	1.0	13th	4.0	21st	1.8
Sixth	1.3	14th	3.0	22nd	1.7
Seventh	1.6	15th	2.8	23rd	1.6
Eighth	3.5	16th	2.6	24th	1.5

of marriage, as appears in the lower part of Figure 7. They show that only 7 per cent of the first births occurred within 8 months of marriage (3.4 among white collar workers and 10.3 among manual workers), as compared with 18 in Italy and 32 in Australia. There is evidently a good deal of variability from country to country. This is partly because of local customs, such as the strong Australian tendency toward premarital conceptions. In addition to this, there is a distinct difference in habits among different social groups, as is evident in Dr. Notestein's data where white collar workers show less tendency than manual workers not only toward premarital conceptions, but also toward conceptions immediately after marriage. The percentage of first births occurring within 1 year of marriage ranges all the way from 23 among white collar workers in New York to 62 in Australia in 1911.

For our present purpose the significant fact is that all these data agree as to one important point. Although first births are especially numerous from the ninth to the twelfth month after marriage, they are spread over a long period, and no one month has much more than 10 per cent of them. On the basis of all the available data we may frame Table 2B, showing the probable distribution of first births in a population where sexual relations before marriage are rather strictly limited and where there is not much birth control.

This is the sort of population in which the season of marriage has the strongest effect upon the seasonal distribution of births. When we apply these figures to Belgium we are probably giving the month of marriage more weight than it actually deserves, but it is better to err on this side than on the other.

Table 2B assumes that 75.6 per cent of the first births occur during the first 2 years after marriage. Table 2A shows that the corresponding percentage is 58 among white collar New Yorkers, 68 in Swiss cities, and 77 or 78 in rural Switzerland and modern Australia. There is no reason to think that the date of marriage has any significant relation to the season of conception of the first children born more than 2 years after marriage, or of the few born before marriage.

On this basis, then, and on that of the known number of marriages each month, Curve D of Figure 6 represents the approximate seasonal distribution of conceptions leading to first births in Belgium. A distinct minimum of first conceptions in January, February, and March coincides with the minimum for all conceptions. The maximum of first conceptions in August and September, however, has no apparent relation to the maximum of later conceptions or to the weather. It apparently depends on the fact that during long centuries the feeling of prosperity engendered by the harvests, and the relief from the heavy work of summer, made late summer and early fall a favorite time for marriages. April, to be sure, has more marriages than any other month because it comes just after Lent, but the great restriction of marriages during Lent itself causes the average for the late winter and spring to be much lower than for the late summer and early autumn.

The seasonal distribution of later births is easily determined by subtracting the first births from all births. The result is seen in Curve C of Figure 6.* This curve is signifi-

---

* No allowance has here been made for childless marriages. If this were done the peak of Curve C would be reduced very slightly, but scarcely enough to be noticeable in the diagram.

cant because it indicates that, when the cultural factor represented by the season of marriage is removed, the seasonal rhythm with its maximum of conceptions in May and its minimum from January to March is accentuated. The range between the highest point in May and the lowest in February becomes nearly 20 per cent instead of 15, as it is when first births are included with later births. The seasonal fluctuations in the later births represent the free expression of the urge toward reproduction. In them the sudden excess of sexual activity which comes when the temperature rises from about 43° F. (6° C.) in March to 58° F. (14.5° C.) in May is accentuated.

The records of Berlin from 1906 to 1910, as published by Gini (1912), agree with what has just been said about Belgium. They show that marriages rise to two sharp peaks in April and October. During those months they are more than twice as numerous as during the rest of the year. Legitimate first births follow a closely similar course 9 months later. They show two maxima, one in January and February with more than the average in March, and the other in July with almost as many in August and more than the average in September. Except for the second maximum the curve of first births is almost like that of all births in Belgium. This suggests that the seasonal distribution of marriages is based to a considerable degree on the physiological rhythm which leads to numerous conceptions in the spring and few in the winter. It is also influenced by economic conditions which make people feel prosperous and give them leisure after the harvest season, thus leading to an autumn maximum as well as one in the spring. In neither Belgium nor Berlin, however, nor in any other place that we have studied, does the season of marriage appear to have more than a minor effect upon the seasonal distribution of births as a whole.

The seasonal distribution of illegitimate births, as well as legitimate births after the first, must be strongly influenced by seasonal variations in the impulse toward reproduction. Unlike legitimate births, however, the illegitimate ones have generally been supposed to reach a maximum in summer because of the opportunities afforded to lovers by the warm, pleasant weather. It seems as if the restrictions imposed by winter weather would limit illegitimate intimacy of the sexes, but have little effect upon legitimate intimacy.

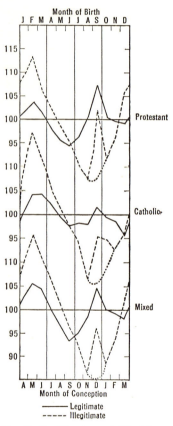

FIG. 8.—Legitimate and Illegitimate Births in Germany.

We shall test this by means of data from Germany and Sweden because data for illegitimacy are not available by months in Belgium. The seasonal distribution of all births in Germany has long been almost the same as in Belgium, except that the September maximum, which we shall examine later, has been more prominent in Germany than in Belgium. It formerly existed in Belgium.

The curves of Figure 8 show that in Germany, before the advent of birth control, the seasonal fluctuations of legitimate and illegitimate births among both Protestants and Catholics, and also in mixed unions, were essentially the same. All six curves show a strong maximum in February. This is much stronger among the illegitimate (the lines of small dashes, not the dots) than among the legitimate. All six also show a second maximum in September, but this, on the contrary, is systematically lower among the illegitimate than among the legitimate births. Nevertheless, the rise to the second maximum is in each case more sudden in the illegitimate than in the legitimate curve. Except among the Roman Catholics the second maximum of the illegitimate curves is limited to the month of September, and represents conceptions in December. To anticipate a later conclusion, this peak of conceptions in December is due mainly, if not wholly, to two causes. One is the return of men who have been working elsewhere, but who come home in winter when there is little work, or at least return for a visit at Christmas time. The other is the license and drunkenness which often accompany the Christmas and New Year festivities.

A comparison of the legitimate and illegitimate curves of Figure 8 indicates that the first cause—the return of the men to their homes—is much more important among the legitimate than among the illegitimate births. All births of both kinds decline in number from February to June, corresponding to conceptions from May to September. This agrees perfectly with what happens in Belgium. In October and November the legitimate conceptions begin to increase because husbands who have been at work away from home during the summer begin to come home. The illegitimate conceptions, however, continue to decline in harmony with the animal rhythm as we have seen it in Belgium. In December, because of the greater number of men who come home, and the greater license of the holidays, both types of conceptions increase, but it is the illegitimate ones that make the biggest jump. Afterward the latter fall off greatly, but the legitimate conceptions, though declining in number, still remain at a fairly high level because so many husbands who will go away in the spring are still at home.

Suppose now that we eliminate the effect of the holiday season. The curves for illegitimate births would then assume the form indicated by the fine dots in Figure 8. This gives curves like those of Belgium except that the minimum of conceptions comes in December instead of February. The range between maximum and minimum is greater than in Belgium, being approximately from 115 to 85 instead of 108 to 92. It is not so great as would appear at first sight, however, for Figure 8 is drawn on a vertical scale twice that of Figure 1. If the effect of the holiday season and of the return home of husbands during the winter were eliminated from the legitimate curves of Figure 8, these, too, would show that the basic animal rhythm has essentially the Belgian form. Thus Figure 8 leads to the conclusion that in Germany two generations ago the births among both Protestants and Catholics followed practically the same seasonal course no matter whether they were legitimate or illegitimate.

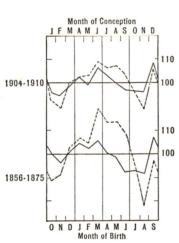

FIG. 9.—Legitimate and Illegitimate Births in Sweden.

The minor differences between the legitimate and illegitimate curves are apparently due to well-known cultural conditions such as the seasonal migrations of the men and the occurrence of festivals. If the effect of these were eliminated all the old German curves would be essentially the same as the recent Belgian curve of births in general.

A comparison of legitimate and illegitimate births in other countries leads to the same conclusion as in Germany. Sweden (Figure 9) illustrates the matter. The Swedish curves, it will be noted, are plotted according to the month of conception rather than birth. They pertain to an early period, 1856-1875, and an intermediate period, 1904-1910. The same two maxima that we found in Germany are evident. The earlier one comes in June rather than May (thus corresponding to births in March) presumably because the Swedish climate is cooler than that of Belgium, as we shall see later. The other maximum comes sharply in December. In their main features the Swedish curves follow those of Germany very closely. In both countries there are two maxima, and in both the illegitimate maximum is higher than the corresponding legitimate maximum in the spring, but lower in

December. In both, the illegitimate curves have the greater range from maximum to minimum; and in both the midwinter minimum of conceptions is not so low among legitimate births as among illegitimate.

In addition to these main resemblances there are three differences between the Swedish and German curves. One of these, the shifting of the earlier maximum from May to June, has already been mentioned. The second is that the Swedish curves, like that of Belgium, have their winter minimum of conceptions in February, or in one case January, instead of December, as would apparently be the case in Germany if it were not for the holidays and the homecomings. The assumed German minimum in December when the days are shortest suggests that the intensity of the light may have an effect upon reproduction. The Swedish and Belgian curves, however, where there is no assumption, suggest that temperature is more important than light. On the other hand, the Swedish maximum in June comes just when the light in that far northern land is strongest and not when the temperature is highest. The truth may be that light, temperature, and perhaps other climatic conditions all play some part in determining the season of maximum conceptions.

The third difference between the Swedish and German curves gives some idea of the reliability of the common idea that illegitimacy increases greatly in warm weather because of the ease with which illicit relations are then possible. The German curves do not support this idea at all. After their maximum in May (births in February according to Figure 8), illegitimate conceptions decline rapidly throughout the entire warm period. In Sweden a similar situation prevails except that in August the two illegitimate curves for that country show a slight bulge. This we may probably ascribe to the opportunities for illicit relations afforded by the summer. The small size of the bulge, however, suggests that the strength of the sexual urge as determined by the rhythm of the seasons is vastly more important than any other factor in determining the seasonal distribution of illegitimacy.

Figure 10 illustrates the same thing in still another way. There the rural curves for Norway (the upper pair) are similar to those of Figure 9 representing Sweden as a whole.

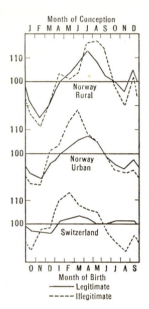

Month of Conception
J F M A M J J A S O N D

110
100
Norway
Rural

110
100
Norway
Urban

110
100
Switzerland

O N D J F M A M J J A S
Month of Birth
——— Legitimate
- - - - Illegitimate

FIG. 10.—Legitimate and Illegitimate Births in Norway and Switzerland.

They are more extreme, to be sure, even though they come from modern times instead of one or two generations ago. The only essential difference is that the maximum of the Norwegian curves comes in July instead of June, as in Sweden. This is presumably appropriate to a more northern climate, for the rural people of Norway live considerably farther north than those of Sweden. The bulge in the curve of illegitimate births in August is like that which comes in July and August in the Swedish curve, and is presumably due to the opportunities for love-making afforded by warm weather in rural districts. The urban curves of Norway resemble the rural curves, but with interesting differences. The illegitimate urban curve, for example, shows a maximum in June instead of July; it shows no bulge during the months of July and August; and there is only the merest hint of a rise in December. Such conditions suggest that in Norwegian cities neither warm weather with its opportunities for the two sexes to meet, nor the return of unmarried absentees at the holiday season, plays much part in determining the seasonal variations of the birth rate. The illegitimate curve there apparently comes very close to representing variations in reproductive activity with only the slightest modification by any conditions except the weather.

A similar statement applies to the Swiss curve of illegitimacy in the lower part of Figure 10. Nevertheless, the Swiss curve, perhaps because it includes a fairly large rural population, shows a slight bulge in August, and a fairly strong minor maximum in December. The contrast between the flattened curve of legitimate births in Switzerland and the sharply defined maximum and minimum of the illegitimate curve is noticeable. Here again the meaning seems to be that the flattened curve is greatly modified by cultural conditions whereas the other curve represents a basic animal rhythm dependent upon physiological conditions, and set in motion by climatic conditions in the form of temperature or sunlight.

A thorough study of the annual rhythm of reproduction must consider not only successful conceptions, but also those that fail to materialize in living births. The failures include abortions, which occur mainly during the first 4 months after conception; miscarriages, which are the same as abortions except that they occur after the sixth month; and stillbirths, which represent deaths at birth. Abortion, as used below, includes miscarriage. It was formerly estimated that 8 or 10 per cent of all pregnancies terminate in spontaneous abortions. This agrees with data collected by Kopp (1934) in the most extensive study of the matter thus far made. In a total of 38,985 pregnancies among New York women she found 3060 spontaneous abortions, or approximately 8 per cent. Williams (1927 [Stander, 1936]), however, states that the actual figure is more nearly 20, since a great many additional abortions take place unnoticed during the first month of pregnancy. The relation of the 3060 spontaneous abortions studied by Kopp to duration of pregnancy is shown in Column A of Table 3.

In a study of the seasonal distribution of births in modern times, allowance must be made for induced abortions as well as those that are spontaneous. According to Tausig (1936), the abortions of all kinds in the cities of the United States probably amount to about 29 per cent of the conceptions (25 per cent of the confinements), while in the rural areas the percentage is about 17 (20 per cent of the confinements). This means that induced abortions are two or even three or four times as numerous as the spontaneous type. In the past, however, the number of induced abortions was less than at present. The period of gestation when induced abor-

TABLE 3

PERCENTAGE OF ABORTIONS ACCORDING TO MONTH OF GESTATION

Month	A 3060 Spontaneous Abortions—Kopp	B 7166 Induced Abortions—Kopp	C 2906 Spontaneous and Induced Abortions at Magdeburg, Germany —Roesle
First..........	9	27	0.4
Second........	42	58	8
Third.........	32	13	34
Fourth........	} 17	} 2	31
Fifth..........			16
Sixth.........			7

tions occur, according to Kopp, is given in Column B of Table 3. Roesle (1930) states that at Magdeburg in Germany the two types show the same relation to gestation, and occur in the percentages indicated in Column C.

In order to obtain the total number of conceptions that fail to produce living births we must also take account of stillbirths. In Belgium these have recently been about 2.7 per cent as numerous as the living births. Taking all things into account we may assume that in Belgium, during the period on which the curve of Figure 1 is based (1927-1933), approximately 25 per cent of all conceptions failed to result in living births and that these are distributed as in Table 4. Even if the percentages there given are in error by as much as 50 per cent the conclusions to be drawn from them will not be altered.

Before we can use Table 4 as a basis for estimating the total number of conceptions each month we must know to what extent the susceptibility of women to abortions, mis-

TABLE 4

ESTIMATED ABORTIONS, MISCARRIAGES, AND STILLBIRTHS AS PERCENTAGES
OF ALL CONCEPTIONS DURING EACH MONTH OF GESTATION

Month	Per-centage	Month	Per-centage	Month	Per-centage
First........	1.9	Fourth......	2.4	Seventh.....	0.6
Second......	8.4	Fifth........	1.5	Eighth......	1.0
Third.......	6.4	Sixth........	0.8	Ninth.......	2.0

carriages, and stillbirths varies from one calendar month to
another. A comparison of Curves *A* and *B* in Figure 11
indicates that in Belgium stillbirths (*B*) show the same sea-

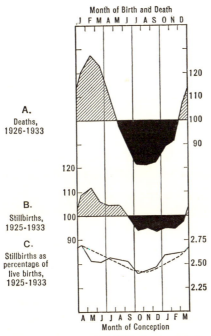

FIG. 11.—Deaths and Stillbirths in Belgium.

sonal variations as do deaths in general (*A*), but vary far less
from season to season. Curve *C* shows that, when the stillbirths are expressed as a percentage of the live births, the
general seasonal trend remains the same. In view of the

fact that under normal conditions the health of pregnant women is better than that of the average population, the variation in the percentage of abortions and miscarriages from season to season may not be any greater than that of stillbirths. Let us see what happens on this assumption (*a*), and also on the assumption (*b*) that the variation is midway between that of stillbirths and deaths in general. Applying these two rates of loss to the number of births in different months and reckoning the losses at different stages of pregnancy at the rates given in Table 4, we get the results shown in Figure 12. There the solid line represents conceptions

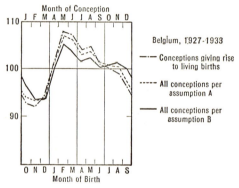

FIG. 12.—Estimate of Total Conceptions in Belgium.

resulting in living births, and is the same as *B* in Figure 6 except that the vertical scale is twice as great. The dotted line represents *all* conceptions according to assumption (*a*), the assumption being that the losses of embryos vary from month to month at the same rate as do stillbirths. The solid and the dotted lines are almost identical, except that the contrast between the seasons is reduced by including the abortions. Even when we make the much more drastic assumption (*b*) that the losses of embryos vary from month to month at rates midway between those of stillbirths and of mortality as a whole, the general form of the curve of conceptions remains unchanged, as appears in the barred line of Figure 12. Hence we conclude that, although abortions, miscarriages, and stillbirths represent a large loss of embryos, their inclusion does not materially alter the general seasonal rhythm of conceptions as inferred from the curve for living births alone.

The net result of our study thus far is that the main features of the seasonal distribution of Belgian births are not in harmony with any hypothesis based either on indirect climatic influences such as diet, or on cultural conditions such as season of marriage. On the other hand, we have found nothing thus far that is out of harmony with the hypothesis of a basic animal rhythm of reproduction which is governed by the weather in such a way that infants are born in greatest numbers at the season when their chances of life are at a maximum.

CHAPTER III

FASTS, FEASTS, AND HUMAN FALLIBILITY: RUSSIA

A Russian curve appears in Figure 1 because Russia affords a pronounced example of statistical inaccuracy and of the effect of religious observances and seasonal migrations. Curve C in Figure 1 shows the seasonal distribution of births as reported from 1870 to 1875 among the Orthodox Christians of four provinces in southeastern Russia. This region is so far in the interior that its climate is very continental. The mean temperature of January ranges from about 3° F. in the northeastern part to 18° F. in the southeast; in July the range is from 70° to 75°. This gives a type of climate very different from that of Belgium or Japan. The whole region is notably poor and backward. Not only does it suffer frequently from drought, and hence from want and even famine, but contrary to the general supposition the amount of cultivated land has long been extremely small in proportion to the agricultural population. Although the majority of the inhabitants belonged to the Orthodox Church before the Soviet revolution, a considerable number were Moslems. The most prosperous and progressive section of the population consisted of Protestants, especially German colonists near the Volga; toward the west Jews formed a part of the city population. Hence in this region it is possible to compare the seasons of birth among people of diverse races and religions.

A period of two generations ago has been selected partly because data for that period happen to be available. Another reason is that in a later chapter we shall inquire how the seasonal distribution of births in general compares with that of persons of unusual eminence. Therefore it is desirable to have data which as nearly as possible represent the time when the eminent people were born. No post-war statistics of births by months in Russia are available.

Since the Russian data are based on the old Julian calendar, the month called January runs from approximately the middle of our January to the middle of our February. For this reason the old Russian data of Figures 1, 14, and 15, are plotted so that the point denoting each month falls at the end of the corresponding month in our calendar, and not in the middle as in the case in other diagrams. In Figures 13 and 16 to 19 where this adjustment has not been made, the reader should mentally shove the Russian curves half a month to the right.

The most extreme feature of the Russian curve in Figure 1 is the small number of births in December (our December-January) and the great number in January. The births in December (71) appear to be only about half as numerous as those in January (124). Much of this difference seems to be due to statistical inaccuracy. One reason for thinking this is that the contrast between December and January becomes greater as one goes from the northwest of Russia, where progress has long been greatest, to the southeast, where there has been least progress. The difference between Livland (now Latvia), near the top at the left in Figure 13, and Astrakan, at the bottom on the right, illustrates this. In Figure 13 the reported births among Orthodox Christians in a number of Russian provinces have been arranged in approximately the positions which the provinces occupy on the map. The number of births for the first and last months of the year, as given in the statistics, is indicated by the dotted lines. The solid lines represent an attempt to correct the statistics.

In a general way the northwestern provinces, where the state of culture has long been the highest, show only a mild contrast between December and January, whereas the contrast increases toward the south and east. The restrictions of our diagram have made it desirable to place the province of Olonetz above Livland so that it wrongly appears to be the most northwestern province, but Olonetz really lies almost as far east as Vologda, which heads the next column of diagrams. Livland is the most northwestern province of Figure 13. It has no dotted line at all, because no excess

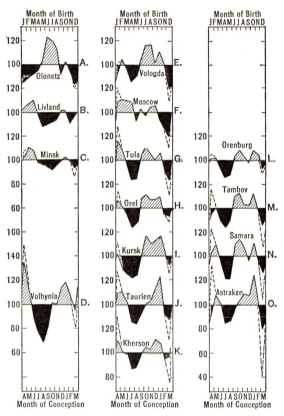

FIG. 13.—Season of Birth among Orthodox Christians in Russia, 1870-1875.

of births in January is indicated. In Astrakan, the most southeastern and most backward province, the contrast between December and January reaches the extraordinary ratio of only 41 reported births in December against 132 in January. This suggests that the ignorant and backward people of Astrakan included a large share of the December births among those reported in January. The only other alternative seems to be that the Lenten season, which will be discussed below, was observed far more rigorously in Astrakan than elsewhere. This supposition is negated by the fact that Astrakan shows no greater response to other fasts

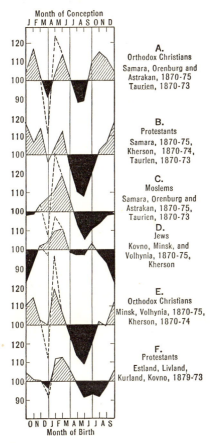

Month of Conception
J F M A M J J A S O N D

A.
Orthodox Christians
Samara, Orenburg and
Astrakan, 1870-75
Taurien, 1870-73

B.
Protestants
Samara, 1870-75,
Kherson, 1870-74,
Taurien, 1870-73

C.
Moslems
Samara, Orenburg and
Astrakan, 1870-75,
Taurien, 1870-73

D.
Jews
Kovno, Minsk, and
Volhynia, 1870-75,
Kherson

E.
Orthodox Christians
Minsk, Volhynia, 1870-75,
Kherson, 1870-74

F.
Protestants
Estland, Livland,
Kurland, Kovno, 1879-73

O N D J F M A M J J A S
Month of Birth

FIG. 14.—Relation of Religion to Season of Birth in Russia.

than do many other provinces. Hence the corrected solid line of the Astrakan curve is very different from the uncorrected dotted line.

Further confirmation of the statistical error in December and January is seen in Figure 14. There the Russian curve of Figure 1 is repeated (*A*), but is plotted according to the month of conception instead of birth. Below it are similar curves for other religious groups. In Figure 14 the *dotted* line in the Orthodox Curve (*A*) shows a tremendous dip in March and an extreme rise in April, but the Protestant curve just below it shows only a moderate difference between the two months. The dotted lines in Figure 14, as in Figure 13, indicate the reported figures, and the corresponding solid lines indicate an attempt to eliminate the error at the end of the year. In Curve *B*, representing Protestants in south-eastern Russia, the contrast between the number of conceptions in March and April (births in December and January) is about the same as among the Orthodox Christians of Liv-

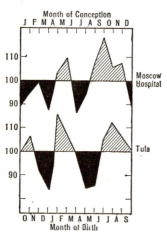

Month of Conception
J F M A M J J A S O N D

110
100 — Moscow Hospital
90

110
100 — Tula
90

O N D J F M A M J J A S
Month of Birth

FIG. 15.—Conceptions in Moscow Hospital and in Province of Tula, 1870-1875.

land as shown in Figure 13. This corresponds with the fact that among the German Protestants of eastern Russia the stage of culture is higher than among the Russians around them, and is much like that of the Orthodox Christians in the most advanced parts of old Russia. Moreover, it is probable that because they did not belong to the established church the Protestants felt obliged to keep their statistics more carefully than did their easy-going Orthodox neighbors.

Still another reason for believing that we are dealing with a statistical error is that neither in Curve *F* of Figure 14, nor in Figure 15, is the contrast between the number of conceptions in March and April extreme. Curve *F* illustrates the conditions among Protestants in northwestern Russia, and may have a slight statistical error. Figure 15, however, has no statistical error in the part based on births in a Moscow hospital.

The curve for the Moslems of southeastern Russia (C in Figure 14) presents a strong contrast to Curve F and to Figure 15. Its dotted portions suggest a contrast between the births in December and January (conceptions in March and April) even greater than that shown in the Orthodox curve. This cannot be due to the fast of Lent, which may be an important element in the form of the Orthodox curve, for the Moslems do not observe Lent. It can, however, be due to failure to report the December births until January, and such an error is likely to be more extreme among the Moslems than among the Christians because the Moslems are more ignorant and also more scattered. If we deduct 20 from the January ratio and add the same amount to December, the Moslem curve of conceptions in Figure 14 rises smoothly from a minimum in December and January to a maximum at the end of May, as indicated by the solid line in Figure 14.

In regions where statistical methods are poorly developed there is a widespread and consistent tendency toward abnormal data in December and January. In old Russia at all times there seems to have been much delay in reporting births, especially in the outlying or more ignorant villages. The central government apparently did not make sufficient allowance for this, but insisted that at the end of the year reports be sent to headquarters even though they were incomplete. The natural result was that many births which occurred in December did not get into the record of the year to which they belonged, but were added to those of the succeeding January. Thus our Russian Orthodox curve in Figure 1 owes part of its low level in December to a statistical error. We have enlarged on this because it is highly important to be on the lookout for such errors. In many cases they can be at least partially eliminated if they are understood. We shall find a different form of year-end error when we come to the early American records. Meanwhile, as already stated, it should be remembered that except in Figure 1 the solid lines for Russia show our estimate of the actual number of births or conceptions; the dotted lines show the number reported.

Religious observances exerted an easily detected influence upon the seasonal distribution of births in old Russia, especially among the Orthodox Christians. This is very clear in Figure 15, which is based on 11,949 births in a Moscow hospital before the World War. The births are here plotted according to the month of conception, and with allowance for the difference between the old Julian calendar and ours. The authority to whom we owe this curve * believes that its three main minima are all due to periods of fasting imposed by the old Orthodox church. He does not make allowance for other conditions, but there seems to be good reason for believing that among the city people who used the Moscow hospital religious observances had a particularly strong effect upon the birth rate. During the religious fasts all marriages were forbidden in old Russia, and an attempt was made to restrict marital intercourse. This was doubtless successful to very different degrees among different parts of the population, but the pre-war Russians as a whole were decidedly devout and superstitious.

The first minimum in the Moscow curve of conceptions occurs in the Russian December. This brings it at both ends of Figure 15, for December of the Julian calendar was equivalent to our period of mid-December to mid-January. The December minimum is the result of the Christmas fast which began early in our December and lasted until about January 6, when the Russian Christmas was celebrated. The next minimum represents the great fast of six weeks in Lent. Its chief effect was to reduce the number of conceptions in our March and thus lead to few births in December. It happens to coincide with the false minimum due to the inaccuracy of the Russian statistics at the end of the year. Therefore, its

---

* The data on which the curve is based were given me by Mr. Leon F. Whitney, but there was no notation as to their source and we have not been able to find it.

form in Figure 15 gives a means of correcting the extreme form which is suggested by the faulty statistics published by the government.

The third and greatest minimum of births in the Moscow hospital curve is ascribed by our Russian authority to a fast of four weeks in midsummer during the Russian June (the last part of our June and the first part of July). This may be correct, but for some unexplained reason—perhaps a statistical error—the province of Moscow as a whole (*F* in Figure 13) does not show such a minimum. It appears in the neighboring province of Tula (the lower curve of Figure 15) at the later date, and is apparently due there and elsewhere to migration, as will appear below.

The peaks of the hospital curve in Figure 15 are quite as important as the depressions. They are doubtless due in part to a reaction against the limitations of the fasts, but the festivities and widespread drunkenness at Christmas, New Year's, Easter, and other festivals which immediately succeeded the fasts do not show the conspicuous results that would be expected. The license which prevailed at such times probably led to a considerable percentage of the illegitimate births which were always numerous in Russian cities under the old regime. In old Russia about 10 per cent of the births reported in the cities of Moscow and St. Petersburg (Leningrad) were illegitimate, whereas in the rest of the country the percentage was only about 3. This may be one reason why the curve of births in the Moscow hospital differs in many ways from the corresponding curves for the population in general. Nevertheless the main maximum of conceptions took place about the first of October, at much the same season as in other parts of Russia. The reason is doubtless the same. In old Russia the women whose children were born in hospitals belonged largely to the lowest social level. Their husbands often went out into the country to find work in summer. When they returned home in the autumn the number of conceptions rose to a high level. Thus the Moscow hospital furnishes an example of the way in which the habits of poor, ignorant, and superstitious people are affected not only by religious fasts and festivals, but also by other social customs.

The seasonal distribution of marriage had no greater effect upon the seasonal distribution of births in old Russia than in Belgium. Nevertheless, the two types of distribution show certain marked similarities which are worth looking into. Fasts, feasts, and agriculture appear to have had an important influence upon both. The prohibition of marriages during fasts naturally led to a great number during the succeeding festivities. The necessities of agriculture made the summer, especially the harvest season, a poor time for marriages. The winter, on the other hand, was favorable because everyone was then at home, and there was plenty of leisure.

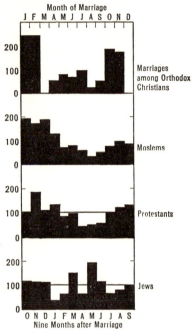

FIG. 16.—Marriages in Russia, 1886, 1889, 1894, and 1897.

Figure 16 shows how these two factors, religion and agriculture—combined to influence the seasonal distribution of marriages among the various religious groups of Russia. It is based on data for individual Russian provinces and separate religious beliefs during later years than have thus far been used—namely, 1886, 1889, 1894, and 1897. These years were chosen simply because reports for them happened to be available. The seasonal distribution of births and marriages respectively is essentially the same in each of the four years, and is like that during the earlier years used previously. It presumably remained about the same throughout the whole of the old regime. If the average number of marriages per day be taken as 100 for each religious group, the Orthodox Christians had 244 marriages per day during their January and February in contrast to practically none in March and December, and only 23 in August. The Mohammedans show a rather regular seasonal swing from 195 in January, when there is little farm work and much leisure, to only 30 in August at harvest time when everyone is busy and many of the young men are away from home. The Protestants show nearly the same seasonal distribution of marriages as the Moslems, but do not go to such great extremes (184 and 43). They had a prolonged period of few marriages at harvest time—July 43, August 45, and September 52. The more urban character of the Jews, and the distinctive seasonal distribution of their religious festivals, caused their marriages to be distributed according to still another pattern.

At first sight it would seem as if a seasonal distribution of marriages so extreme as that of the Orthodox Christians ought to have an appreciable effect upon the seasonal distribution of births. Our suspicion that such may be the case appears to be strengthened when we see how closely the curves of marriages (dotted line) and conceptions (solid line) agree in Section *A* of Figure 17. The dotted lines there show marriages and are the same as the heavy bars in Figure 16. A line is used instead of bars merely to facilitate comparison with conceptions. The solid lines of Figure 17 show the number of conceptions giving rise to living births. Among these Orthodox Christians the seasonal distribution of marriages and conceptions is much alike except that the maximum of conceptions in April is only faintly matched in the curve of marriages, and the latter has a slight peak in July which finds no parallel in conceptions. Part of this discrepancy between the two curves, however, is due to the error in the January statistics, a condition to which attention is called by the asterisks in Figure 17. Among people of other religious faiths the resemblance between the curves of marriages and of conceptions is not quite so strong as among the Orthodox, but Figure 17 shows that among Russians of all faiths except the Jews marriages and conceptions both sank to a minimum in summer.

This does not mean that the small number of marriages

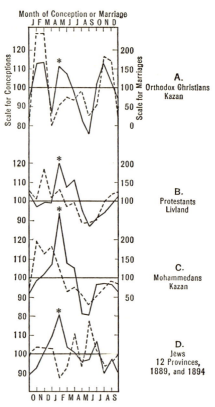

Fig. 17.—Births in Russia, by Religions, 1886, 1889, 1894, 1897. (Plotted according to Gregorian Calendar.)

is the cause of the small number of conceptions. It merely means that the same conditions limited both marriage and reproduction. The small effect of the season of marriage upon the seasonal curve of births is evident in Figure 18. The solid line shows the seasonal distribution of all Orthodox births, while the dotted line shows that of later births when first births occurring within a year of marriage are eliminated. The elimination has been made on the assumption that there are no births during the first 7 months of marriage, and that 5 per cent occur during the eighth

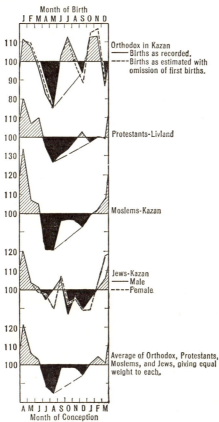

FIG. 18.—Births in Russia by Religions. (Plotted according to old Julian Calendar.)

month, 15 per cent during the ninth and also the 10th, 10 per cent during the eleventh, and 5 per cent during the twelfth. Thus 50 per cent of all first births are assumed to be concentrated within 5 months. This is a much greater concentration than occurs in the other countries for which we have data (see Table 2, page 48), and is presumably

much greater than actually occurred in Russia. Nevertheless, even with so extreme a concentration, the elimination of
the first births does not tend to flatten the seasonal curve.
On the contrary, it intensifies it.

From this we conclude that among the Orthodox Christians of old Russia the seasonal distribution of marriages was
of little or no importance as a cause of the peculiar seasonal
distribution of births. It was merely one of several results
which arose from the combined action of the climate, the
religion, the seasonal distribution of labor, and certain other
factors which we shall shortly discuss. All these caused variations in reproduction so great that in Kazan, according to
Figure 17, the births per day among Orthodox Christians
in October and November (conceptions in January and
February) were approximately 50 per cent more numerous
than in May. The causes which produced such variations
in conceptions led to a corresponding seasonal variation in
marriages.

Figure 17 indicates that among people of other religious
faiths the relation between the seasonal distribution of births
and marriages is not so close as among the Orthodox Christians. The seasons of marriage, however, have no more effect
upon those of births among these other groups than among
the Orthodox. In a word, even in an extreme case like
Russia the seasonal distribution of marriages is almost negligible as a factor in the seasonal distribution of births. It
is more likely to reduce than to increase the fluctuations of
the curve of births.

Having eliminated marriages, and being able to make allowance for statistical inaccuracy and religious or social oc-
currences in the form of fasts and festivals, let us next examine our Russian curves to see how far they show the basic
annual rhythm which we have seen in Belgium, Sweden,
Germany, Norway and Switzerland. Look back at all the
Russian curves of Figures 1 and 13, and see how far they
agree as to births during the 6 months from November
to April. Do the same for Figures 14, 15, and 17, but

bear in mind that they are plotted according to the month of conception. In their corrected form more than half (13) of the 25 different curves in these figures indicate a maximum of births in February. Most of the rest (10) show a maximum in January, but in several of these the maximum would shift to February if they were corrected for the statistical error at the end of the year. Only the curves for Olonetz and Livland in the left-hand column of Figure 13 fail to show maxima in these two months. In Livland the maximum comes in March, but February stands almost as high. Only Olonetz, with a June maximum, departs far from the general rule. That province lies in the far north and we shall see later that it is the exception which proves the rule.

From all this it seems possible to draw a definite conclusion. Throughout the vast country of Russia, except in the extreme north, a maximum of births occurs among all races and religions in the late winter, generally in February. Put in terms of our calendar, this means that a maximum of conceptions occurs systematically in late May and early June. The regularity of this maximum can be judged by turning back to Figure 14 (page 65), where people of four religious faiths in different parts of Russia are compared. Curve *A* represents Orthodox Christians in southeastern Russia; curves *B* and *C* respectively represent Protestants (mainly Germans) and Mohammedans (largely Tartars) in the same region; *D* represents Jews in a region overlapping the Protestant area, but farther west; *E* is based on Orthodox Christians in the same southwestern area as *D*; and *F* is the curve for Protestants in the Baltic provinces farther to the northwest. It is impossible to use the same provinces for all four religions, because all are nowhere found together in sufficient numbers.

A glance at these 6 curves makes it clear that the most nearly uniform feature of the whole series is a maximum of conceptions in the late spring at approximately the first of our June. The rise in conceptions which precedes this maximum begins in every case at least as early as the beginning of our April. The succeeding decline lasts until the beginning of our September, and September in every case shows an increase. Thus for 6 months, from April to September, there is almost perfect harmony in the fluctuations of reproduction in all parts of Russia from the Baltic to the Caspian and among all of the four main religious and racial groups. Moreover, this maximum of conceptions in late May and early June agrees with what we have found in Belgium, Germany, and elsewhere. It indicates that in Russia, also, conceptions take place in great numbers during the late spring when the temperature averages about 55° in the cooler Baltic regions and 60° to 65° in the warmer southeast. This should be compared with corresponding temperatures of about 58° F. to 63° F. in Belgium and the neighboring countries of Germany, Switzerland, Norway, and Sweden. It brings a maximum of births at the season which we have already found to be presumably the best for infants. Apparently Russia is like Belgium and Japan in showing strong evidence of a basic seasonal rhythm of reproduction like that of animals.

The other 6 months, from October to March, are much more puzzling because of the diversity of the curves in Figure 14. In general, to be sure, the number of conceptions increases during the autumn. A second maximum, however, is reached in September among the Jews (Curve D); in October among the Orthodox Christians of southeastern Russia (A); and not till December among their Protestant neighbors (B) and also among the Protestants of the Baltic region (F). A corresponding maximum appears still later (in January) among the southwestern Orthodox (E). It should be noted, however, that this maximum agrees with a third maximum among the Orthodox of the southeast (A), while the pronounced October maximum of the latter is reflected in a very small maximum among the western Orthodox of curve E. And finally the Moslem curve (C) shows only a single maximum and a single minimum. But this differs only a little from the northwestern Protestant curves (F).

All this is very confusing, but one point stands out clearly. In this half of the year from October to March the various Russian curves show much diversity, whereas in the other half they show a high degree of uniformity. We have already concluded that this uniformity suggests that the maximum of conceptions in our May or June not only in Russia, but also in other countries, indicates a widespread cause acting in the same way in many lands. The only such cause that we can find is climate. On the other hand, the diverse form of the seasonal curves showing conceptions in Russia from September or October to April seems to indicate that the fluctuations during that period are due to cultural conditions which vary widely from place to place, or from one type of people to another. The fact that the two Orthodox curves of Figure 17 have a family likeness, and that the two Protestant curves behave similarly, while the Jewish and Mohammedan curves behave differently, points strongly to this conclusion. We have already seen that fasts and feasts are cultural factors to which part of the departure of the curves of birth from the basic annual rhythm is due, but they do not offer a complete explanation. In the following paragraphs we shall look for still other cultural conditions which influence the season of birth.

In our search for other causes of the irregularities of the Russian curves of birth, let us turn again to Figure 17. There we have curves for four religions in individual provinces. The data employed are the latest at our disposal. American libraries, by the way, are woefully lacking in the statistical records of other countries. In all four curves of Figure 17 the most regular feature aside from the maximum of births in January is a minimum in May. The January maximum of births, when corrected for the year-end error and for the old Julian calendar, it will be remembered, becomes a maximum of conceptions in April or May. The minimum in May, when corrected for the old calendar, becomes a minimum of conceptions in August and September.

In order to get rid of minor fluctuations, let us smooth

the curves of Figure 17. The result appears in Figure 19, where the smoothed curves are plotted according to the month of birth rather than of conception in order to facilitate comparison with Belgium. To this same end dotted lines have been added which indicate the basic annual rhythm. If allowance could be made for the year-end error,

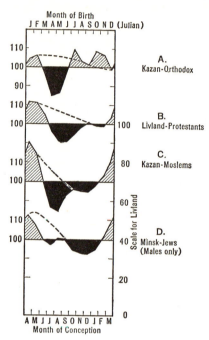

FIG. 19.—Smoothed Curves of Births in Russia by Religions (Julian Calendar).

the maximum of all the curves might come in February, but we cannot be positive about this.

The process of smoothing largely eliminates the effect of fasts and feasts except in the Orthodox curve at the top of Figure 19. With the help of the dotted lines it brings out the fact that a large portion of each of the other curves conforms fairly well with the Belgian model. And, finally, it shows that the main feature still remaining unexplained is a pronounced drop in births which usually begins in March and ends at various times from June to August. In other words, beginning in June, or in May among the Jews, there is a pronounced deficiency of conceptions in comparison with what would be expected on the basis of the fundamental annual rhythm. This continues through September, or even through November among the Protestants.

A minor cause of this decline of reproduction during the summer is perhaps found in the strenuousness of agricultural labor, but this does not apply to the Jews, who rarely lived on the land. Among the Orthodox, Protestants, and Moslems, who were overwhelmingly peasants, the harvest season from July to September was by far the busiest time of the year. Earlier in the season, to be sure, the plowing and sowing oblige the men to work to the point of exhaustion. This may be one reason why the peak of reproduction comes in April (births in January), rather than in May or June as one would expect from the temperature and sunlight. The women take little part in the plowing. During the harvest season, however, everyone is hard at work in the fields, women and children as well as men. This heavy labor may diminish the number of conceptions. Both men and women work extremely long hours, for the daylight lasts far into the evening. At night people are so weary that they drop asleep almost as soon as they finish the evening chores. How greatly this diminishes the number of conceptions it is impossible to say, but the weariness due to agricultural labor is at least a factor to be considered. By the first of September (the middle of our September) the work begins to slacken, and in October and November there is very little outdoor work. The men, in fact, often have only one or two hours of work per day. Although no exact data are available, it seems probable that the cessation of work stimulates reproduction not merely because of leisure and freedom from weariness, but also because the work of the summer has given vigor to everyone.

By far the most important cause of the reduced number of conceptions in summer is the absence of many of the men, especially the young men. In old Russia this tendency was accentuated by the system of living in large families. Married sons often lived with their parents, brothers continued to live together after the death of their father, and many other combinations of relatives were made. This was a genuine economic advantage. In spite of the common opinion to the contrary, the amount of arable land in Russia is small in comparison with the population. In the old days the fields allotted to the individual peasants by the "mirs," or village councils, were often too small to occupy the whole of a man's time. If there were two men in the family, one, with the help of the women, could cultivate two shares. The other went off and worked for one of the large landowners. In some cases where there was only one man in a family, the women did all the work in the home village, and the man went away because that was the only chance to get a little real money. In old Russia a vast amount of land was held in great estates which hired many men during the summer. The young men were especially likely to go away in this fashion, leaving their wives at home. Naturally the rate of reproduction fell to a low level. When the men came home in the fall it increased, and the general level during the winter was high compared with summer.

In Figure 19 it is very interesting to see how clearly the diminution in reproduction during summer conforms to the social and economic conditions of the four religious groups. The Jewish curve begins to sag below the dotted line in May and remains below until August, provided we employ the date of conception as given at the bottom of Figure 19. This probably indicates the extent to which Jewish merchants went out among the villages. In the late spring, as soon as the roads were passable, they loaded themselves with merchandise to supply the needs which had remained unsatisfied during the long winter and the muddy early springtime. When the harvest season arrived the peasants were too busy to buy much. So even in August most of the itinerant Jews had returned home, and Curve D shows a minor maximum of conceptions. Thereafter the conceptions diminished in harmony with the basic animal rhythm, just as in Belgium.

Among the Moslems of Kazan some of the men doubtless left home for the plowing in May, which may perhaps be one reason why the maximum of conceptions occurred in April rather than later. The number of men who could plow, however, was limited by the number of horses. Most of the men were away from home only during the harvest season from about the first of our July to the middle of September. The great decline in conceptions at this time may be due partly to hot weather, for Kazan lies fairly far south in Russia, but it must be due mainly to the seasonal migration of the men.

The upper curve of Figure 19 shows that in summer the Orthodox Christians of Kazan behaved about like their Moslem neighbors. It is greatly complicated by feasts and fasts, however, and the high level of conceptions during January and February (births in October and November) is note-worthy. The Protestant curve of Figure 19 suggests that in Livland (modern Latvia) the men began leaving home earlier than in Kazan, and stayed away much later. This may be partly because they were more industrious. A more important reason is that the men left home for two types of work instead of one. Lumbering is a main industry in Latvia. Therefore many men not only work on the farms in summer, but remain away from home during the autumn to cut trees in the forest. Therefore the dotted line for Livland remains above the solid line till December, according to the scale for conceptions as given at the bottom of Figure 19.

Taken as a whole, the Russian curves discussed in this chapter present a good example of the main influences which determine the seasonal distribution of births. They display four main elements. The most conspicuous is a statistical error by which the number of recorded births is too low in December and too high in January. This is very noticeable in the curves for the earlier of the two periods here used, in the 1870's, and is still clearly evident in the later statistics for the 1890's. The second element is the fundamental annual rhythm like that of animals. In practically every Russian curve it takes the form of a maximum of births in January or February; but, when allowance is made for statistical errors and for seasonal migration, it appears that the normal date is the Russian February. This corresponds to our mid-February to mid-March and is the result of conceptions from the middle of May to the middle of June according to our calendar. The third element consists of irregular fluctuations dependent on religious and social customs. These vary from region to region, and from one religious or social group to another. They are one of the most puzzling features of our problem. The fourth element is seasonal migrations due to the demands of various kinds of occupations. Agriculture is the chief occupation to be considered, but lumbering and trade also play their parts. In addition to these four elements the Russian curves show evidence of being influenced more or less by the temperature of the summer, but the discussion of this is postponed to a later chapter. The whole matter may be summed up by saying that the Russian curves present an extraordinary example of the way in which seasonal curves of birth are influenced by weather, work, social customs, and human fallability.

CHAPTER IV

CLIMATIC EXTREMES AND MIGRATION: JAPAN AND MASSACHUSETTS

JAPAN COMPARED WITH BELGIUM

The basic annual rhythm of reproduction is greatly modified as one goes from region to region. This is well illustrated by the contrast between the curves of birth in Japan and Belgium as given in Figure 1 (page 30). Hiroshima, the Japanese province there used, is in the far south of the main island of Japan. The curve of birth is not so regular as that of Belgium, but it becomes more regular if two statistical errors are eliminated. One is like the Russian error at the end of the year. In certain curves for other Japanese provinces, which we shall examine later, it is quite prominent. In the present case, however, it is so slight that we may neglect it. The other error is large. It arises from a condition which Gini (1934) points out in a report dealing with errors in the statistics of Italy. In Japan the parents covet the privilege of sending their children to the state schools at as early an age as possible. At the opening of any given school year those children are eligible who have attained a certain age before the preceding March. Hence many parents whose children are born in April, or even in May, succeed in having their children recorded as born the preceding March. This is especially true in relatively remote provinces such as Hiroshima. Therefore, the true maximum of the Japanese curve in Figure 1 almost certainly comes in February, and the excess of births in March should be added to April and May. For our present purposes this makes no appreciable change in the curve except to throw the maximum into February instead of March, as may be seen in Figure 34 (page 150).

83

Recognizing this change in the maximum, we find that the Japanese curve of Figure 1 agrees with the Belgian curve in two respects. First, it shows an almost uninterrupted seasonal swing with a sharply defined maximum and minimum. Second, the maximum in February (conceptions in May) comes at approximately the same time as in Belgium. The differences between the two curves are quite as noticeable as the resemblances. In the first place, the Japanese curve shows a pronounced minimum in June (conceptions in September), which has no parallel in Belgium. In the second place, there is a minor Japanese maximum in September (conceptions in December). This finds no parallel in the modern curve of Belgium, but is closely paralleled in earlier Belgian curves, and in Germany, Sweden, and other countries. It is apparently due to the midwinter homecoming of absentees. Even though Christmas has no significance in Japan, the shortest days of the year and the diminution of agricultural work are natural reasons for the return of absent husbands. A third difference between the two curves is that the Japanese curve shows far greater variation from maximum to minimum than does the Belgian curve. From a maximum of 138 in February (disregarding the false maximum in March) it catapults down to 96 in April (July conceptions) and only 63 in June (September).

In seeking an explanation of the differences between Japan and Belgium we can promptly dismiss most of the factors already considered in respect to the latter country. Diet cannot be an important element in shaping the Japanese curve because the conceptions drop tremendously during the summer at just the season when the Japanese enjoy a really good diet instead of the very monotonous diet of rice on which they mainly subsist the rest of the year. Illegitimacy, feasts, fasts, and seasons of marriage are all ruled out for two reasons. First, there is no evidence that any of them produces much effect upon the seasonal distribution of births in Japan. Second, even if all of them happened to work in the same direction, they could not possibly account for a change which reduces the number of births by more than 50 per cent between February and June. Seasonal migration may account for the minor maximum in September, but it cannot account for the great contrast between winter and summer. The overwhelming majority of the Japanese stay at home throughout the year. The weariness and exhaustion due to agricultural labor cannot produce the observed effect, for the number of conceptions rises rapidly during the season of heavy work in April and May, and is at a very low ebb in the less strenuous time from August through November, during at least half of which the work is no heavier than in the spring. June and July, when the rice is being transplanted, are the most strenuous and tiring months. Conceptions do indeed decline at that time, but they are far above their lowest ebb, especially when births recorded in April, and representing July conceptions, are supplemented by their fair share of those recorded in March.

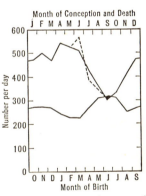

Fig. 20.—Conceptions and Deaths in Japan, 1901-1910.

Turning to the weather, and to the related conditions of health and dress, we find quite a different situation. The character of the weather appears to agree perfectly with the number of conceptions that give rise to living births. This is illustrated in Figure 20, where the upper curve represents births from 1901 to 1910 in Japan as a whole. The births have been plotted according to the time of conception and have been expressed in terms of their actual numbers. The dotted line represents the actual record, and the solid line our estimate of the allowance to be made for excess registration in March. The lower curve in Figure 20 shows the number of deaths. It is evident at a glance that conceptions and deaths follow almost opposite courses. In May and June, when deaths are at a minimum, conceptions are near the maximum. In September the opposite is the case. Conceptions are so few and deaths so many that the population actually declines. The best explanation of this remarkable condition seems to be that the hot, humid summer saps the vitality of the Japanese to such an extent that they are physically unfit for reproduction. The women suffer especially, not only because they have to cook and do housework in the midst of flies and other discomforts, but also because their heavy dress with its tight sash makes them insufferably hot. Moreover, when they go out in the pouring rain, as they frequently do, the long full skirts drag them down with a load of water. Anyone who has spent a summer in Japan knows that one is wet with rain or perspiration most of the time.

Until the second half of June the temperature, even in southern Japan, does not average above 70° F. for night and day together, and there are many fresh clear days in spite of the heavy rain. Then the southeast monsoon becomes well established and brings a most uncomfortable combination of heavy rain, extreme humidity, and temperatures averaging from 75° to 82° for night and day together over the region where most of the Japanese are found. Professor Okada of the Japanese Central Observatory describes this season thus, as quoted by Kendrew (1922):

> In Japan proper . . . we usually have a rainy season beginning towards the middle of June and extending through the first half of July. During this season the sky remains wholly overcast with clouds, and more or less rain falls every day. The air is so moist that walls, pavements, etc., become damp, and furniture and clothes get mouldy. The weather is indeed depressing and unpleasant. This rainy season . . . is the most important period for the cultivation of rice. The copious rainfall . . . soaks the rice field and makes it just right for transplanting the rice seedlings.

Although the heavy clouds keep the mean temperature from rising much above 75° during this period, the noonday thermometer often goes above 80°, and the night temperature is not far from 70°. In the middle of July the rain slackens, although still heavy, and the temperature rises to an average of about 80° with nights that rarely fall below 75°. This continues through August, which is generally the hottest month. September is about as hot as early July and is again a period of very heavy rain. Thus the discomfort of the long, humid summer culminates in September. Thereafter, in the most densely populated parts of Japan the weather is delightful until December. Only in January does it become uncomfortably cool, and the cool period is short. It is succeeded by a long spring during which the climate is almost ideal.

The responses of human reproduction to this sequence of seasons seems to be in complete harmony with what we have seen in Belgium. Speaking in terms of conceptions, and following the year from its beginning, we find that January with a mean temperature of 39° F. at Hiroshima is a little too cool. The death rate rises a little higher than in November, and the number of conceptions drops somewhat, so that the Hiroshima curve in Figure 1 (page 30) shows a minor minimum in October. In February and March the conditions of health change but little, as is clear in Figure 20, and the conceptions increase only slightly. With the advent of April, however, the death rate falls somewhat, and the number of conceptions rises to a high level which is almost maintained in May. This period is the most delightful season of the year—cherry-blossom time and iris time, when everyone is cheerful and the love of beauty expresses itself most fully. By the end of June, however, the mean temperature has risen above 70° and the humidity has become extreme. Then the death rate rises rapidly, and the number of conceptions falls even more rapidly.

According to Mills (1930) this hot, wet period of poor health is not marked by any diminution of sexual activity. He bases his statement on the fact that houses of prostitution in Tokyo are reported to be as much frequented at that time as at others. It is quite possible, however, that men who do not frequent such houses as a rule go there in summer because their wives do not feel sexually inclined. It is also possible that conceptions are as numerous as usual in summer, but that the weakness and lassitude of the women cause a huge number of early abortions. That this is at least partially true is indicated by the preponderance of male births arising from conceptions in summer, as will appear in a later chapter. It must be remembered that in Japan the women suffer greatly from the heat—far more than do the men. Many work indoors or over fires; many others share in the very arduous work of standing in the mud and water of the rice fields all day long while they stoop over from the hips and set out the rice plants. Their clothing is peculiarly unfit for such work, for even when their thick skirts are tied around their waists, they become heavy and uncomfortable because they are soaked with water from the rice fields or the rain. It is not pleasant to be a young woman, especially a peasant, during the hot, humid Japanese summer.

When the heat and humidity of September are past, the Japanese recover their strength, the death rate begins to fall, and conceptions increase. This desirable condition continues with only a little check throughout the winter. There is, to be sure, a slight increase of deaths in midwinter. Corresponding to this there is a slight drop in the number of conceptions during January and February. In the Hiroshima curve of Figure 1 the peak of births in September may be due only in part to the return of absent husbands in December. It may be due in equal or greater measure to the fact that in January the stimulus of cooler weather gives place to a reduction in vigor because the lowering of the temperature has gone too far. As soon as the cool weather is past, however, the number of conceptions begins to increase rapidly. This agrees with what we were led to suspect in Belgium, namely, that a drop toward the optimum temperature may stimulate reproduction, even though it may not be so effective as a rise from lower temperature. Another way of putting the matter is that the Japanese conditions agree with a conclusion based on measurements of factory work in both Japan and America as set forth by Yagi (1933) and Huntington (1924, 1935). The conclusion is that after a period of very hot weather a lowering of temperature is of great value to health, but the return to full physical vigor is very slow, so that the effect of a hot summer may still be evident after 3 or 4 months. On the other hand, the Japanese winter, especially in southern provinces such as Hiroshima, is so mild that people recover from its slightly depressing effect very speedily. Thus the Japanese come to the delightful weather of spring with excellent health, and in such a physical condition that the rise to the optimum temperature acts as a powerful stimulant to reproduction.

All this agrees excellently with what we have seen in Belgium. We shall assume that the reader accepts the conclusion that the apparent Japanese maximum of births in March is false, and that the real maximum comes in February. If such is the case, the optimum temperature for conception in Hiroshima is 63° F. (17° C.) in comparison with 58° F. (14.4° C.) in Belgium. This is a small difference in view of the fact that the people of Hiroshima have lived for many centuries in a climate where the hottest month averages 80° F. (26.7° C.), whereas the Belgians have lived equally long where the corresponding temperature is only 63° F. (17° C.). The Japanese, through long generations in their particular type of climate, have doubtless become at least partially adjusted to it, as have the Belgians to theirs. Nevertheless, the optimum temperature of the two racial groups has become only slightly differentiated. Since we find a similar relationship between health and temperature as well as between reproduction and temperature not only in these two countries, but also in many others, we seem to be led to two conclusions. First, the Japanese curve of Figure 1 is mainly an expression of the effect of the climate upon health and hence upon reproduction. Second, there is a close connection between the optimum temperature and the maximum rate of reproduction.

So far as we can yet see, the general climatic hypothesis which fits the outstanding and permanent features of the seasonal distribution of births in Belgium, Germany, and Sweden is also applicable to Japan. It requires only such changes as are inevitable because of the differences in climate. The climatic hypothesis, however, does not exclude other hypotheses, for the seasonal distribution of births is undoubtedly the result of the interaction of many factors. In Japan the heavy clothing of the women and the arduous labor of the rice fields during June and July are probably the main modifiers or exaggerators of the effect of climate. Nevertheless, this probably explains only a small part of the tremendous decline in conceptions in July. So let us apply to Japan what seems thus far to be our most fundamental hypothesis, namely, that man has acquired an innate reproductive rhythm which is set in motion by the weather or by related conditions such as sunlight and diet, and which is so adjusted that the young are born in greatest numbers at the season when their chances of survival are greatest. With this goes the supplementary hypothesis that after many generations in a given type of climate people's reproductive processes become more or less modified so that the maximum climatic stimulus to reproduction occurs under conditions which tend to cause births to be especially numerous at seasons which are favorable for the survival of infants in that particular climate. In southern Japan a child born in January, February, or March has from 5 to 3 favorable months ahead of it before the deadly part of the summer arrives. It also has before it the season when its mother will be best fed, and will be increasingly able to nourish it. When the summer arrives it is not yet old enough to eat anything except its mother's milk and to that extent it is in less danger than it will be later from the bacterial infections which are the bane of Japanese summers. A year later, in its second summer, the child is old enough to be past the most susceptible stage, although the danger is still great. The child born in May, June, July, or August, on the contrary, meets extreme dangers while it is still very young. Even though its mother is better fed than in winter she is likely to be greatly strained by the heat and humidity, by her very poor type of clothing, by exhausting work in the rice fields, and by using food or water which carry bacterial parasites, especially those causing digestive troubles. The child itself is very likely to be upset not only by its mother's milk but also by the heat which makes it uncomfortable and fretful. Thus, the Japanese summer is a very bad time in which to be born.

The autumn is better, but not so good as the winter and early spring. The child born during the period from October to December, let us say, has the advantage of a long period before the dangers of the first summer arrive, but it faces a little danger from the cool winter on its own account, and a greater danger from the fact that during its early months its mother lives more and more exclusively on polished rice, which is a very poor source of vitamins and other nourishing products. Moreover, by the time the depressing summer arrives, the child is old enough to be eating some food aside from milk so that it is in especially great danger from the digestive troubles which are the chief bane of early childhood. Hence it appears that the seasonal distribution of births in Japan is such as to preserve the maximum number of children. The Japanese and Belgian curves of Figure 1 seem to point to identically the same hypothesis.

BIRTHS IN MASSACHUSETTS

In its seasonal distribution of births Massachusetts has certain features in common with Belgium, Russia, and Japan. Although the curve of births in that state nearly a hundred years ago (Curve D in Figure 1) looks quite different from those of the other countries, it has a similar although very small maximum near the beginning of the year. Thus in a mild way it agrees with the hypothesis that human reproduction, like that of animals, is subject to an annual rhythm which tends toward a maximum of births in the late winter or early spring at the time most favorable for the survival of the young. Two months after this maximum, early Massachusetts, like Japan, shows a minimum corresponding to conceptions during the warmest part of the year. Then comes another maximum from August to October. This agrees with a major maximum in Russia and with a minor one in Japan. In comparison with the earlier maximum, however, it is much more pronounced than in the other countries.

Before analyzing these main features of the Massachusetts curve, let us examine the minor maximum in December. This appears to be a statistical inaccuracy. It is the kind characteristic of a stage of statistical development higher than that of Russia, but not equal to that of modern Belgium. In early Massachusetts a few of the later births in each month seem usually to have been recorded during the succeeding month, and therefore to have been counted as belonging to that month. At the end of the year, however, before the annual reports were sent to headquarters, a special effort was presumably made to complete the record. Hence December apparently includes all its own births and some belonging to November. Thus a false but minor maximum is indicated. January, on the other hand, does not get full credit for its own births and has no compensation through births occurring in late December. We shall probably come close to the truth if we eliminate the false December maximum by transferring to January 6 per cent of the births recorded in December.

Our next problem is to explain why the number of conceptions begins to increase in September, attains a high level in November, stays at nearly the same level through January, and then declines to a minimum in April. We shall omit for the present a considerable fraction of this maximum which is probably climatic. In Russia we found that a similar autumn maximum was due largely to the migration of agricultural laborers. A similar explanation applies in part to early Massachusetts, but in a more complex form. There are several reasons why in Massachusetts a century ago many more men were at home in winter than in summer. Some went away during the warmer months to work on farms or in factories. A considerable number were in process of migrating west. They came home in the winter to visit their families, who were waiting till the new home was well established before moving west.

Another form of migration also tended to raise the birth rate every autumn. Each summer, in those days, there came to Massachusetts a large number of immigrants from Europe. Most of these were relatively young. Perhaps the most common type of woman was the young bride of a few months. Since most of the immigrants arrived in the spring and summer, this meant that in the succeeding months the number of infants was materially increased by births among people who did not live in America the previous spring. In Massachusetts, just as in Russia, there may be other factors which have not been considered. Nevertheless, migration within the country and immigration from without seem to account for at least part of the 12 per cent higher rate of conception from October to January (births from July to October) than from April to September (births, January to June.)

The effect of climate and mode of life must not be overlooked in explaining the seasonal curve of births in Massachusetts. Even the children born there in July have a good chance of survival. They experience really hot weather during only a few days of earliest infancy, especially near the coast. Their mothers are unusually well fed, and continue to be so throughout practically the whole winter. In this respect early New England with its abundant apples, cabbages, root crops, milk, and meat was far superior to any except the most-favored bits of Europe. Moreover, the conditions of clothing and housing are of the best. The contrast between the death rates of summer and winter is, therefore, much less than in many milder regions such as Italy, as is shown in *World Power and Evolution* (Huntington, 1919). Hence two conditions may increase the birth rate from July to October. First, excellent conditions of housing and diet, as well as the stimulus of autumn weather, may help to maintain a high level of conceptions from October to January. Second, these same conditions may reduce the number of abortions and thus increase the number of births from July to September. We shall return to this problem in later pages.

Whether the preceding conclusion is true or not, Massachusetts, Russia, and Japan all appear to be significant as examples of the way in which cultural conditions modify the normal seasonal rhythm of reproduction. Belgium, on the contrary, appears to be an outstanding example of the almost unadulterated effect of climate.

Chapter V

SECULAR CHANGES IN SEASON OF BIRTH

The season at which children are born may change from generation to generation. Belgium illustrates this, as appears in Figure 21. The two post-war curves at the top show little except the pure annual rhythm, which is especially smooth from 1921 to 1926. Previous to the World War, however, a minor maximum in September (conceptions in December) becomes more and more evident as we go backward in time, and a dip appears in July corresponding to conceptions in October. The range from the main maximum in February or March to the main minimum also becomes much more pronounced, and this minimum shifts from November to July.

The explanation of these changes probably lies mainly in the cultural transformation whereby Belgium has become more urban, more industrial, better fed, more able to protect itself from adverse weather, and more fully committed to the limitation of families. The minor maximum of births shown by the early curves in September suggests that for-

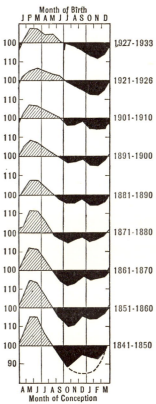

FIG. 21.—Secular Changes in Seasons of Birth in Belgium.

95

merly more men than at present worked away from home during part of the year, but came back in the winter, especially at Christmas time. This would be expected in view of the modern decline in the importance of agriculture, and the improvement of transportation. The better heating of houses, the better diet, and the better medical care of modern times would all, we should suppose, tend to reduce the contrast between the summer and winter, and thus lessen the seasonal contrast in births. The modern practice of limiting families would presumably work in the same way.

The change in the seasonal course of births with the progress of time is by no means confined to Belgium. Figure 22 shows what has happened in western Europe. The curves on the left represent seasonal fluctuations in the Nineteenth century; those on the right show the recent situation. In every case the tendency is much the same as in Belgium. In Norway the early curve on the left shows the normal annual or animal cycle except that this is strongly interrupted by a great excess of births in September. This corresponds to conceptions at Christmas. It confirms our hypothesis that the September maximum of births is due to the return of men who have been away from home. In practically no other country are so many seafaring men, fishermen, and others away from home for long periods. A great number of these make it a point to come home in midwinter, especially in time for the Christmas and New Year's festivities. In modern Norway this tendency is still evident, but has become much less pronounced. This is what one would expect now that modern transportation makes it easy to come home frequently, and occupations such as seafaring and deep-sea fishing have become relatively less important than formerly.

In Scotland the situation is much the same as in Norway, but a great many men were formerly at home for 3 months in winter. In both of these northern countries the modern maximum of births occurs in April, corresponding to conceptions in July. Evidently in such cold countries the heat of summer does not hinder reproduction. Passing down through the other countries of Figure 22, we see in Denmark essentially the same thing as in Norway and Scotland, but the difference between the past and the present is less. In the Netherlands the early curve shows a great depression in

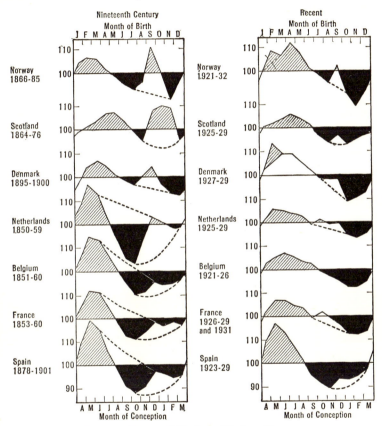

FIG. 22.—Season of Birth in Western Europe.

summer which probably indicates that a large number of seafaring men, boatmen, and laborers were away from home from June or July to November. The suddenness with which the births increase in August and September apparently indicates that a great number of men returned home during November and December. In the modern curve the situation is like that of Belgium and France except that there is slightly more irregularity. In all three cases the modern curves have almost the perfect form of the animal rhythm.

Figure 22 shows that in modern Spain the summer minimum of births and the September maximum still existed in 1926-1928, but were much reduced in comparison with 1878-1901. In the modern curve the minor maximum in September is less pronounced than formerly, which apparently means that the farm laborers leave home less now than formerly, and are absent mainly during the grape and olive harvests in October and November. It should also be noted that in both of the Spanish curves the downward swing from April to July (conceptions from July to October) is steep and deep. This resembles the situation in Japan. It may have some connection with the great length and enervating quality of the summers in those two countries. If this is the case, it means that the extreme heat produces a weakening effect from which it requires several months to recover. We shall return to this later.

Figure 23 provides another illustration of secular change in the seasonal distribution of births. Here we have the countries of central Europe arranged in order from north to south. On each side the upper curve represents Finland, then come two sections of Sweden, and so on down to the 3 lower ones for sections of Italy. In each curve on both sides the spring maximum is evident, although it may occur in any month from January to March, and is negligible in modern Finland. In the older curves the September maximum is likewise clearly evident as far south as northern Italy. It is barely visible in central Italy and disappears in southern Italy. This agrees with what we know as to seasonal migrations. Northern Italy, for example, with its pronounced peak of births in September, has long been well known for the extent to which its laborers migrate to France and elsewhere in summer. The southern Italians, on the contrary, stay at home or else migrate far away to America.

In the modern curves of Figure 23 the September maximum, corresponding to conceptions in December, has almost disappeared, and in Switzerland it is completely gone.   This

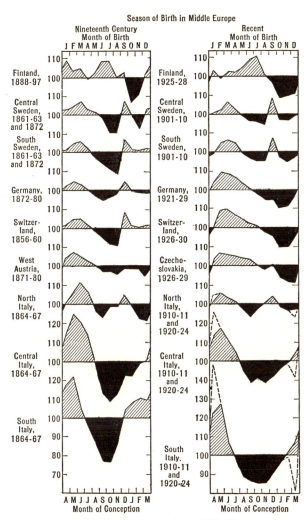

FIG. 23.—Season of Birth in Middle Europe.

illustrates the fact that all these countries have been through the same process of industrialization and urbanization which has been so pronounced in Belgium.   Agriculture and the tendency for men to go away for the summer and return in the winter have both declined. So, too, have the excesses and drunkenness connected with the holiday festivities. Thus in all these northern countries of central Europe the change is almost identical with that which we have observed in Belgium, and there is evidently a very strong tendency toward the typical curve of the animal rhythm of reproduction.

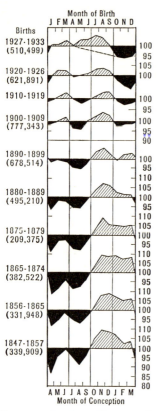

FIG. 24.—Secular Changes in Seasonal Distribution of Births in Massachusetts.

In Italy, however, the case is different. Northern Italy shows some diminution in the September maximum, and the curves for the center and south retain almost their old form, or at least they do this when the solid lines are used. The dotted lines, however, indicate the births as reported, but a correction is necessary in Italy as in Russia. At the time of these statistics Italy had taken a backward step, which has since been corrected. The curves for central and southern Italy dip very deeply in summer, just as in Spain and Japan where there are also long hot summers.

The secular change in the season of birth in Massachusetts (Figure 24) has been more complex than in Belgium. Taking the Massachusetts curves as a whole, maxima in February or March and again in July, August, or September have been prominent features for nearly a century. There is, however, a decided change in their relative importance. As time has passed, the late winter maximum has become progressively higher. In the early curves it is far below the average, but from 1919 to 1926 it rises almost as high as the summer maximum. The latter has suffered less change than the winter maximum. At all times it has been a fairly constant feature. Although it is not so high now as formerly, it is almost as important in relation to the fluctuations of the curve as a whole. In late years it has occurred in July instead of August, thus indicating the greatest number of conceptions in October instead of November. The minor maximum in December, which we have ascribed to statistical error, disappears after 1900.

During the course of time the two main minima of Figure 24 have changed as markedly as the maxima. In the oldest curve the deepest minimum comes in January. Its depth is partly due to the statistical error discussed above. As time goes on, this minimum is thrown back and becomes longer. From 1900 onward it embraces the whole of the months of October, November, and December, but not January. Since 1920 the births in the latter month have been about average in number. The other minimum changes somewhat differently. In the oldest curves it comes in May and is very low, Later it occurs sometimes in May and sometimes in April, and becomes much less prominent. In the most recent curve (1927-1933) it has largely disappeared, and at its lowest point is above the average for the year as a whole.

Massachusetts is by no means the only state where such changes in the season of birth have occurred. Figure 25 shows a similar situation in Michigan. Other data indicate that the same general conditions prevail in the intervening states and in the entire northeastern part of the United States. In Figure 25 the seasonal distribution of conceptions, rather than births, is shown for Michigan in the solid lines and for Massachusetts in the dotted lines of Section A for recent times and Section B for 60 years earlier. The resemblance between the two states is obvious, even though the Michigan curves display greater extremes. Equally obvious is the strong contrast between the curves dating back to about 1870 and those of two generations later.

The full explanation of the changes in the seasonal distribution of births in the northeastern United States is not yet evident. The general tendency has been toward a curve like that of Belgium, as appears in the dotted line in the upper part of Figure 24. But this tendency is forcibly inter-

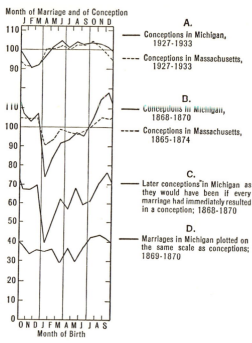

FIG. 25.—Conceptions and Marriages in Michigan Compared with Massachusetts.

rupted from April to September. It is as if at that time a wave of births were superposed upon the steady seasonal swing arising from the basic animal rhythm. When we consider the modern curves of Massachusetts and Michigan from the standpoint of conceptions (*A*, Figure 25), we see that conceptions are least numerous in the winter, that is, from January through March, at the time when the general conditions of health are least favorable. Then they rise to a maximum in June and decline very slightly in July. All this agrees with the basic animal rhythm and with conditions of health. The subsequent rise, however, to a higher or longer maximum from August to October departs from the animal rhythm which we have found in Europe.

One possible explanation of this is that, if the temperature rises sufficiently high in summer and thus imposes a serious check upon reproduction, a drop to the optimum temperature stimulates reproduction. This appears to be true in Japan (Figure 1), Spain (Figure 22), and Italy (Figure 23), and we shall find further evidence of it later. In early June the temperature of both Boston and Detroit is close to the optimum, which is approximately 63° F. This same temperature prevails again toward the middle of September. In earlier times, as is clear in Figure 24, there was always a decided drop in the number of conceptions during the warm months between these two periods of optimum temperature. This suggests that the number of conceptions varies from season to season in harmony with the health and vigor of the parents regardless of the welfare of the infants. But why, then, has the old minimum of conceptions in July so nearly disappeared? The answer may be that in modern times such improvements as pasteurized milk, plenty of clean fresh vegetables, screened houses, outdoor life, vacations, opportunities for recreation, and the elimination of diseases such as dysentery and malaria have caused the summer to be the most healthful time of the year. August is generally the month of lowest mortality. Thus the tendency toward conception in summer has apparently been strengthened, while the danger to the children conceived in summer and born shortly before the advent of the following summer has greatly diminished.

A comparison with Japan will make the matter clearer. We have seen that in that country the mildness of the winter seems to leave people in such good physical condition that the death rate falls very low and the reproductive rate rises very high during the succeeding spring with its marvelously delightful climate. The depressing summer, on the contrary, leaves people so enfeebled that they do not recover their full strength for a long time. In the northern United States the rôles of the seasons are the reverse of what they are in Japan. The winter is the bad season and the summer the good season, as a rule, and this has become more so since the modern development of sanitation, hygiene, medicine, and diet. Therefore the Americans not only have a low reproductive rate and a high death rate in winter, but are slow in reaching the opposite condition in the spring. In summer, on the contrary, the harm done by extreme weather is slight, and as soon as the more favorable condi-

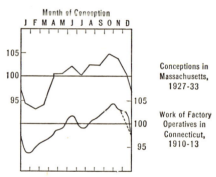

FIG. 26.—Conceptions and Human Efficiency.

tions of the late summer or early fall arrive, people feel a stimulation which lasts well toward winter.

The measured work of factory operatives affords independent evidence that the months from August to November are a period of unusual vigor in the northeastern United States. This is illustrated in Figure 26. One of the curves there is the curve of conceptions in Massachusetts from 1927 to 1933. That is, it is the upper curve of Figure 24 plotted according to the month of conception. The lower curve of Figure 26 shows the efficiency of piece workers in Connecticut factories from 1910 to 1913. It furnishes perhaps the best available measure of seasonal fluctuations in vigor among healthy young people in the northeastern United States. An almost

identical curve for Pittsburgh is also available.   The close
resemblance between the two curves of Figure 26 is evident.
Abundant data from other regions, including Japan as well
as the United States and Europe, leave little doubt that
factory work is a genuine measure of physical vigor and that
it fluctuates in harmony with the weather.   Hence it seems
clear that in modern Massachusetts and Michigan, just as in
Japan and more than in Belgium, the number of conceptions
fluctuates in harmony with the physical vigor of the people.
One curious thing about all this is the speed with which
the conquest of the diseases of summer appears to have
brought with it an immediate change in the seasonal distribution of births.

The reader may ask why the Massachusetts curve differs
so much from that of Belgium. The answer is twofold. First,
the winter in Belgium in very mild so that it does not involve
a severe physical strain like that imposed by the American
winter and still more by the Japanese summer. Therefore
the arrival of spring has a much more immediate stimulating
effect than in Massachusetts. There is little to be overcome
in the way of arrears of weakness. In the second place, the
Belgian summer has essentially the optimum temperature.
In the autumn the temperature falls very slowly compared
with what happens in Massachusetts, and the stimulus afforded thereby is correspondingly small. This may not be
the full explanation, but it at least affords a suggestion of
one of the lines along which a fuller explanation may be
sought.

A comparison of conceptions and deaths month by month
for many years throws much light on the changing relation
of births and deaths to one another and to health, climate,
and human progress. In each section of Figures 27 and 28
the upper curve shows the number of conceptions resulting
in live births each month in Massachusetts. The lower curve
shows the number of deaths in the same period. The scale
on the left indicates the number of conceptions or death as
it would have been if all the months had exactly 30 days,

thus eliminating the irregularities due to the varying length of the months. The shaded area between the two curves visualizes the extent to which conceptions leading to live births exceeded deaths, and is a measure of natural growth of population. Solid shading indicates excess of deaths over births. Dotted lines have been added to each curve to bring out the degree to which the summer as well as the winter is associated with a reduction of conceptions and an increase in deaths. In examining all these diagrams it must be remembered that the curves are plotted according to the actual num-

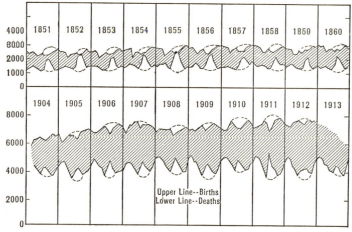

FIG. 27.—Births and Deaths in Massachusetts, 1851–1860 and 1904–1913.

ber of people and not on the basis of ratios. Therefore a fluctuation of a given magnitude is much more important in 1860, when the population of Massachusetts numbered only 1,231,000, than in 1910, when it numbered 3,366,000, or in 1930, when it had reached 4,250,000.

In the period from 1851 to 1860 (upper part of Figure 27), the deaths in Massachusetts rose regularly each year to a minor maximum associated with cold weather and to a major maximum associated with hot weather. The minor maximum usually occurred in March, but in 1855 it was delayed till April, while in 1860 it came in January. There was none in 1858 because the maximum for the winter of 1857-1858 came in December.   This winter maximum was due largely to the deaths of older people rather than children, although there were of course many deaths among the latter.   The summer maximum in the middle of the last century was much more regular and impressive than the winter maximum.   In some years (1852, 1855, 1856) the deaths rose to almost twice the ordinary level of the winter.   The excess of deaths above the dotted line was due chiefly to digestive disorders among young children.   Among adults the deaths

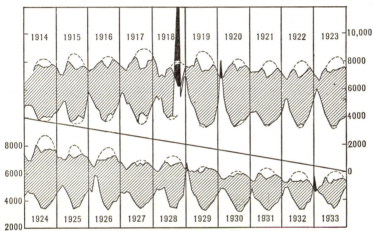

Fig. 28.—Births and Deaths in Massachusetts, 1914–1933.

usually increased relatively little in summer, and in some cases followed approximately the course of the dotted line.

In these modern days it is hard to realize the extraordinary contrast which formerly existed between the seasonal distribution of deaths among young children and older people.   This is illustrated in Figure 29, which is based on about 900 children under 5 years of age, and nearly 2800 persons over that age is recorded in the Huntington Genealogical Memoir (1915.)   Most of these people were born between 1800 and 1890.   They supply a fair sample of the general conditions prevailing in New England, and also all over the United States and in many other countries, before the advent of modern preventive medicine. The solid lines shows that among persons who had passed the critical period of early childhood the deaths reached a distinct maximum in March, fell to a minimum in July, and then rose in August and especially September. They fell off a little in November, but rose again in December. The dotted line attached to the solid line shows the approximate course of events today. The space between this line and the solid line represents the extent to which modern sanitation and medical practice have altered the seasonal incidence of deaths among adults by reducing the fatalities from such diseases as typhoid fever and dysentery. The main line of dashes, with its high peak in August, is the most notable feature of Figure 29. It shows that from November to June the deaths among young children used to follow about the same course as among older people. Beginning in July, however, and culminating in August, they shot upward to almost double their previous level. September was almost as bad as August, and the deaths did not return to what may be called their normal level until November. The dotted line attached to the line of dashes shows the course of events today. The space between the two lines illustrates the enormous gain to early childhood as a result of modern methods of diet and prophylaxis.

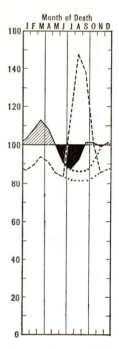

FIG. 29.—Seasonal Distribution of Deaths in Early New England.

Turning back now to Figure 27, we see that, in spite of the comparatively good health of the adults in summer, each period of hot weather saw a decline in the number of conceptions giving rise to living births. Such declines, or at least failures to maintain the previous rate of increase, coincide approximately with the periods when the deaths of the children increased, as is evident from the dotted lines. Thus, in 1852 the upper dotted line shows a deficiency of conceptions from August to October and the lower an excess of deaths from July to October. Judging from Figure 27 alone one might surmise that the enormous increase in deaths among young children, which became extreme in August and usually culminated in September, frightened the parents and made them decide not to have more children. This is not the case, however, because the drop in conceptions almost invariably begins in July at the same time as the rise in deaths, and is well established before the deaths are numerous enough to attract attention. Moreover, in modern times, although the summer maximum of deaths has disappeared, the summer decline in conceptions continues.

One of the most impressive facts about Figure 27 is the way in which the upper curve, showing conceptions, fluctuates in a fashion almost opposite to that of the deaths in the lower curve. Note how the maximum of deaths each winter is accompanied (1855, 1860) or immediately followed by a distinct minimum of conceptions. The summer maxima of deaths are also accompanied by minima of conceptions. In some years (1852, 1855) the deaths were so numerous and the conceptions so few that deaths exceeded conceptions. Note, too, how the dotted lines attached to the curve of conceptions begin in June in every year except 1852 and usually end in November. This means that the months from July to October inclusive formed a period of diminished reproduction. In practically every case the duration of this period is essentially the same as that of the corresponding period of increased mortality. Note, also, how the dotted lines of the curve of conceptions slope upward more than those of the mortality curve. At this period in the history of Massachusetts an excess of conceptions occurred each year with perfect regularity in the late fall and early winter.

From all this it seems evident that during the 10 years from 1851 to 1860 the following sequence of events was normal: During the winter the deaths increased until March and the conceptions diminished until April. Then in the spring a reversal occurred so that deaths diminished and conceptions increased until May or June, when the temperature averaged a little above 60° F. With the coming of hot weather in July the deaths among young children increased rapidly, and the conceptions declined, but not at so great a rate. In September the deaths were usually at a maximum, but even before that, in August, when the temperature dropped only a little, the conceptions had usually begun to increase. In November, as a rule, the deaths had dropped to a minimum, but not so low as in June, and conceptions had risen to almost the highest point of the year. In view of all this, it seems quite clear that the march of the seasons was the basic factor in the fluctuations of both conceptions and deaths. Low temperatures and high temperatures were both accompanied by many deaths and few conceptions. Periods when the temperature was rising toward 60° F. and when it was falling from 65° or so toward 45° or even 40° were marked by few deaths and many conceptions. These conditions of the weather were obviously associated with other conditions of health, work, and social customs which influenced both deaths and conceptions.

Now let us see how far these same conditions prevail in later times. The lower part of Figure 27 and the two sections of Figure 28 carry the record of births and deaths from 1904 through 1933. These 30 years are especially interesting because they were a time of great transition. Figure 27 shows that at the beginning the births, or rather the conceptions, were increasing rapidly because of the growth of the population. This continued until about 1917 (Figure 28), but thereafter the rate of increase became progressively less because birth control and other conditions began to reduce the birth rate drastically. Up to 1917 the absolute number of deaths as well as births continued to increase because of the growth of population, but the spread of medical knowledge, sanitation, and hygiene lowered the deaths in proportion to the population. Hence the general level of deaths—that is, the total number—increased less rapidly than the births, and the period from 1905 to 1917 was one of great natural increase of population as is evident from the breadth of the shaded band in Figures 27 and 28. After the World War the number of deaths declined a little, but not at any such rate as the births. As a consequence, the two curves have again begun to cross one another. January, 1929 and 1933, and February, 1934, as well as the influenza periods of 1918 and 1920, are examples of months when deaths exceeded conceptions that resulted in live births. It is noticeable that in recent times it is the winter months which show an excess of deaths, and not the summer months as was true in the middle of the last century.

Since 1900 the seasonal curves of both deaths and births have changed their form conspicuously. Even by 1904, at the beginning of the lower section of Figure 27, the curve of deaths was decidedly different from what it had been half a century earlier. The summer maximum, although still strongly developed, had diminished in size. Medical care, the pasteurization of children's milk, a more healthful diet, and other improvements had reduced the summer death rate so that in many years it was less than that of winter, and only in extremely hot summers like 1911 did it exceed the winter maximum even for a month. From 1912 onward the summer maximum becomes of very minor proportions. In 1919 it can scarcely be detected, and from 1924 onward (the lower part of Figure 28) it practically disappears. At the same time the winter maximum of deaths becomes more and more prominent. In January, 1929, there were twice as many deaths as in the preceding July, August, or September. Even in ordinary years such as 1930 to 1932 the deaths per day were about 50 per cent more numerous in February than in July and August.

This excess of deaths in winter is quite different from the situation from 1850 to 1860, even if we consider only the adults and assume that their death rate followed the dotted lines in Figure 27. In the old days the deaths at the worst season, which came in March, rather than January or February as has happened lately, were rarely as much as 50 per cent in excess of the hypothetical summer minimum. In Figure 29 the excess is only about 33 per cent. Of course the difference between the old conditions and the new was less than appears when one first glances at Figures 27 and 28, because the far greater population in the later period raises and magnifies its entire curve. Nevertheless, there is a real difference. It is as if in these modern days we were saving people's lives in summer only to sacrifice them in winter. It might seem as if our modern methods of heating our houses, using well-warmed bathrooms instead of unheated privies, driving in closed and heated cars during stormy weather, wearing waterproof coats, taking winter vacations in the south, and otherwise protecting ourselves from the elements would reduce the winter death rate. Little of the kind has happened in Massachusetts, however. Relatively speaking, the winter peak of deaths is higher today than at any other time since statistics were available. We may reasonably expect that the next great step in medical progress will be to round off the winter peak of deaths, so that even the bad years will be no worse than 1927.

The changes in the form of the curve of conceptions (the upper curve of Figures 27 and 28) are more complex and difficult to understand than those in the curve of deaths. In the first few years of the present century the curve of conceptions still showed the same form as 50 years earlier. It was rising rapidly, and the autumn maximum was higher than that of the spring. From 1904 to 1906 this was especially true. Thereafter a change becomes evident. The two maxima become more nearly equal, with sometimes one and sometimes the other the larger. The birth rate was declining in the years before the World War, but not sufficiently to counteract the growth in population or to prevent a steady rise in births until 1917. In June of that year and in January, 1918, conceptions reached the highest level ever known in Massachusetts. This June maximum was due in

part to the many war-marriages which took place before
young men went into the army. The same cause, together
with furloughs at Christmas time, undoubtedly caused the
maximum of the following winter to occur in January instead
of November. So, too, the absence of the soldiers caused the
succeeding minimum in the spring of 1918 to be very low,
and co-operated with the influenza epidemic to produce an
excessively low level in the autumn of that year. A little
later the coming home of the soldiers and the marriage of
many of them produced an unusually sharp peak of conceptions in May, 1919. Still another outstanding fact is the
way in which the number of conceptions dropped to a low
level at the time not only of the main influenza epidemic in
1918, but in the second epidemic early in 1920.

Interesting as such details are, they are far less important
than the rapid decline in the birth rate which becomes evident after the war. So swift has been the descent that with
increasing frequency Massachusetts is now experiencing
months during which deaths are more numerous than conceptions. Accompanying this decline there has been a distinct change in the form of the curve of conceptions during
the summer. Previous to 1923 the curve almost always displays a distinct and more or less symmetrical dip culminating in a low point during July or August. This same form
occurs in some later years such as 1925, 1928, and 1931. In
1923, 1926, and 1932, however, and to a certain extent in
other years, the curve of conceptions forms an almost straight
line from May, or even April, to November or December.
The winter depression remains the same as ever, but the rest
of the year is being flattened out, and the summer minimum
is disappearing. In 1932 the conceptions remained at almost exactly the same level from January to November, aside
from April. Such a condition is unparalleled at any earlier
date. It indicates a drastic change of habits.

This change is analogous to that which has occurred in the
seasonal distribution of deaths. Man's interference with the
so-called normal course of events has changed the late sum-

mer and early autumn from the most deadly to the most healthful season for young children, and from an unfavorable to a favorable season even among adults.   The corresponding interference with births appears to be in process of eliminating the summer minimum, but years like 1931 and 1933 still show the old form.   In explanation of this there may be a possibility that a change in the extent to which men are absent from home in summer has something to do with the matter.   Between 1860 and 1930 there has undoubtedly been a change in this respect.   At the earlier date the proportion of young men who left home to go out west, or work on farms elsewhere was much greater than now, but between 1910 and 1930 there was little change in this respect.   By far the most notable change in habits affecting reproduction has been the rapid spread of birth control, especially since the World War.   Such a drastic change can scarcely fail to have an effect upon the old seasonal swing of conceptions.   What the final result will be is not yet evident. We have already seen reason to suspect that equilibrium may ultimately be reached with a seasonal distribution of births like that of Belgium and the other countries of western Europe, but as yet the change since the beginning of the present century has carried us only about half way to such a result.

This study of conceptions and deaths from month to month over a long period of years confirms the hypotheses which have previously seemed most probable.   The intimate interplay of climatic influences on the one hand and cultural influences on the other is everywhere evident.   Each season of the year is associated with its own particular kind of physiological response in the way of disease, death, and reproduction.   Man, however, is able to modify these responses and even to eliminate some of them, as in the case of the summer diseases of children.   That he can entirely eliminate the effect of the seasons and cause the death rate to be uniform throughout the year does not yet seem possible.   In the same way the seasonal distribution of conceptions in Massachusetts appears to have been greatly modified by internal migration, by changes in immigration from abroad, by the modern tendency toward the limitation of families, and perhaps by the growing luxury of our mode of life. Thus certain features such as the high rate of conception in the late fall and winter have disappeared. Nevertheless, the effect of the weather is still evident in the spring maximum of conceptions, the late winter minimum, and perhaps also in the fall maximum. Cultural and climatic conditions must evidently be studied with equal care if the factors that control the seasonal distribution of both births and deaths are to be understood.

CHAPTER VI

AMERICAN VARIATIONS IN SEASON OF BIRTH

Geographical variations in the season of birth are no less important than variations during the course of time. For the United States and southern Canada this is illustrated in Figure 30. There many states and provinces are arranged approximately as they appear upon a map. On the right, seven regions near the Atlantic coast extend from Manitoba

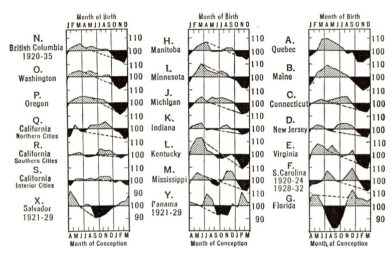

FIG. 30.—Months of Birth in United States and Canada, 1926–1932, and Central America, 1921–1929.

to Mississippi, and on the left six Pacific coast regions from British Columbia to southern California.

The eastern series is the most impressive. There the Quebec curve (*A*) is an almost perfect replica of the corre-sponding curves for Sweden, Norway, early Belgium, Germany, and other countries of western Europe. The maximum in March and April, due to conceptions in June and July, is perfectly developed, as is the minimum in October and November due to conceptions in January and February. Even the minor maximum in September on account of the return of the absent menfolk at Christmas time assumes its usual form. In Maine (*B*) a similar situation prevails, but the curve is even more perfect with its maximum in April (conceptions in July) and its minimum in November (February). The September maximum has vanished just as in modern Belgium.

In Connecticut (Curve *C* of Figure 30) the standard annual rhythm is clearly present, as becomes more evident when the dotted line is added. It is much flattened, however, in comparison with Maine and Quebec, and the maximum in March is comparatively inconspicuous. A new feature is added in the form of a prominent bulge beginning in May and rising to a major maximum in August. This means that in comparison with what would be expected according to the basic animal rhythm (the dotted line) conceptions are especially numerous from August through November, just as we have seen to be the case in Massachusetts. In New Jersey a similar situation prevails, and the bulge is even more pronounced than in Connecticut. The number of births exceeds what would be expected by almost equal amounts in each month from June through September (conceptions from September through December). In a previous chapter we have seen reason to associate a similar bulge in the most recent curves of Massachusetts with the "climatic" energy which factory operatives display in the fall. The matter is so important that we shall return to it after finishing our survey of Figure 30.

The Virginia curve (*E*) in Figure 30 shows the basic rhythm in steeper form than in New Jersey, but with two pronounced departures. One is the September maximum due to conceptions in December. Search as we will, it seems impossible to find any satisfactory explanation for this except the one so often mentioned, namely, the holiday return of men who have been away from home. The other is a minor maximum in May (conceptions in August). What seems to be the same maximum reappears in greater force in South Carolina (*F*, Figure 30), but is there pushed back to April (conceptions in July). The extreme size of the September maximum and the low level of the curve from January through March make the South Carolina curve so different from the others that one's first impulse is to wonder whether the data are wrong. This question is more likely to arise because, during the period covered by Figure 30, South Carolina was dropped from the birth-registration area for a time because its statistics did not reach the required standard of accuracy. North Carolina, however, where the statistics are more accurate, shows the same features in a form midway between Virginia and South Carolina.

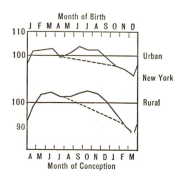

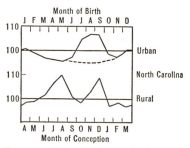

FIG. 31.—Urban and Rural Births in New York State, 1923-1926, 1928, and in North Carolina, 1922-1926, 1928.

The lower part of Figure 31 shows that in North Carolina the maxima in May and September and the low level from January to March are primarily associated with the rural districts and not with the cities, and the same is doubtless true in South Carolina and Virginia. In both North Carolina and Virginia the spring maximum is delayed until May as befits their position north of South Carolina. The seasonal distribution of agricultural work and the itinerant character of Negro labor appear to be the reasons for this spring maximum of births. These three states contain a large percentage of Negroes, 27 per cent in Virginia, 29 in North Carolina, and 46 in South Carolina. The Negroes are mainly rural and poor, and many are landless. Seasonal migrations of the men in search of work are as much the rule among them as among the old Russians. The rural curve of North Carolina in Figure 31 and the curves for South Carolina and to a less extent for Virginia in Figure 30 suggest that a considerable fraction of the men are away from home during April, May, and June. That is the season of spring plowing and of the planting of cotton and tobacco which demand much labor. In July and August the laborers apparently come home for a while and there are many conceptions, but in September and October they are again in the cotton fields. Then in November they begin to come home, and all are at home in December. Thus in the South, just as in Russia, the form of the seasonal curves of births is a complex mixture of the direct effects of climate plus the indirect effects through agriculture and social customs.

The urban curve of North Carolina in Figure 31 resembles the normal curve of the animal rhythm more than does the rural curve. The winter maximum, however, is pushed back as far as January or even December. There is also a pronounced bulge during July, August, and September. This seems to indicate that a great many city men are away during much of the year, but come home from October to December. In studying this diagram, and most of the others, it is easy to exaggerate their significance because the zero levels of the various curves are not shown. The zero of the urban curve of Figure 31 lies far below the bottom of the figure. The difference between the lowest and highest points of the curve is 12 per cent. Although this is a considerable amount, it is not so much as might appear at first glance when one may unconsciously assume that the bottom of the diagram represents zero. In Figures 1, 19, and 29 (pages 30, 78, and 108), the zero for at least part of the curves is shown, and one can judge the real amplitudes more fairly.

Among the curves of Figure 30 the one for Florida is unique. The normal maximum is visible near the beginning of the year, but has been shoved back into January and

February. The most pronounced feature is a great depression of the birth rate culminating in May and June (conceptions in August and September). Can this be due to seasonal migration? The greatest migration is that of the hundreds of thousands of northerners who flock to Florida in the winter. Is their influx sufficient to account for the high level of births during the entire winter, especially in January and February, and for the very low level in May and June? This is scarcely possible. In the first place, even if we omit the peak in September, the high level of winter begins in October. At that time only the merest vanguard of winter visitors has arrived.

On the other hand, the greatest exodus of visitors from Florida takes place in March and April at just the time when the birth rate falls most rapidly. The index number of births declines from 108 in February to 83 in May. If such a drop were due wholly to winter visitors it would mean not only that a quarter of the people went away, as might easily happen, but that a quarter of all the pregnant women went away. Such a condition is out of the question. Only a very small percentage of the hundreds of thousands of persons who visit Florida in winter consists of expectant mothers. They are the ones most likely to stay in their more northern homes, or at least to be in their northern homes when their babies are born. Mothers from the north have little effect on the Florida birth rate. Moreover, after the minimum in May and June the number of births increases very rapidly in July and August, but that is the very time when women from other states most carefully avoid Florida. It is also the time when the few Florida women who can afford to do so are most likely to go to some cooler place for the sake of their expected babies.

If the drop in the Florida curve in summer cannot be due to women who visit Florida in winter, can it be due to migrations of the men among the permanent residents? To a certain extent this is possible. The curve in Figure 30 indicates that conceptions are at a minimum in August and September. At that time there is relatively little work on the truck farms and in the orange groves of Florida. On the other hand, there is a good demand for cheap labor farther north in the cotton fields of Georgia and Alabama. Florida itself, by reason of heavy summer rains, has practically no cotton fields, and the same is true of the neighboring part of Georgia. Thus the distance to be traversed to the cotton fields puts a check on the number of men who go there. So does the fact that before the cotton season ends the truck farms and orange groves farther south and on the coast supply another reason for going away from home. Even though most of the Florida Negroes live in the northern part of their state they certainly do not pick cotton in anything like the same proportion as the Negroes of South Carolina. Nevertheless, the summer dip in the Florida curve is several times as great as in the South Carolina curve. Moreover, the Florida curve shows no peak like that of both North and South Carolina in July (births in April), and the conceptions in Florida begin to turn sharply upward in October just when the cotton-picking season is in full swing.

Then, too, there is another Negro migration in Florida. This is a southward movement in winter, especially among young women who go to the great resorts as servants. This would tend to reduce the conceptions from December to April at exactly the time when they are high. In most countries the September peak is a good indication of the extent to which the men of a region work away from home during part of the year. In comparison with the succeeding months it is comparatively small in Florida, and far smaller than in the Carolinas. Thus many lines of evidence combine to indicate that migrations offer little help in explaining the great summer dip in the curve of births in Florida.

In order to explain the summer depression and winter high level of the Florida curve it is not necessary to appeal to migration. Southern Spain, Italy, Egypt, and Japan all have less migration of laborers than has Florida. Nevertheless, they all show the same general decline in conceptions during hot weather, especially toward its end and immediately afterward. At Jacksonville during the period when conceptions are most numerous the temperature averages 68° in April and 74° in May. The May temperature is too high for the best health among white people. It may not do much harm to Negroes, but even for them it appears to be above the optimum. In June the temperature averages 79°, July and August 81°, and even September 78°. Most of Florida is still hotter. Only in October does the temperature at Jacksonville (70°) return to a level which is comfortable and healthful even for Negroes. Thus the period of few conceptions coincides very closely with that of depressingly high temperatures, but the conceptions lag a little after the heat, as would naturally be expected.

The conclusion to which we thus seem forced is that in Florida the summer depression of the curve of conceptions is mainly due to hot weather and only secondarily to migration, whereas in old Russia a similar depression was due primarily to migration and only secondarily to hot weather. In both cases the fundamental factor is the seasonal rhythm of the weather, but this rhythm may act directly or indirectly. The contrast in Figure 30 between the concave curve of Florida and the convex curve of Maine appears to be a vivid example of the diverse ways in which the seasonal distribution of births is influenced by hot summers as opposed to those that are just warm enough to be delightful.

The rest of the Florida curve, the high part from September through January, resembles most of the other curves that we have studied. The familiar holiday maximum in September is clearly evident. So, too, is the minor minimum from October to December which indicates a falling off of conceptions during the cool months from January to March. This minimum, however, is well above the average for the whole year and only a trifle lower than the maximum in January and February. This maximum is what one would expect on the basis of the climate. The temperature at Jacksonville averages 55° in January, 58° in February, and 62°

in March. These are very desirable temperatures. In fact for northerners they are better than those of April and May when conceptions are most numerous. But perhaps they are not quite so good for the natives of Florida. Nevertheless, they are very good even for them. The true state of affairs seems to become evident when one draws the dotted line attached to the Florida curve in Figure 30. That line suggests the same sort of annual rhythm as in Belgium and Maine, but with its maximum more nearly in winter. It also suggests that the normal annual rhythm is almost obliterated by a great depression of conceptions during the six months of greatest heat.

If we look, now, at the entire series of curves for the eastern United States in Figure 30, several generalizations seem justified. First, the basic animal rhythm is everywhere evident. Second, it is much modified by cultural conditions, as in South Carolina, and by climatic extremes, as in Florida. Third, the effect of the summer upon conceptions changes steadily as one goes from north to south. In Quebec and Maine conceptions are most numerous in June, July, August and September. In Connecticut there is a slight decline in July. In New Jersey this is more pronounced and lasts through August. In Virginia and South Carolina the summer drop in conceptions disappears because of the peculiar seasonal distribution of agricultural labor and the spell of little work in July or August. The urban curve of North Carolina, however, indicates a minimum of conceptions from July through September. In Florida we find a tremendous drop at this same period. Thus as we go from cool to hot regions the summer changes gradually from the season of greatest reproduction to that of least reproduction. Another way of stating the case is that, although extreme cold and great heat are both detrimental to reproduction, the effect of heat is much the worse. A similar relationship is evident in respect to health and mortality. In Quebec and the north the summer is the season of best health; in southern Florida it is the worst part of the year.

A fourth conclusion is that as one goes from north to south the maximum of births occurs earlier in the season. This, of course, is a necessary consequence of the changing effect of the summer. The month of maximum births is April in Quebec and Maine; March in Connecticut; February but almost March in New Jersey; February most unequivocally in Virginia; and finally January and February on equal terms in Florida. South Carolina is not really an exception, for we have seen that the low level of its curve in January and February is due to the cotton picking in October and November. The city curve of North Carolina fills the gap left by South Carolina. Its maximum so far as the basic annual rhythm is concerned comes in January, with December almost as high. It is probable, however, that here, too, seasonal migrations of the Negroes, and perhaps of whites, enter into the matter. Otherwise it is difficult to account for the high level of the North Carolina urban curve from July to September (conceptions from October to December).

Our fifth conclusion is that, if there were no complications due to migrations and other cultural factors, the month of maximum conceptions would have almost the same temperature everywhere. The mean temperatures of the chief city or capital of each state or province at the time of the spring maximum are as follows: Quebec (Montreal) 67°; Maine (Portland) 67°; Connecticut (Hartford) 67°; New Jersey (Trenton) 66°; Virginia (Richmond) 66°; North Carolina (Raleigh) 56°, but it is not certain that the December-January maximum of births in the urban portion of Figure 30 really represents the maximum according to the basic animal curve; Florida (average of Jacksonville and Tampa) 72°. Taking all these things together the general conclusion is that in the eastern United States and Canada the variation in the seasonal distribution of births depends mainly upon climate, but is strongly modified culturally.

This conclusion is strengthened by a study of the curves for the central and western sections of the country. The dotted lines of the central and western sections of Figure 30 show that the basic animal rhythm is everywhere present except perhaps in the south and interior of California (Curves *Q* and *R*). There the curves become very flat, as is natural in so uniform a climate. In each section of the United States there is also a tendency for the spring maximum of births to occur relatively late in the north and early in the south. Manitoba (curve *H*) has its maximum in April; Minnesota (*I*), Michigan (*J*), and Indiana (*K*) in March; Kentucky (*L*) from mid-February to mid-March; and Mississippi (*M*) in February. On the west coast there is only a hint of this tendency, but this is not surprising in view of the fact that the July temperature at San Diego (65° F.) is only 3° higher than at Vancouver, British Columbia, more than 1200 miles farther north.

Another outstanding feature of Figure 30 is the uniformity in the date of the main minimum in contrast to the variability in that of the main maximum. Except in Florida and the interior of California every one of the 19 curves in Figure 30 has its main minimum in November or December. Even in Florida, December shows a minor minimum which seems to represent the minimum according to the standard annual rhythm which is there broken down by the long hot summers. The curve for the interior of California may be disregarded so far as its minor fluctuations are concerned. It is based only on Stockton, Fresno, Bakersfield, and a few still smaller cities in the dry interior valley, and is far less valid than the other curves of Figure 30. When it is smoothed, however, by our standard formula, $\dfrac{a+2b+c}{4}=b'$, and the minor irregularities are thus eliminated, its main minimum is found in December. Hence we seem to be justified in concluding that except where the summers are very long and warm the minimum number of births in the United States and Canada occurs in November and December and corresponds to a minimum of conceptions in February and March. Those are the months when winter weather and its attendant ills cause physical vigor to be at its lowest and the death rate at its highest.

It seems strange that the season of greatest physical depression and fewest conceptions should also be the time when births are most numerous in a large part of the United States. Such a coincidence suggests that from the standpoint of the survival of the race the condition of the mother at the time of the child's birth is less important than either of two other conditions. One is the physical condition of the parents at the time of conception; the other, the hazards to which the child will be exposed during the early stages after birth. We shall return to this subject later.

Having examined the curves of Figure 30 from north to south, let us clinch the matter by looking at them from east to west. In doing this we shall pay special attention to two features which do not agree with the basic animal rhythm. One of these is the minor minimum of births in the spring or early summer, and the other is the maximum in summer which we have already discussed in respect to Connecticut and New Jersey. Beginning at the top in Figure 30 we find that among the three northern curves those of Quebec (A) and Manitoba (H) would be much alike were it not that, after the main maximum in April, the Manitoba curve takes a slump. From August to October something reduces the number of conceptions in Manitoba but not in Quebec. A similar situation prevails in Minnesota (I) as compared with Maine (B). A comparison of these four curves with the dotted lines indicating the basic animal rhythm suggests that in the central plains of North America some special cause depresses the number of conceptions in the summer and early autumn, and raises it thereafter.

Can this cause be the heat of summer in the interior? A July temperature of 68° at Portland, Maine, versus 72° at St. Paul, perhaps affords a little support of this idea, but July temperatures of 66° at Quebec and 69° at Montreal in the province of Quebec, *versus* 66° at Winnipeg in Mani-

toba, argue equally strongly in the other direction. Therefore, we conclude that we must search for a cultural cause.
This appears to be found in the migration of laborers during the summer. Because of the small size of the farms,
the type of crops, and the conservative habits of people in
Maine and Quebec, very few farm hands are employed away
from their homes. In Winnipeg and Manitoba the big
wheat farms employ many itinerant helpers during the harvest season. Thus both the summer depression of conceptions and the autumn peak in the central plains seem to be
explained. The situation is like that of Russia only less
extreme. The only question is whether there are enough
summer migrants to explain a drop of 6 or 8 per cent in
the birth rate. The British Columbia curve (N) is so much
like that of Washington (O) that it does not require separate discussion.

The curves in the second row from the top in Figure 30
all show a family resemblance, but each has its own individual quality. The Maine curve (B) is very regular;
Minnesota (I) shows a dip in the spring and a rise in the
summer which are presumably due to the migration of farm
laborers as in Manitoba. The Washington curve (O) shows
a strong bulge from May to September much like that of
Connecticut, but more prolonged and flatter as befits a more
uniform climate. In the next line, Oregon (P) has a curve
like that of Washington, but smoother, while Michigan
comes very close to the Washington-Connecticut type. In
the next line the curves for New Jersey (D), Indiana (K),
and the northern cities of California (Q) all show (1) a
maximum early in the year; (2) a distinct but minor minimum in the spring; (3) a bulge which is small and short in
Indiana but lasts from May to November in California; and
(4) a main minimum at the end of the year. The parallelism between the three curves in this latitude is curious,
as is the general parallelism in any given latitude or type of
climate all over the world.

In the present case the resemblance between northern California and New Jersey is particularly interesting because of the climatic differences between the two places. In both regions the outstanding fact is the highly favorable character of the autumn. The spring maximum of births due to conceptions in May is followed by a minimum due to a decline in conceptions in July. In the mild summers of California the conception rate begins to rise even in August; in the hotter New Jersey summer the rise is delayed till September; and after the very hot summers of Indiana the rise does not begin until October. Thereafter, in each case, the autumn is a highly favorable time for conceptions, just as in Washington, Michigan, and Connecticut. In general the size of the autumn bulge of conceptions (summer bulge of births) is inversely proportional to the severity of the preceding summer.

In the lower lines of Figure 30 these same features are still apparent, but in a changed or diminished form. In California the bulge due to autumn conceptions is small in the south (R) and insignificant in the interior cities (S). The flatness of these two curves may be due partly to the uniform climate, but the almost universal practise of birth control may also be important. It will be remembered that in Massachusetts (Figure 28, page 107) we found a recent flattening of the curves of birth for which we could find no explanation unless it be birth control. In California birth control has gone so far that the state needs 50 per cent more children in order that natural increase may maintain the present population.

The curves for Kentucky (L) and Mississippi (M) are of the same general type as those of their neighbors farther east. Kentucky, to be sure, does not show the May maximum of Virginia (August conceptions), perhaps because itinerant Negro laborers are less numerous. Kentucky's percentage of Negroes (9) is only one third that of Virginia. Both states, however, are alike in having a very steeply inclined curve representing the basic annual rhythm. The curve for Mississippi differs from that of South Carolina in having a maximum in February at the time when one would expect it.

We can explain this only on the supposition that during the cotton-planting season from April to June the South Carolina Negroes go away from home much more than do those of Mississippi. On the other hand, the Mississippi Negroes, who form 50 per cent of the population of that state, apparently go away in large numbers during the picking season and return in November and December. The way in which both of these states show a September maximum of births higher than the spring maximum is interesting. It is another of the many features which show how sensitive the seasonal distribution of births is not only to climate but also to human habits of work and play.

Let us now turn back once more to the summer bulge of births first noted in Connecticut and later found highly developed in New Jersey, Michigan, and the Pacific regions from San Francisco north. A similar bulge is seen in many of the Russian curves of Figure 13, but there at least part of it is quite clearly due to the migration of farm laborers. It certainly is not due to any such cause in the United States, for farmers form only 15 per cent of the occupied men in Michigan, 7 per cent in Connecticut, and 5 per cent in New Jersey, and there are practically none in the cities of California. We are evidently dealing with a case where wholly different causes lead to apparently similar results. In Europe a similar bulge is seen in the modern curves for Holland and France, but it is very small, and there is no hint of it in Scotland and Belgium. It seems evident, then, that we are dealing with a condition which is especially developed in America and is not due to migration.

This condition has two distinctive characteristics. First, it is limited to the most healthful and stimulating climatic regions; second, it is new. In Figure 30 the bulge is large and strong on the Atlantic coast from southern New England to New Jersey. The upper curves of Figure 24 show that it is well developed in Massachusetts, but it is absent in Maine (Figure 30). It extends westward along the Great Lakes strip, and it is characteristic of the cool Pacific coast.

In other words, it occurs in just the regions where many lines of investigation indicate the best climate from the standpoint of health and activity. The newness of this bulge is evident in Figure 24. During the nineteenth century May and June were months of very few births in Massachusetts, whereas now they stand close to the top. They have reached this position only since the World War. Our problem is to discover what changes have occurred since about 1915 in the most progressive parts of America in such a way as to cause a notable increase in the percentage of conceptions during August, September, and to a lesss extent October.

The chief changes to be considered seem to be as follows: (1) the rapid spread of birth control; (2) the use of automobiles; (3) a great reduction in death rates; (4) a great increase in summer vacations and sports, especially among the younger generation; (5) improvements in diet, especially through the increased use of vegetables and fruits. Numbers 3, 4, and 5 really belong together, for they are all parts of a widespread improvement in health.

It is almost impossible to determine the exact effect of birth control on the seasonal distribution of births. We saw in Figure 28, however, that in Massachusetts birth control seems to be associated with a tendency to flatten the curve of births. Some confirmation of this is found in the upper part of Figure 31 (page 118) where the curves of rural and urban New York State are compared. Between 1923 and 1928 birth control had already made rapid strides in the city, but was little practised in the rural districts of upstate New York. Figure 32 shows that the curves for these two regions are alike except that the city curve is flattened on both peaks, whereas the rural curve, although based on only about one-sixth as many births, is well rounded. Moreover, in April the rural curve stands above the average, while the city curve dips to the average. This agrees with the Massachusetts data in suggesting that birth control tends to cut down the peaks in the seasonal curves of births, but does not have much effect on the depressions. In New York City the low level

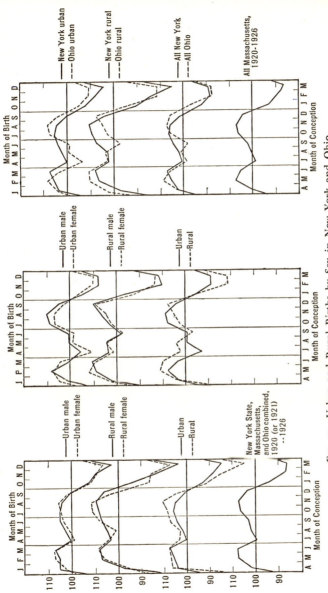

Fig. 32.—Urban and Rural Births by Sex in New York and Ohio.

of births in April (conceptions in July) apparently means that conceptions still drop off in hot weather, whereas farther north in the cooler rural districts this does not happen to so great a degree. The essential point, however, is that, so far as the evidence now goes, birth control does not appear to be responsible for the increase in conceptions during August and September.

The effect of automobiles and of our present great mobility is problematical. It is difficult, however, to see how the seasonal distribution of births could be changed by automobiles except through their effect on health and vacations. Before the advent of the automobile a good many husbands and wives were separated during part of the summer because the wife took the children away to the seashore or country, while the husband stayed in the city and worked. The automobile has reduced this considerably. It has probably also made for better health. Thus it may have helped to bring the conceptions in summer to a higher level. It cannot explain our problem, however, because so far as vacations are concerned its effect must be greatest in July and very small in September. Figure 24 (page 100) shows that in July the change in conceptions has been much smaller than in August, and no greater than in September. Moreover, there has been a relative increase of births in October, so that that month now shows a maximum of conceptions even though it is not helped out by the homeward migration of farm laborers and others in any such way as formerly.

When we turn directly to health, our problem seems to be solved. Figure 29 (page 108) shows two conditions which presumably increase the number of conceptions during August, September, and October. First, it shows that those are the months during which modern medicine has had the most effect in improving the health of adults. In former times the adults of the northern United States enjoyed very good health in July, as appears from the low level of the black shading in Figure 29. In August the death rate rose, and during September and October it was slightly above the average for the year. All this has now been changed. August and September are the best time of the whole year for adults as well as infants, as appears from the upper line of dots in Figure 29. Therefore it is natural that conceptions in those months and in the ones immediately afterward should reach a high level. The other change illustrated by Figure 29 is pyschological, and we are not sure of its importance. In the old days the deaths of children reached an appalling peak in August and continued at a high level in September. Under such conditions thoughtful people might well hesitate about having children. They might also say that they would defer the birth of children so that they would not be born when the death rate was so high. There is no longer any need for such caution.

This brings us back to the main conclusion to which everything seems to point. When cultural factors such as migrations, fasts, and festivals are eliminated the number of children conceived at various seasons of the year appears to depend primarily upon the health and vigor of the parents. Mankind seems to be normally adjusted to climate in such a way that people have the best health and greatest vigor at the season which will give the infants the best chance of life. If improvements in medicine, hygiene, diet, and sanitation change the seasonal incidence of disease and weakness, the seasonal distribution of births changes also. If this brings births at a season unfavorable for the infants, the result is bad. In the case of the northern United States, however, this has not happened because with the change in the seasonal conditions of health among adults there has gone a still greater change in that of infants, so that summer is now highly favorable to them as well as to their parents. In a climate like that of the United States, the greatest vigor of all comes now at the end of the period of lowest mortality, or during the period immediately thereafter. Therefore factory workers do the most work per hour and conceptions are most numerous in October or November. Persons who are physically weak may begin to suffer a little from ill health in those months, but vigorous people are stimulated to the highest degree as the weather becomes cool but not cold. This stimulating effect is particularly noticeable in the United States, presumably because of cool waves that accompany cyclonic storms. This is perhaps the reason why the bulge that we have been discussing is so much more prominent in America than in Europe, but we find it there among certain classes, as will appear later. Thus the summer bulge in the curves of birth from Massachusetts to the Great Lakes and on the Pacific coast seems to be due to conceptions which were stimulated by autumn weather following a summer which now improves human health instead of handicapping it. It therefore seems to be of climatic origin, just as are the spring maximum in Quebec, which results from conceptions in midsummer, and the deep depression during the spring in Florida which results from the heat of the preceding summer.

Chapter VII

OTHER GEOGRAPHICAL VARIATIONS

In other parts of the world the seasonal variations in births are adjusted to climate in essentially the same way as in the United States and Canada. We have already seen that Figure 22 (page 97) provides important evidence as to changes from the past to the present. It is equally significant as an example of geographical variations from north to south. Dotted portions have been added to some of the curves to represent the presumable distribution of births if cultural factors could be eliminated. The dashed lines represent alternative, but less probable, interpretations of the same sort. For our present purpose the curves on the right of Figure 22 are especially important because in modern times the cultural factors that influence season of birth have been reduced to small proportions, making it possible to study the climatic relationships of births without being confused by purely cultural irregularities.

The most outstanding feature of Figure 22 is the obvious presence of the basic annual rhythm in each curve for western Europe, just as in North America. The next feature is that the rhythm reaches its maximum later in the north than in the south. Modern Norway and Scotland show maxima in April (conceptions in July), while modern Spain, far to the south, has a very sharp maximum in February (conceptions in May). Although the modern Danish curve also has a peak in February, we suspect that the true physiological, or climatic, maximum comes in March and April. The February peak looks as if it were cultural as does the similar but smaller peak in Norway, and the very faint maximum in the Netherlands at the same time. In modern Belgium the maximum comes distinctly in March, while in France the months of February and March stand equally high. If we are right in assigning a cultural cause to the February peak in Norway, Denmark, and the Netherlands, the maximum of the basic physiological curve of birth changes regularly from April in the north to February in the south. In other words, the month of maximum conceptions changes steadily from July in Norway and Scotland to May in Spain. Even as the curves stand in Figure 22 this transition is clearly evident, although irregular.

The older curves from western Europe, on the left of Figure 22, show a similar transition. The three most northern countries, Norway, Scotland, and Denmark, show a tendency toward delaying the maximum until March, or even April and May in the case of Scotland. The next three, the Netherlands, Belgium, and France, have theirs in February with March as a very close second in two cases; and Spain has the sharpest of February maxima. In evaluating this change from north to south it must be remembered that the climatic contrast between Norway and Spain is less than that between Quebec and Florida. Oslo is colder than Madrid by 16° F. in January, and 14° F. in July; the corresponding difference between Montreal and Jacksonville are 41° and 12°. Hence we should expect the change in the seasons of birth from north to south to be more distinct in eastern North America than in western Europe.

The next point to note in Figure 22 is the shape of the curves in summer. In the old days the births fell off greatly during the summer in the Netherlands, Belgium, France, and Spain, but not in the three more northern countries, Norway, Scotland, and Denmark. The question at once arises whether this decline in summer is climatic or cultural in origin. Let us assume for the moment that it is climatic. In that case the dashed lines at the bottom of the diagrams for Belgium, France, and Spain, may indicate the true course of the normal animal rhythm. If we use the dashed lines, all the old curves become alike in showing a bulge which begins in August, culminates in September, and continues into

October or November. We believe, however, that the dotted lines more nearly represent the basic rhythm. This, to be sure, suggests that different methods of reasoning are used for the three northern and the four more southerly countries respectively, but this is not really the case.

There are two main reasons for choosing the dotted lines. In the first place, they give curves which quite closely resemble the much smoother modern curves, even when the latter are not corrected for cultural irregularities. This is especially conspicuous in Scotland, the Netherlands, Beligum, and France. The dashed lines, on the contrary, except in Spain, give curves quite different from the modern ones. In the second place, the seasonal distribution of absences from home for the sake of work is different in the north and in the south of western Europe. In Norway, Scotland, and to a less degree Denmark, the men who formerly went away from home to find work were mainly fishermen, sailors, or overseas emigrants, whereas in Belgium, France, and Spain they were largely agricultural laborers. In Norway upwards of 80,000 men—a tenth of the entire number of male workers—are employed in the cod fisheries alone. Little Denmark, with a twelfth the population of France, catches fish worth from one-fourth to one-third as much as those caught by the larger country. Fishing, especially cod fishing, is an occupation for winter as well as summer, great quantities of fish being needed in cold weather not only because they keep well then, but also because Lent creates a great demand for fish in Catholic countries. In former times, before methods of refrigeration were perfected, cool weather was almost essential to deep-sea fishing, far away from home, for otherwise the fish would spoil. Nevertheless, midwinter storms check the fisheries, and for a time the fishermen stay at home, especially at the holiday season. Sailors, who are numerous in these northern countries, also tend to be away at all seasons, but are more likely to come home in winter than at any other time. Hence in countries where fishermen and sailors are numerous the births follow the normal rhythm most of the year, but show a sudden increase due to the return of the men in midwinter. Overseas emigrants also come home mainly in winter because that is the time when there is least work. In Scotland, during the middle of the last century, the combined effect of these causes, and perhaps others, was to produce an extremely high birth rate during September, October, and November by reason of conceptions in December, January, and February.

From the Netherlands southward, fishing has always been relatively much less important than in Scotland, Norway, and Denmark. Agriculture, on the contrary, especially the raising of grain instead of cattle, has been vastly more important. Hence, it was formerly the custom, and is still in less-advanced regions, for agricultural laborers to live at home much of the year, but go away in summer, especially at harvest time. While they are at home the curve of conceptions follows the normal rhythm, but when they go away it shows a sudden drop. Thus it seems only logical to assume that the effect of migration upon the seasonal distribution of births is different in the northern countries of Figure 22 from what it is in the others. Hence, the dotted lines, and not those shown in dashes, appear to be the ones which truly represent the basic annual rhythm in the older as well as the newer curves of Figure 22.

Using, then, the dotted lines, we find that western Europe agrees with North America in other respects, as well as in the shifting of the month of maximum births as one goes from north to south. In the modern curves on the right of Figure 22 the steepness of the curves diminishes as one goes southward from Norway. It reaches a minimum in the flat curve of the Netherlands, and then increases until it is about as steep in Spain as in Norway. This agrees with what we have already found in America. The fact that the modern European curves fail to show any such summer minimum of conceptions as we have seen in Florida is also in agreement with the American conditions. Although southern Spain is very hot in summer, the heat is by no means so prolonged as in Florida.   Moreover, the major part of Spain lies at a considerable elevation on a plateau so that it is only moderately hot in summer.   Tampa, in Florida, has 6 months with a mean temperature of at least 75° F. (23.3° C.), whereas Madrid has only 2, and even Seville in the hottest part of Spain has only 4.   Thus we should expect that when cultural irregularities are eliminated the seasonal curve of births in Spain would resemble the curves of states like Virginia, Kentucky, and Mississippi, and that is what we find on comparing Figures 21 (page 95), and 30 (page 116).

Central Europe (Figure 23, page 99) largely repeats the conditions already seen in western Europe, but several features are more extreme.   One of these is the September peak which is prominent in most of the early curves, and is still evident in some of the modern ones.   In the older curves Finland has a decided maximum in January, corresponding to conceptions in April; and the same is true in northern Sweden, the curve of which is not here given.   At first sight, so early a maximum seems inappropriate to such cold countries, but here, as in so many other cases, local customs offer an explanation.   Lumbering is one of the great occupations of these forested regions.   Hence, many men are away from home during the winter, but return home when the snow melts in March and April.   This apparently accounts for the high level of both the Swedish and Finnish curves from December through February.   If this cultural feature is eliminated, the physiological maximum of births comes in March and represents conceptions in June.   Still another extreme feature of Figure 23 is the great excess of births in Finland during the summer.   In the following discussion we shall speak as if this did not exist, but shall return to it later.

The same general features of geographical variation which we have seen in North America and western Europe are evident in central Europe, especially when allowance is made for the features mentioned in the last paragraph.   As we go from north to south the physiological maximum is pushed back toward the earliest portion of the year.   In the north, in all parts of Sweden, it occurs in June (births in March). The same is true of modern Germany, but the older German curve shows the maximum a little earlier, as appears when one uses the scale of months at the bottom of Figure 23. In Switzerland, May and June vie with one another for supremacy. Italy presents some peculiar features. In old Italy the northern section shows a maximm of conceptions in June, while in the south and center this shifts back to May (births in February). In the modern Italian curves, if one uses the reported data as shown by the dotted lines, the corresponding maxima appear to come a month earlier—May in the north and April in the south. This, however, is not really the case, for modern Italy displays a year-end error somewhat like that of old Russia, but with an interesting difference. Many births of boys born in November and especially December are not reported till January in order that military service may be postponed a year. This error increases from north to south in harmony with the decline in culture, as is evident when the dotted corrections are compared with the solid lines showing the data as reported. Probably the maximum of conceptions in all parts of modern Italy comes in May, leading to a maximum of births in February, but the intensity of this maximum increases toward the south. Because of this statistical error we cannot speak so surely about central Europe as about western Europe and North America. Nevertheless, even in central Europe the tendency toward an earlier maximum of reproduction as one goes toward the south is evident.

Two other general features follow the American example quite closely. One is the steepness of the basic curves in the north and the south, and their flattening in the center. Compare old western Austria, on the left, or modern Czechoslovakia, on the right, with Sweden or southern Italy. The other tendency is toward an exaggerated depression of the curve of births during the summer in the far south. This is evident in both central and southern Italy no matter whether the older or the newer curves be employed. In the far south the modern curve shows a broad, flat minimum of births from May through August. This means few conceptions from August through November. The similar minimum of conceptions in Florida occurs during August and September. In Italy, unlike Spain as a whole (Figure 22) the hot summer seems to be the cause of a depression of vitality such as occurs in Florida and Japan. The depression begins in May and continues into September. It should be noted, however, that southern Italy is not much hotter than central Spain, and even the hottest part of Sicily is not so hot as Seville. The full significance of this will appear shortly when we look at curves for various sections of Spain. Meanwhile our conclusion is that the part of Europe in central longitudes from northern Sweden to Sicily resembles western Europe and still more the United States in (1) the universal presence of an annual rhythm, (2) the tendency toward an earlier maximum of births as one goes from north to south, (3) a flattening of the curves in the most favorable middle latitudes, and (4) a tendency for extreme heat to cause a great decline in conceptions during or after the summer in the far south.

Let us turn now to two exceptional features of Figure 23, one being in northern Italy and the other in Finland. The two curves for northern Italy are distinctly different from those for the rest of Italy, but are a good deal like those for old Switzerland and Germany, and modern Sweden. Each shows two maxima which in both size and shape are nearly equal, especially in the modern curve. The maximum of births in February or March is merely the normal maximum according to the basic animal rhythm. The shape and size of the other maximum agree with the idea that it is due to the return of migrant laborers from France or elsewhere, which begins in October and naturally culminates at the holiday time in December. France receives a flood of Italian laborers each summer. It is interesting to note that Hungarian data, at least from 1900 to 1902 as given by Gini (1912), show almost the same features as those of North Italy.

Central and southern Italy, on the contrary, show little evidence of seasonal migrations.

Before discussing the Finnish curve with its maximum of births in July (conceptions in October) let us glance again at Russia as illustrated in Figure 13 (page 64). Because of the great statistical inaccuracy in December and January we cannot be sure of the exact month of either the maximum or the minimum of the basic annual rhythm. Using the solid lines, however, we note that in the western (left-hand) row of diagrams Olonetz far to the north shows a maximum of births in June; Livland, farther south, shows it in March; Minsk in February, and Volhynia in January. In the middle row of curves we find two February maxima in the north; all the rest, except Taurien, are in January. The February maximum of Taurien may possibly be due to over-correction of the excess of births recorded in January. In the eastern row of diagrams all the maxima assignable to the basic rhythm come in January in the uncorrected curves, and in February in the corrected curves. In evaluating the Russian data it must be remembered that all parts of Russia are cold. Even at Odessa in the far south the seasonal range of temperature is about like that of Chicago and Detroit. Therefore, we cannot expect that the climate will cause great variations in the curves representing the basic animal rhythm. Bearing in mind this fact, as well as the statistical limitations of the Russian material, we conclude that in old Russia there was a general tendency for the maximum of conceptions to occur earlier in the season as one goes farther south. Thus the geographical variations in the season of birth agree with what we have found in central and western Europe and North America.

The prominent maximum of births which occurs during the summer in far northern Russia (Olonetz, Figure 13) is repeated in both of the Finnish curves of Figure 23. The old Finnish curve has such a maximum in June and July; the new one has it in July; the Olonetz curve, from a Russian province a little east of Finland, shows it in June, and

Vologda (Figure 13), farther east, has a maximum in July and August. These are cold regions where the warmest month has a mean temperature of not more than 60 to 63° F. Their curves, especially those of modern Finland and Olonetz, show that during September and October the number of conceptions is much higher than would be expected. Even in modern Finland, where the data are much the most reliable, those months have from 20 to 25 per cent more conceptions than January, February, and March. This is interesting because the modern Finnish curve resembles those of modern Massachusetts, Connecticut, and California. In the American curves we ascribed the autumn maximum of conceptions to the stimulating effect of bracing autumn weather following a summer which under modern conditions depresses vitality very little. We were led to do this by the close resemblance between curves of conception and those of work in factories. Are we justified in ascribing a similar origin to the similar maximum in the old curves for Finland and far northern Russia? This brings up a question with which we are continually faced. In a problem such as the seasonal distribution of births are we justified in ascribing almost identical results to different causes? If we do this are we merely dodging the main issue and thereby demonstrating that none of the hypotheses thus far suggested is valid?

These questions are so important that we may well devote a few paragraphs to them, even at the risk of repetition. In the first place, seemingly identical results often spring from highly diverse causes. Tremors of the earth's crust result from explosions of dynamite, from volcanic eruptions, from faulting of the solid rocks, from the impact of large meteors, from the passage of heavy trucks over the rocks, and doubtless from other causes. A tree may die from drought because of extreme cold, unduly porous soil, the deflection of a stream, or the cutting of a root, as well as from lack of rain. Insanity may arise from fear, from specific diseases, from exposure, from shell shock, and from many other causes. Even the most skilled psychiatrist may be unable to detect the cause so long as he does not know the entire history of the patient. Hundreds of other examples might be cited to show that seemingly identical results flow from highly diverse causes. In fact, the only sound scientific procedure is to recognize this fact, and be ready to use whatever hypothesis best fits the case, provided it does not conflict with other facts elsewhere. This last is the important point. It is dangerous to use one hypothesis here and another there to explain similar facts, unless all the hypotheses are applied equally to all cases, and every hypothesis is eliminated which conflicts with any known facts.

The next point to emphasize is that in testing hypotheses it is advisable to begin with the simplest and most easily tested. In the problem now before us the three main causes of fluctuations in the curves of birth stand in the following order in this respect: (1) the degree to which husbands and wives are separated at different seasons, (2) the physical condition of the parents at one season as compared with another, and (3) the effect of the various seasons upon the survival of the infants. The separation of husbands and wives may be due to actual physical distance, or to social customs such as the Russian fasts. In modern Finland (Figure 23) and in Olonetz (Figure 13) this last cause of seasonal fluctuations in the birth rate can be eliminated. We know of no social custom which would produce the observed curves of births if the husbands were at home all the time. As for physical separation, the pertinent facts depend mainly upon the low temperature, the presence of forests, and the necessity of relying on other occupations in addition to agriculture. Finland, and still more Olonetz lie on the very northern edge of the region where agriculture is possible. In Olonetz, to quote the encyclopedia, "the chief source of wealth is timber, next to which come fishing and hunting. More than one-fifth of the entire male population leave their homes every year in search of temporary employment." Here in two sentences we find a seemingly complete explanation of a good deal of the peculiar quality of the Olonetz curve of births.   In summer, especially during August and September, the absentees tend to come home to take care of the main business of agriculture, that is, the harvesting.   They stay at home two or three months, but as winter comes on and the ground becomes covered with snow they go away again, or at least they did under the old regime.   Some went into the forest for lumber or furs; others went to St. Petersburg or other cities to pick up odd jobs.   In November a great many were away, but some came back at Christmas time.   Almost the same number were apparently at home through the Russian December, January, and February.   The Olonetz curve of Figure 13 suggests that in March a considerable number went away once more, and that most of them stayed away at least through April, May, and June.

In view of all this we conclude that the main features of the Olonetz curve were determined by the highly migratory habits which the men adopted because of the peculiar climatic characteristics of that province.   If we discover elsewhere, as we do, that the various seasons alter the urge toward reproduction, we may safely assume that the same is true in Olonetz.   The migration of one-fifth of the men, however, and probably of more than one-fifth of the young husbands, was so potent an influence upon the birth rate that it largely obliterated other influences.   It caused the births to vary from only about 85, according to our index numbers, up to 122.   This means that births in June (conceptions in September) show an excess of about 42 per cent over those in December and January (conceptions in March and April).

In northern Finland the occupational conditions are much the same as in Olonetz, but in southern Finland they are less extreme.   The chief reason for the homecoming of absentees is the harvest in August and September, thus causing the greatest number of men to be at home in September and October, and the greatest number of births to take place the following June and July.   The chief reason for being away from home is the very extensive lumber industry, which calls away the lumbermen as soon as the ground is covered with snow, and keeps them away until the snow melts. Thus the number of conceptions declines rapidly in November, December, and January, and remains low through March. Judging by other regions, such a decline would take place, even if all the men remained at home, for it seems to be the regular result of cold weather. But in Finland the effects of cold weather are re-enforced by migration.

In Connecticut, on the other hand, a distinctly different type of climate seems to produce a strong physiological stimulus in the autumn at just the time when the most men are at home in Finland. Then winter produces its normal restraining influence upon reproduction. We cannot find any type of separation of husband and wives which explains the facts in Connecticut, but we do find independent evidence of physical vigor as shown in factory work.

In neither of these cases does the survival of the children enter into the matter. Nevertheless, the hypothesis of a survival value in birth at certain seasons seems to be the only explanation of the very widespread occurrence of a late winter or early spring maximum of births. Thus when our three main hypotheses as to seasonal variations in the birth rate are applied in the correct order they seem to explain all the facts thus far observed. They do so without contradicting one another, and they supplement one another at the required points. Thus in a curve like that of the Moscow hospitals (Figure 15) the most obvious effect is that of social customs, which keep the two sexes apart, even though the other three types of factors are also operating. In Olonetz (Figure 13) the dominant effect is that of occupational migration. In Connecticut neither of these produces any effect that we have been able to recognize, and the most noticeable feature is the effect of stimulating weather. And finally, in the Belgian type of curve we come back to the animal rhythm, based on the survival of the infants and presumably underlying all the other curves. This rhythm appears to be dominant in Belgium merely because social customs and migration have no appreciable effect, and the climate does not cause the basic seasonal rhythm to produce any unfavorable effect.

Let us next examine the seasonal distribution of births in the various sections of Spain. In the main part of Figure 33 ten Spanish provinces are arranged in the order of their temperature. First, on the left, come three cool provinces—Corunna, Oviedo, and Santander, on the northwest coast. There the temperature averages below 67° F. even in July, and from 44° to 47° in January. The next province, Lugo, lies on this same coast, but a larger portion of it extends inland so that it is slightly warmer than the others in summer and cooler in winter. Barcelona, on the east coast, but still in the north, comes next. Its winter temperature is about like that of the other northern provinces, but in July the average temperature rises to 75° F. The next four provinces lie along the southeast coast and are arranged in the order of their location. Valencia is located close to the central latitude of Spain; then come Alicante and Malaga, while Cadiz is in the extreme south. In these provinces the mean temperatures of January range from 50° to 54° F., and that of July from 75° to 79°. Seville is placed last in Figure 33 because its inland location and low altitude make it warmer than Cadiz and Malaga, even though it lies farther north. Its mean monthly temperatures range from 52° in January to 85° in July.

Notice how the spring maximum retreats as one goes from north to south in Figure 33, or rather from cooler to warmer regions. In Corunna, which lies at the very northwest corner of Spain and is fully exposed to cool winds from the Atlantic, it comes in April. In Oviedo and Santander, farther east and not so cool, March and April stand about equally high. In Lugo, close to Oviedo, but with less seacoast and a larger proportion of warm inland territory, the maximum comes in February. Barcelona also shows its maximum in February, but with January as a close rival. Among the remaining five provinces, all of which lie in the warmer parts of Spain, two show maxima in February and three in

January. If it were not for the February maxima of Valencia and Cadiz the tendency toward an earlier maximum as one goes from cooler to warmer regions would be almost perfect.

Another noteworthy point is the much greater range from maximum to minimum in the warm southern regions than

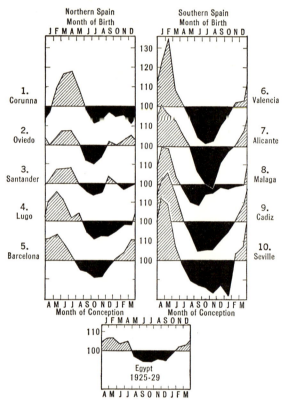

FIG. 33.—Births in Spanish Provinces, 1863–1867 and 1878–1882, and Egypt, 1925–1929.

in the mild regions of the north. In Seville the range is from 132 to 82; in Santander from 107 to 93, or less than one-third as much.

Again, there is a gradual, although not perfectly regular, change from the Belgian type of curve in the northwest to the Florida type in the south. In Corunna the climate is much like that of Belgium except that it is warmer in winter. There, just as in Belgium, the animal rhythm is dominant, with a maximum in March and April and a minimum in December. This is broken, to be sure, by a depression during the summer, due to a deficiency of conceptions in October and November. This may be due to the absence of the men from home, some being fishermen, and some going south to assist in the olive harvest. The presence of a little peak in September in the curves for Oviedo and Santander as well as Corunna is almost certain evidence of the migration of laborers. Otherwise there would not be a return of absentees at Christmas time. Aside from the maximum in late winter or early spring, however, the details of the Spanish curves are not easy to interpret without exact knowledge as to local peculiarities of occupations and customs.

On the other hand, the situation is very clear in respect to the deepening and lengthening of the summer minimum as one goes toward warmer regions. It is marvelous to see how rapidly the number of births in the province of Seville drops from February to March and then not quite so fast from April to June. This means a very rapid drop in conceptions from May, when the temperature averages 70°, to June (75°), July (84°), and August (85°). Even after the maximum heat is passed, the decline in conceptions continues at a diminished rate through September (80°), October (69°), and November (60°). Then comes a rise during December and a further drop during January. These two features lead us to wonder whether the elimination of migration among laborers would cause the curve of births in Seville to assume a form more like that of Malaga with a minimum in June due to deficiency of conceptions in September. Or perhaps the great heat of summer causes so much debility that the Seville curve would be more like that of Valencia with a minimum of conceptions in October. The regularity of the Valencia curve and the absence in it of any hint of a September maximum due to homecomings in December suggests that there the curve depends almost wholly on climate with little modification by migration. The February peak in this curve indicates a maximum of conceptions in May when the tempera-

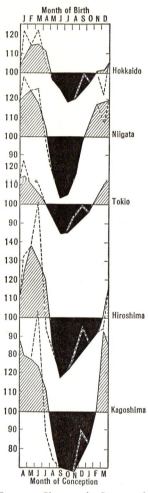

Month of Birth
J F M A M J J A S O N D

Hokkaido

Niigata

Tokio

Hiroshima

Kagoshima

A M J J A S O N D J F M
Month of Conception

FIG. 34.—Changes in Season of Birth from North to South in Japan, by Provinces, 1899, 1900, 1902-1907.

ture averages 64°, which is approximately the optimum for physical health among Europeans.

Turning now to Japan, Figure 34 shows curves of birth for five provinces distributed from the northern island of Hokkaido, or Yezo, to the southern part of the southern island of Kiushu. In all these curves the original data as published by the government are indicated by the dotted lines. The corresponding solid lines represent our attempt to make corrections for the two types of error mentioned when the curve for Hiroshima was discussed in Chapter IV (page 83). One of these is a correction because the births of December have not all been recorded when the returns are sent to the central office at the beginning of the new year. Hence December appears to have less than its true number of births and January has too many. It is interesting to note that this error is great in the north, diminishes southward, and disappears in the far south. The only explanation which we can think of is that in the far north where Hokkaido is located, and also in the mountainous parts of Niigata on the west side of the main island, a cold winter and considerable snow much restrict and delay communication with outlying villages. In the central provinces of Tokyo and Hiroshima there is very little snow, and the outlying villages are less isolated. This agrees with the degree to which the records appear to ascribe too few births to December and too many to January. With its apparent excess of births in December, Kagoshima in the far south falls so far out of line with what one would expect on the basis of its climate that we suspect a misprint or some such error in its data as here used.

The other error is the one whereby births occurring after March are ascribed to that month in order that the children may enter school a year earlier than would otherwise be possible. This error varies in close harmony with the degree of progress. It is fairly large in the rather backward northern island, less marked in the western province of Niigata, and almost disappears in the metropolitan province of Tokyo. Farther south, where culture again declines, the error becomes acute, and is greatest of all in Kagoshima. Curiously enough this particular error tends to be greater in Tokyo city than in the rest of that province, as may be seen by comparing the left side of Figure 35 with Tokyo province in Figure 34.

The correction of these two types of error, as made in the solid lines of Figure 34, is inevitably arbitrary. In one case a certain number of births is taken from January and added to December; in the other case births are taken from March and added partly to April and in smaller measure to May. The reader can see for himself how this has been done. So far as the conclusions of this book are concerned any reasonable adjustment of these errors would have the same effect. There is scarcely room for doubt that the elimination of the apparent minor minimum of births in December is in harmony with the facts. It seems equally clear that, the farther south we go in Japan, the more reason there is to reduce or eliminate the maximum in March.

A third type of change is also indicated by the dotted lines in Figure 34. This takes the form of the elimination of the September maximum. In Chapter IV we gave reasons for thinking that this is mainly cultural. This conclusion is strengthened by the fact that no such maximum occurs in the Niigata curve of Figure 34, or in four of the six curves of Figure 35. If the maximum is not cultural it must be cli-

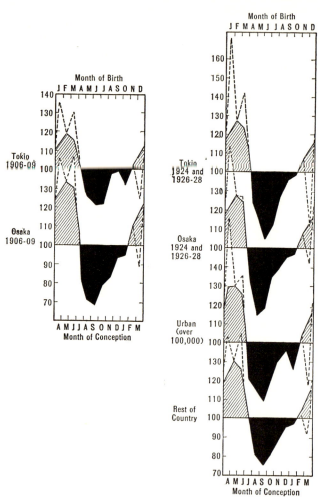

FIG. 35.—Season of Birth in Japanese Cities and Rural Areas, 1923, 1924, 1926, 1927, and 1928.

matic, and must be due to the prevalence of stimulating conditions of weather up to December, followed by depressing conditions during January. If this were the case the

September maximum ought to be strongly developed in Hokkaido where the mean temperature of January is only 27° F. at Hakodate and 21° at Sapporo. It also ought to be well developed in Niigata where the January mean for the city is 35° and that of the more elevated parts of the province considerably lower. But the September maximum is less pronounced in Hokkaido than in Hiroshima and Kagoshima far to the south, and it is entirely missing in Niigata. Such variation is possible in a cultural factor; it is impossible in a climatic factor. Hence we conclude that in order to show the true course of the purely physiological rhythm in Japan we ought to eliminate the September maximum as well as the excess of records during January and March. It may seem as though we were greatly altering the form of the Japanese curves by substituting the solid for the dotted lines, but the fundamental features of a late winter or early spring maximum and a deep midsummer minimum are not affected. Moreover, as we have already indicated, some correction of March and December is obviously needed, as Gini has well pointed out, and no reasonable method of correction will give results differing essentially from ours.

Assuming then that the solid lines represent approximately the true course of the physiological conditions which cause seasonal variations in the birth rate, let us analyze Figure 34. The analysis is comparatively simple. It starts in the same way as that of the United States, western Europe, central Europe, Russia, Spain, and Italy. In other words, it calls attention to the fact that the main maximum of all the Japanese curves comes in the late winter or early spring, and occurs earlier in the season as one goes southward. Thus in Hokkaido it comes in March and corresponds to conceptions in June. In Niigata and Hiroshima it occurs in February. Tokyo, with its maximum in January, falls a little out of line. This may represent a permanent condition, but it may also arise from some fault in our method of correction, or from some exceptional condition during the special years here employed. In Figure 35 both an early and a late curve for Tokyo city, in distinction from Tokyo province, show their corrected maxima in February. Finally, in the most southerly (Kagoshima) curve of Figure 34 the corrected maximum comes in December, corresponding to conceptions in March. If this is an error, as has been suggested above, the maximum probably comes in January; but in either case, the general fact of an earlier date for the winter maximum as one goes toward the south remains unchanged.

Another agreement between the Japanese curves and those of other regions is the fact that in the most progressive part, which is also the part where the climatic advantages are on the whole the greatest, the curves tend to flatten. The Tokyo curve is flatter than those above or below it. Even in the relatively flat Hokkaido curve the range from maximum to minimum is 30 per cent (115 to 85) in comparison with 26 (85 to 111) in Tokyo. Still a third main agreement with other regions is that the dip in the curves during the summer becomes broader as well as deeper in the south.

In the southern hemisphere births have the same relation to the seasons as in the northern. In Figure 36 a number of

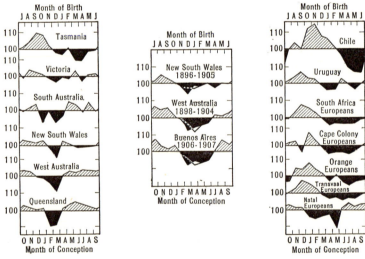

Fig. 36.—Seasonal Distribution of Births in the Southern Hemisphere, 1921–1929.

southern curves have been plotted so that July replaces January as the first month on the left, thus eliminating the difference in the seasons on the two sides of the equator.   Their
general form is like that of the curves of regions with similar
temperatures in the northern hemisphere.   Except for Chile
every one of these 16 curves has a maximum in July, August,
or September, corresponding to January, February, or March
in the North.   New South Wales, however, and the Europeans of Cape Colony and Orange have equal or higher
maxima in October.   Aside from Chile and Natal all these
curves also show a minimum in December or January, corresponding to June or July.   In some cases there appears to
be a year-end error such as we have found in other countries.
In the three central curves of Figures 36, based on old data
taken from Gini (1912), allowance has been made for this,
thus bringing the minima in December, which corresponds
to the northern June.   It is noticeable that, although September sometimes shows a maximum of births which might
be attributed to the homecoming of husbands at Christmas,
there is no regularity about this.   This is normal, for Christmas is the harvest season in several of the warm wheat-rais-
ing regions of Figure 36, and it is a busy season everywhere.
On the other hand, the Chileans and the Europeans of
Orange and especially Cape Colony show a depression of
births in September.   This may be accidental, but in Cape
Colony, at least, one wonders whether visits to England by
one member of a family during the holiday season may actually lower the birth rate the following September.   We do
not feel at all sure of this, and have no data by which to
test it.

Chile and Tasmania, at the top of Figure 36, are the coolest
regions there represented.   It is of interest that they show
pronounced maxima rather late in the season in the same
fashion as the cooler regions of the northern hemisphere.
Thus in all their main features these curves for the southern hemisphere are in harmony with those for corresponding
climates north of the equator.

As a final test of geographical variations in season of birth and their relation to the weather let us turn to the tropics. Unfortunately data as to births by months in tropical countries are not only very scarce, but also very unreliable. Moreover, in countries where the temperature is always above the optimum the seasonal responses of reproduction are presumably different from those in temperate countries. Let us begin with Mexico, which lies within the tropics but

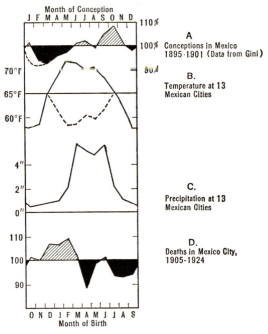

FIG. 37.—Conceptions, Deaths, and Weather in Mexico.

consists so largely of highlands that most of the people live at temperatures not far from the optimum. We shall use birth data supplied by Gini (1912), but we do not vouch for the accuracy of Mexican statistics nor do we know how completely they represent the whole country.

Curve *A* in Figure 37 illustrates the seasonal distribution of conceptions leading to legitimate births in Mexico as a whole. Other data published by Gini show that in the

southeastern provinces of the country and among illegitimate births the seasonal variations are the same as among
legitimate births except that the maxima in October and
especially January are more pronounced. The suddenness
with which the January peak rises in the illegitimate curve
(not here reproduced) and its variability from one curve to
another suggest that in both the legitimate and illegitimate
curves it is of cultural origin. Its most probable cause appears to be the prolonged New Year festivities with their
homecomings and drunkenness. Hence we may disregard
it, and assume that in Section *A* of Figure 37 the dotted
line represents the true annual rhythm. This rhythm is like
that of Belgium except that the seasons of maxima and minima are almost reversed. The question at once arises whether
such a reversal is due to the climate or to some peculiar social
conditions. We cannot think of any social or cultural condition which would produce such a result. On the borders of
the United States there is a seasonal migration of laborers
into Texas, but this would not cause an excess of men at
home in September and October, nor is it of sufficient size
to be of much effect. On the whole the Mexicans tend
strongly to stay at home at all seasons.

Turning now to climate, Curves *B* and *C* of Figure 37 illustrate the average temperature and rainfall at 13 stations so
chosen as to represent the general distribution of the Mexican population. Because most of the Mexicans live upon a
high plateau, the average temperature is 18.7° C. (65.6° F.),
which is almost the optimum for Europeans. Essentially
this same temperature is the average for October, which is
the month when conceptions are most numerous.

At first sight, however, neither temperature nor rainfall
seems to have much to do with the rhythm of reproduction,
but taken together, they may be significant, especially when
their relation to diet is also considered. To begin with
temperature, the dotted line attached to Curve *B* is the same
as the solid curve above it, but reversed. It shows the amount
by which the temperature departs from 65° F. It brings out

the fact that during the six months from May to October the rate at which the temperature falls is closely parallel to the rate at which conceptions (Curve *A*) increase. Even the minor dip in August appears in both curves. After reaching a maximum when the temperature averages 65° conceptions decline as the temperature drops below that level. Thus from May to December they agree with the extent to which the temperature departs from 65°, which appears to be the optimum.

In general the period of many conceptions is one of few deaths. The minor maximum of deaths in September (Curve *D*), when conceptions are numerous, appears to be due in considerable measure to deaths from dysentery and malaria, which become abundant toward the end of the dry season. On the dry plateau fresh fruit and vegetables then become fairly abundant although extremely rare during much of the year. This must be of great benefit to the health of the population as a whole, but in some places such as Mexico City and Yucatan it is accompanied by considerable dysentery. Malaria also becomes abundant at this time in the drier parts of the country where water stands in pools during the later part of the wet season. Dysentery and malaria, however, may not have much influence upon the number of conceptions, as will appear when we discuss India. When allowance is made for these diseases, the course of the death rate from May to December is probably almost the opposite of that of conceptions. In other words, good health and many conceptions go together. They follow the course that would be expected on the basis of the departure of the temperature from the optimum and the quality of the diet.

From January to May a different situation prevails. The death rate rises rapidly, whereas conceptions drop to a minimum in February and March, and then increase. These things happen in spite of the fact that the temperature is rising toward the optimum during the first half of this period and is not very high even at the end. The average for 13 cities is then 72° F., but of course there are great variations from city to city and too much faith must not be placed on averages. One reason for this spring rise in the death rate may be the dryness, dust, and monotonous character of the weather during the dry season. The unfavorable relationship between dryness and health is rarely appreciated, although the records of millions of deaths make it clear (Huntington, 1919, 1921, 1930). Another reason may be the poor diet of corn and beans, with practically no meat, milk, fruit, or vegetables, upon which most of the Mexicans subsist during the dry period.

In the well-populated parts of Mexico the dry period from November to April appears to do much harm. At that time the rainfall averages less than 1 inch per month. Such conditions are accompanied by bad health not only in Mexico, but in India, Egypt, South Africa, and elsewhere. The highest death rates in the world are found in dry cities such as Mexico City and Johannesburg, and especially in those such as Cairo and Lucknow, that are hot as well as dry. Moist, hot cities such as Madras, Bombay, Calcutta, and Vera Cruz have better health than the corresponding dry cities. In Mexico City, as is evident in Curve D of Figure 37, the death rate rises steadily from the beginning of the dry season in November until the wet season begins in May. Part of the increase is due to malaria, which becomes common in the lower and wetter parts of Mexico in the earlier phases of the dry season which there begins later than on the plateau. At Mexico City, however, the high death rate during the dry season is apparently due partly to the very poor diet, partly to the dryness, and partly to the temperature, which is there lower than in Curve C.

When the rains become abundant in June, the deaths decline rapidly. This happens in spite of the fact that April, May, and June, with mean temperatures of 64°, 65° and 64° F. at Mexico City, are almost ideal in this respect. The coming of the rain with the attendant cloudiness, atmospheric humidity, variability, freedom from dust, and better diet seems to cause a great improvement in health. Hence deaths fall to their lowest level in July. In the lowlands, however, the situation is different, for Vera Cruz has its lowest death rate in April before the very hot weather begins, and its maximum in December, thus almost agreeing with Bengal in India, as we shall soon see.

We may now sum up the most probable relationship of conceptions and weather in Mexico, but must remember that more accurate data as to both births and deaths are needed. The probable reasons for the low level of conceptions from February to April include the extremely bad diet of practically nothing except corn and beans on which the people subsist for many months, and the dryness, dust, and consequent ill health of the dry season. The probable reasons why conceptions increase rapidly on the return of the rainy season include a drop toward the most favorable temperature, a desirable condition of variability and atmospheric humidity, and a diet which becomes increasingly healthful until about October. The whole matter needs much more study, but the Mexican data do not appear to be out of harmony with our general hypothesis.

The relation between births and the seasons is even more complicated in India than in Mexico, but leads to the same conclusion. In a later chapter, where we deal with people of eminence and employ a limited body of very accurate data, we shall find a truly extraordinary agreement between births and temperature in India. This is not so clear in Figure 38. The first thing that strikes us there is the fact that the seasonal distribution of conceptions (A) disagrees with that of deaths (D).

Let us examine the factors which appear to influence the seasonal variation in conception. The chief cultural factor of this kind in India is festivals in March and September which are accompanied by a high degree of sexual license. At those times, more certainly than at others, husbands visit their wives who still live with the wife's parents, as is a common custom in India. Curve A shows that at the time of the March festival there are many conceptions; in September, very few. This suggests that the festivals cannot be more than a minor factor in determining the number of conceptions.

Can diet be the cause of the difference between March and September? In March the Bengalis are comparatively well fed, although the vast majority are almost always under-

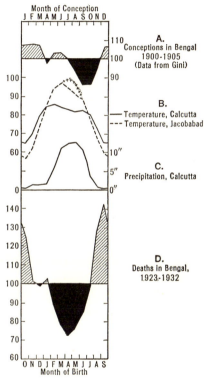

FIG. 38.—Conceptions, Deaths, and Weather in India.

nourished. The main rice crop is harvested in January, thus giving a relatively ample supply of food for a while. From December to March fresh vegetables are available more abundantly than at other seasons, although they are always scarce. From April to July the diet deteriorates, partly because the supply of rice is likely to run low, and partly because the heat and then the very heavy rain (Curve *C*)

prevent the growth of fresh vegetables. July, when conceptions are at the average level, is probably the worst month
from the standpoint of diet. The winter rice has by that time
been mostly eaten, the mango crop is coming to an end, and
other kinds of food are scarce. In September the diet becomes more abundant because the summer rice has been harvested, but the continued downpour of rain—11 or 12 inches
per month—makes fresh food more scarce than ever. Conceptions fall to a minimum at this time, and this may be
due in part to a delayed effect of poor nutrition. Thus diet
may be a factor in the low rate of conceptions in summer
as well as in the high rate in winter.

Let us now see whether conceptions show any relation to
temperature. The solid line in Section *B* of Figure 38 shows
the temperature at Calcutta, which may be used to represent
Bengal. Only in winter does it fall low enough (65° F.) to
be anywhere near the optimum as determined in cooler countries, and it remains there only during December and January. In summer it rises very high, and would rise still
higher if the clouds and rain brought by the southwest monsoon did not cool the air. The possible course of the temperature, if there were no monsoon, is suggested by the dotted
line in Section *B*, which shows the actual condition at Jacobabad a little farther north than Calcutta and much farther
west near Baluchistan. Jacobabad lies in a desert. Therefore the rise of temperature is unchecked by cloudiness and
rain except as indicated by the departure of the dotted line
from the line of little crosses. Since Calcutta lies under a
vertical sun for many weeks, its temperature would doubtless rise even higher than the line of crosses, were it not that
the sunlight is intercepted by clouds and the air is cooled by
rain.

Conceptions are at a maximum from December to March
when the mean temperature ranges from 65° to 79°. On the
basis of temperature alone we should expect conceptions to
be at a maximum in December and January. When allowance is made, however, for marriages, festivals, the home-

coming of husbands in March, and the good diet of the winter, it is not surprising that the period of most abundant
conceptions begins in those months and continues into February and even March when the average temperature has
risen to 79° F. Although this period is rainless, proximity
to the sea and an abundance of water in rivers and irriga-
tion ditches prevent the atmospheric humidity from falling
as low as in Mexico, but they do not prevent dust. With the
coming of hot weather (85° in April), the number of conceptions declines, as would be expected on the basis of temperature. In May and June, however, it rises once more,
which is contrary to what we should expect at first thought.
But in Section *B* of Figure 38 notice the difference between
the curves of temperature at Calcutta (the solid line) and
Jacobabad (dotted). At Calcutta, May is less than 1° F.
warmer than April; and June, July, and August are actually
cooler. So far as people's feelings are concerned the difference is much greater. The coming of the monsoon in May
with its clouds and rain not only brings relief from the
vertical sun, but lays the dust and makes life far more pleasant. The wind also becomes much stronger, which is a great
relief after the stagnant heat of April. The effect is essentially the same as that of a drop of temperature. We should
therefore expect an increase in conceptions, and that is just
what we find. In spite of the relief thus afforded by the
monsoon at first, the summer is very hot, moist, and sticky.
As it continues, the first effect wears off, the wind becomes
weaker and more fitful, the air is stagnant, and people dread
its later stages. In harmony with this, and with the added
impetus of poor diet, conceptions drop to a minimum in
September and October. Not till November does the temperature fall below 80°. In that month a temperature of
72° is accompanied by a sharp increase in conceptions, which
continues in December, when the temperature has fallen to
an average of 65°.

Taking the year as a whole, the major seasonal course of
conceptions in Bengal seems to follow the temperature quite

closely. Nevertheless, it appears to be modified somewhat by three other factors. One of these is social customs in the form of feasts, which probably account for the sharp angle of Curve *A* in Figure 38 in March. A second is diet, which probably tends to raise the level from December to March and to lower it from August to October. It is not easy to separate the effect of diet from that of the weather. Nevertheless, the apparent effect of our next factor seems to indicate that the weather is much more important than the diet. This next factor is the combination of breezes, cloudiness, rain, and relief from the hot sun which accompanies the first onset of the southwest monsoon.

Although there is a close relationship between health and reproduction, the seasonal curves of conceptions and mortality by no means always agree. This is pre-eminently the case in Bengal. There the mortality curve (*D*) does not follow the course that one would expect on the basis of either diet or weather. Part of the discrepancy may be due to the unreliable character of the mortality statistics, but that must be only a minor factor. According to the Indian Census of 1921 the omissions in recording deaths in Bengal may be as great as 50 per cent in some districts and average about 20 per cent year after year in large sections. There is no certainty, however, that the errors are much greater at one season than at another. In summer, many deaths may fail to be recorded because great heat and humidity make everyone feel wilted, and heavy rains convert the broad plains into an impassable sea of mud. In winter, the pleasant temperature makes people feel energetic and the dryness makes it easy for officials to move around and keep informed of what is happening, but malaria makes many an official too feeble to care about his records. Curve *D* ought, perhaps, to be flatter than it is, but there is no doubt that the death rate rises rapidly in the late fall and early winter.

The main cause of the maximum of deaths in December is "fevers," as the census calls them. These are rife at that time, and account for three-quarters of all deaths during the year as a whole. The full establishment of the dry season in November (Curve *C*) permits the formation of a multitude of stagnant pools all over the flat plain. In these the mosquitoes breed by billions, and spread malaria everywhere. Even if malaria does not kill people, it opens the way for other diseases. Hence in October the death rate rises to the average (Curve *D*), and in November it shoots up terrifically, becoming higher than in any month except December.

It is sometimes said that this high death rate is due to cool weather, but that must be a very minor factor. In November the average temperature for day and night together at Calcutta is 72° F., which is about like July in New York. A drop to that level from 80° in the preceding month can scarcely cause a great increase in deaths even among people such as the Bengalis who have practically no means of protecting themselves from the cold. It is still less probable that a drop of 2° from September to October (82° to 80°) can be injurious to health, but the death rate rises very rapidly at that time. Moreover, if a mean temperature of 72° were very harmful in November, a temperature of 65° in December ought to make the death rate rise faster from November to December than from October to November. There ought also to be a still further rise in January (65°) and at least a continuance of high death rates in February, for that month, with a mean temperature of 70°, is 2° cooler than November. Curve *D*, on the contrary, shows that January has a lower death rate than either November or December, and in February the deaths drop suddenly to the average level for the year as a whole.

The relative abundance of both rice and vegetables from January to March, as we have seen, probably helps to bring about this improvement in health, but the decline in malaria is far more important. As the stagnant pools dry up during the almost rainless winter, the mosquitoes gradually disappear, and malaria diminishes greatly after its peak in December. By April, however, the heat becomes extreme, and the death rate again tends to rise—more, perhaps, than Curve *D* indicates. Then comes the monsoon season with its clouds and rain. These lower the death rate considerably, even though the temperature is very high and the humidity great.

Deaths in Bengal fall to their lowest level in July when the summer rains have become well established. One would expect the poor diet at that time to raise the death rate, but any effect of this sort is completely overshadowed by other and more favorable conditions. One of those may be that the accumulated filth which was washed into the streams and even the wells at the first coming of the rains has now been carried away. A much more important condition is that most of the mosquito larvae have also been washed away, so that malaria is at a low ebb. A high degree of cloudiness also helps by providing relief from the hot sun. Cooling breezes are common, and finally there is no dust. With the coming of the dry season in October or November, as we have already seen, all this is changed. Innumerable stagnant pools are left as the rains decline, and soon swarm with malarial mosquitoes. There is not much wind to cool the air and blow away the mosquitoes. Hence malaria gradually assumes alarming proportions. At the same time another bad condition arises. Each village becomes a center of filth. Most Indian villages have no toilet facilities aside from the open fields or the more sheltered parts of the streets. This is bad enough in wet weather, but when the faeces become dry and powdery, they are blown everywhere by the wind and carry infection far and wide. Moreover, the unbroken sunshine day after day, and the uniformity of the weather week in and week out, are not favorable to health (Huntington, 1930).

This brings us back to the main lesson of our Indian data. The seasonal distribution of conceptions there seems to depend mainly on temperature, or at least on people's feelings as to comfort when mean temperature, humidity, wind, cloudiness, sunshine, and rain are all taken into account. In other words, it follows the course that would be expected from our study of other regions. The people of India appear to be stimulated to reproduction by essentially the same conditions of bodily comfort which characterize the optimum in cooler countries. Such factors as diet appear to play only a subordinate rôle. Conceptions, however, follow a seasonal course quite different from that of deaths. This seems to be at variance with the idea that reproduction varies in harmony with health. The seeming contradiction arises from the fact that there are at least three distinct types of seasonal fluctuations in health. One is due to the more or less direct effect of the weather upon the nervous and glandular systems and thus upon metabolism, reproduction, and the course of certain types of diseases. All parts of the population are presumably affected by this almost equally. A second type is due to the indirect effect of the climate through diet. The effect of this varies greatly according to people's economic status, occupation, and mode of life. A third type of fluctuation in health is due to epidemic diseases. These may produce a high death rate among certain parts of the population at a time when the health of the great majority is excellent. Conceptions apparently tend to follow the directly climatic type of fluctuation more closely than either of the others, although dietary fluctuations appear to add their own distinct contribution. The epidemics, on the contrary, appear to have much less effect upon conceptions than would be expected, although they have a great effect upon deaths. Even so tremendous an epidemic as that of influenza in 1918 influenced conceptions only mildly in comparison with its effect on deaths (Figure 28, page 107).

The way in which the three types of influences combine to determine the seasonal course of the death rate is well illustrated in New York and New England. In Figure 39 (page 168), for example, the inhabitants of New York City two or three generations ago, regardless of age or sex, experienced a distinct maximum of deaths in February or March. Among older people this was prolonged into April. This maximum was apparently due partly to the direct effect of the weather, partly to its indirect effect through epidemics and other diseases, and partly to dietary deficiencies. Another maximum, due mainly to digestive parasites, but partly to the direct effect of heat, appeared among persons of all ages in July and August. It was very extreme among children 1 and 2 years old, and very mild among those aged 5 to 10.

Except among very old people two minima of deaths are also evident in Figure 39, one in May or June and the other in October, November, or even December. The spring

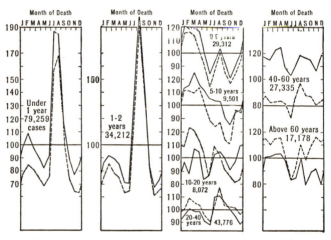

Fig. 39.—Deaths in New York City, 1854–1863 and 1865 by Month, Age, and Sex. Solid lines male; dotted, female.

minimum is closely connected with the optimum temperature and the main period of reproduction. It also occurs at a time when the rather unfavorable diet which formerly prevailed in winter began to be improved by such foods as dandelion greens, rhubarb, asparagus, and strawberries. How much the diet had to do with the decline in the number of deaths it is hard to say. The return of the death rate from its high summer level to the second minimum began with the return of the temperature to the optimum and also with the time (September) when diet was probably at its best among our predecessors of 70 or 80 years ago. The fact that in general this minimum is lower than the one in May and June may well be due to the fact that it follows a long summer during which the diet steadily improves.

Now that the deaths due to epidemic diseases in summer have been almost completely eliminated, the best health is experienced in August or September when diet and temperature apparently combine to produce the best physiological environment of the year. Thus today the lowest death rate for the population as a whole comes at almost the season when the death rate for all ages used to be highest. The seasonal distribution of health is now much more like that of conceptions than formerly, although there are still differences, and the present distribution is doubtless susceptible of further modification. As a result the curve of health and the curve of reproduction will probably become even more alike than they are today. In other words, the more completely man is able to eliminate or control specific diseases, the more completely the seasonal distribution of deaths appears to agree with the seasonal distribution of conceptions, provided the latter is not artificially restricted.

When we apply the lesson of New York to India we see that in India epidemic diseases, especially malaria, account for so large a share of the deaths that they produce a huge peak in winter. This peak is like the old summer peak of New York. If hygiene and medicine were sufficiently advanced, it would probably disappear. The Indian curve of mortality might be completely reversed, as has almost happened in New York, and might thus become closely similar to the curve of conceptions. It is obvious that the seasonal distribution of both births and deaths in tropical countries needs vastly more investigation on the basis of far more reliable statistics than are now available. Nevertheless, our study of Mexico and Bengal indicates that even in such diverse types of tropical countries the seasonal distribution of births appears to bear a closer relation to the weather and especially to temperature than to any other factor. Moreover, the relation in these countries is in harmony with that which we have found in all the other countries that we have been able to investigate. In every case there appears to be a basic annual rhythm of births which depends primarily upon the degree to which the temperature at the time of conception approaches an optimum not far from 60° or 65° F.

CHAPTER VIII

LENGTH OF LIFE

In previous chapters we have seen reason to believe that the basic annual rhythm of births owes its origin to seasonal fluctuations in the reproductive vigor of the parents. We have also seen that the children born at the maximum of this rhythm appear to have the best chance of survival. It is therefore logical to inquire whether the children born at the maximum of the seasonal cycle display any more vigor than those born at other times. The available data permit us to test this in at least three ways—by longevity, by the relative numbers of the two sexes, and by achievements. The present chapter considers longevity.

Our data as to length of life come from two chief sources—biographical reference books and family histories. Two biographical books have been employed, namely, the *Dictionary of American Biography* and *Who Was Who,* a British publication which gives brief biographies of persons who were included in the British *Who's Who* and died between 1897 and 1928. In using the American book only persons born in what is now the United States were included. Most of the births date from 1750 to 1870, the great majority being in the first half of the nineteenth century. In the British book only persons born in Great Britain and Ireland were included. Most of these also were born in the first half of the nineteenth century. In both books deaths due to violence or to epidemics such as yellow fever were omitted when there was a record to this effect. A number of soldiers who died young were also omitted, especially British officers who died from 1914 to 1918. Even though the cause of death was not stated, it seems reasonable to suppose that they died because of the war.

The biographical dictionaries unfortunately record very few deaths of young people. Practically no children are included, and very few persons who die before the age of 40. In a sample consisting of about 2000 persons from *Who Was Who* only 0.8 per cent were under 40 years of age, and only 4.6 per cent under 50. Moreover, there are many reasons for believing that people who distinguish themselves are on the whole more vigorous and live longer than those who do not win distinction. More than 56 per cent of the sample just mentioned lived to be over 70 years of age. Therefore, whatever differences there may be in the vigor of persons born in different months are largely concealed by the fact that we are dealing with a very long-lived group in which the great majority possess a constitution better than the average. Then, too, these more or less distinguished people live more comfortably than the average, have better medical care, and are less exposed to risks. All these conditions presumably tend to neutralize, or at least lessen, whatever differences there may be because of the season of birth.

In using the genealogical books, or "family histories," these difficulties are partly obviated. The deaths of persons of all ages are recorded. Nevertheless, the deaths of children and young people are omitted more frequently than those of older people. The deaths of poor, insignificant, ignorant, and neglected people also tend to be omitted because such people leave few records. Therefore even in the data from the family histories there is some selection of the stronger, more successful, and longer-lived types. This by no means obliterates whatever differences there may be by reason of season of birth, but it probably renders them less distinct than they would otherwise be. No deaths of children under 1 year of age have been included. Hence whatever differences we may find represent the vigor of the children after the dangers of the first year of life have been successfully met.

The results of our tabulation of longevity are shown in Figure 40. The upper curve of Section I shows the length of life of 10,890 persons in the *Dictionary of American Biography*. The average for all, regardless of the month of birth, is 68.9 years. Those born in February died at an average age of 69.7 years, and those born in June at 67.8 years. With so large a number of cases, nearly 1000 per month, such a difference is significant, as will appear later. It becomes still more significant when we note that from February to June the curve of longevity declines steadily. Then the curve rises again, and after a minor irregularity in September, reaches a secondary maximum in October and November.

The lower curve in Section I shows the number of births each month among the persons whose length of life is shown in the upper curve. It is constructed according to our regular method; 100 is the average number of births per day during the year as a whole, and the births per day each month are expressed as percentages of this average. The two curves of Section I are alike in the following respects: (1) a maximum in winter—January in the case of births, and February in that of longevity; (2) a minimum in June; and (3) a secondary maximum in October. They are unlike chiefly by reason of a minor maximum in the longevity curve during July and August, and a high level of births as opposed to a low level of longevity in December. The resemblances are much greater than the differences. This suggests that even among long-lived groups, such as the most eminent Americans, the length of life varies not only according to *season* of birth, but more or less closely in harmony with the *number* of births. In other words, one of the factors which determine length of life appears to be something which is closely connected with the basic annual rhythm of reproduction. Persons born at the time when this rhythm is at its maximum appear to be relatively long-lived; those born at the minimum of the reproductive cycle appear to be relatively short-lived.

The hypothesis stated in the last two sentences receives strong support from the remaining sections of Figure 40, aside from the British section (II). Leaving the latter for future study, let us examine Sections III to VII. These are based on ordinary Americans whose length of life has been ascertained by Mr. Charles L. Ziegler from the genealogical memoirs of some 80 families. Section III represents nearly

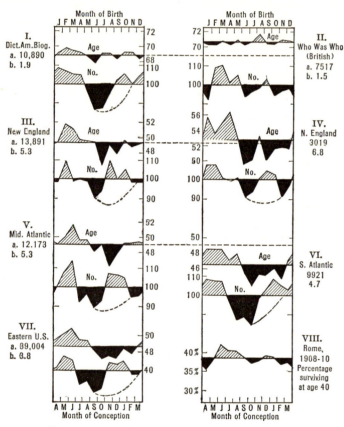

FIG. 40.—Longevity according to Month of Birth.

14,000 people, mainly New Englanders, with the addition of some New Yorkers and a few from other parts of the northeastern United States. Section IV is based entirely on New Englanders—3000 of them—belonging to families not included in Section III. Section V comprises 12,000 persons born in the Middle Atlantic States of New York, New Jersey, and Pennsylvania; and Section VI, which required a search in some 50 genealogical books, consists of 10,000 persons born in the Southern States. Maryland and Virginia supplied most of the southerners, but some came from the Carolinas and a few from states farther south or west. Finally Section VII includes all four of the preceding sections, and serves as a summary of the whole situation.

A highly significant fact about these five sections of Figure 40 is that all the "age" or longevity curves show that people born in February or March live decidedly longer than those born in July or August. It is equally significant that, in spite of irregularities in the longevity curves, there is a fairly regular trend from a single winter maximum to a summer minimum and back again. A third significant fact is that in every case the curves of longevity and those below them, which show the number of births, vary in fairly close harmony during the first six or seven months of the year, but diverge later, as is suggested by the dotted lines. The agreement and the divergence are both in accord with the hypothesis that the winter maximum of births is primarily a biological phenomenon, whereas the second maximum, at a later season, is probably due at least in part to cultural factors such as migration and high standards of living, as will appear more fully later. In winter both the birth rate and the longevity of the persons born at that time conform to the basic animal rhythm. In summer and early autumn, on the contrary, the curves of birth all depart from the basic rhythm and rise to a pronounced secondary maximum. Thus length of life seems to vary in close harmony with the basic annual rhythm of reproduction (the dotted lines), but is influenced relatively little by purely cultural conditions such as migrations and standards of living.

The Italian section (VIII) of Figure 40 is compiled in a different way from the others, but points to the same conclusion. It is based on data from Gini (1912) as to the percentage of persons born in Rome who survived at the age of 40 years in 1908 to 1910. It has the same general form as the other curves of longevity, including a maximum in March, a minimum in July, and a minor maximum in September and October. It differs from corresponding American curves chiefly in having a more pronounced minimum in January. The curve of births in northern Italy (Figure 23, page 99) is closely similar to the Roman curve of Figure 40, but the curve for central Italy differs. It lacks the minor maximum in September. The essential point, however, is that the Italian curves, like those of America, show the basic animal rhythm not only in reproduction but in the longevity of persons born at different seasons.

Before we examine the British section of Figure 40, which differs from all the others, let us inquire how reliable our seasonal curves of longevity really are. In earlier chapters we have not attempted to calculate probable errors, or to apply exact mathematical methods such as correlation coefficients. Such a procedure has been unnecessary because the seasonal differences with which we have been dealing have been so large that by common consent there is no doubt of their significance. The uniformity with which the same seasonal curve of births is repeated year after year in any given country, the systematic and gradual way in which changes in the form of the seasonal curves take place from decade to decade and also from region to region, the magnitude of the differences between one season and another, and the close resemblances between the curves of neighboring regions all make it certain that we are dealing with systematic variations and not with accidents. Therefore thus far our problem has been to determine the conditions which lead to seasonal variations in the birth rate. Now, however, we are confronted by a problem in which it is important to determine whether the variations in longevity of which we have found evidence are mathematically significant. The facts on which to base a conclusion are given in Table 5.

The table shows that in the longevity curve of Section I (Figure 40) the average length of life of 894 eminent Ameri-

TABLE 5

LONGEVITY AND MONTH OF BIRTH

A Section in Fig. 40	B No. of Cases	C Group of People	Month and Average Age		Difference between		
			D Maximum	E Minimum	F Actual	G Probable	H Ratio F/G
I	10,890	Eminent Americans	Feb. 69.67	June 67.84	1.83	±0.38	4.8
III	13,891	New Englanders	Feb. 51.7	July 46.4	5.3	±0.71	7.5
IV	3,019	New Englanders	Apr. 56.4	June 49.6	6.8	±1.62	4.2
V	12,173	Middle Atlantic	Mar. 51.5	Aug. 51.5	5.3	±0.71	7.5
VI	9,921	South Atlantic	Jan.-Mar. 48.5	July 43.8	4.7	±0.77	6.1
VII	39,004	Groups III–VI	Mar. 50.8	Aug. 47.0	3.8	±0.30	9.0

cans born in February was 69.67 years, whereas that of the 773 born in June averaged only 67.84 years. According to ordinary statistical methods, it is possible to determine the "probable error" of any such averages. This means two equal values, one above and one below the average, which are of such magnitude that it is equally probable that the true value lies within or without these limits. Thus if the average is 100 and the probable error is ± 1, there is 1 chance in 2 that the true value lies between 99 and 101, and 1 chance that it lies somewhere beyond these limits.

If two averages are to be compared, it is possible to compute their "probable difference." If the actual difference is the same as the probable difference, there is 1 chance in 2 that the observed difference is accidental. As the ratio of the actual difference to the probable difference increases, the probability that the difference is accidental diminishes very rapidly. If the ratio is 4, there is only 1 chance in 142 that the observed difference is accidental. In Section I of Figure 40 the probable error of the average of the persons born in February is ± .25 and that of those born in June is ± .27. This means that the probable difference between the two averages on the basis of chance alone is ± 0.38. Inasmuch as the actual difference is 1.83, or 4.8 times the probable difference, the chances that so great a difference is due to mere accident are only about 1 in 1000. Therefore we are fairly safe in assuming that some definite factor causes eminent people born in February to live longer than those born in June. The fact that there is a steady decline in average longevity from people born in February to those born in June makes it still less probable that we are dealing with accidental differences.

Sections III to VI in Table 5 indicate that among four distinct groups of ordinary Americans living in different parts of the country the actual differences between the longevity of those born in winter and summer range from 4.7 to 6.8 years and are from 4.2 to 7.5 times as great as the probable differences. A ratio of 7.5 means that there is only 1 chance in about 1,000,000 that we are dealing with a purely accidental difference. When the four groups of Americans are put together, as in Section VII, the difference between February and July still amounts to 3.8 years. The ratio between this number and the probable difference increases to 9.0, because we are now dealing with 39,000 persons. Such a ratio means that there is only 1 chance in 100,-000,000 that we are being misled by accidental coincidences.

The data from Rome and the systematic way in which the average length of life varies from a maximum among people born in February to a minimum among those born in July must also be considered in estimating the reliability of our results. When this is done, the chances of being misled by mere accidents become only 1 in untold billions. In other words, it is practically certain that on an average the Americans born in February and March during the last century lived at least 3 years longer than those born in July, August, and September. This of course tells us nothing as to the cause of the variation in length of life. It merely tells us that such a variation is an established fact. The similarity of the longevity curves, however, to the portions of the curves of births due to biological rather than cultural causes tells us that longevity is somehow connected with the conditions which cause a maximum of births in the late winter or spring.

In view of all this it is puzzling to find that the British data in Figure 40 (Section II) do not agree with those from America and Italy. In fact the British curve of longevity, ✓ based on 7517 persons in *Who Was Who,* fluctuates in almost the opposite way from the corresponding American curve (Section I). From a minimum of 70.2 years in January it rises irregularly to 71.7 in August, and there is a second maximum of 71.0 in December. Incidentally it is of interest that the average length of life among all these British leaders is 70.7 years in comparison with 68.9 for the corresponding Americans. This difference of 1.8 years may be due to the less trying as well as less stimulating quality of the British climate, and to the way in which the climate is conducive to healthful outdoor exercise. Or perhaps it is due to the less strenuous life in Britain, a condition which may be interpreted either socially or climatically.

To return to the average ages of the six hundred British born in January and August respectively the probable error of these averages is ± 0.31 in both cases. This means that the probable difference on the basis of pure chance is 0.44. The actual difference is 3.3 times the probable difference. Hence there is 1 chance in about 50 that we are dealing with a difference due to accident.

In order to get a true estimate of the reliability of a curve as sinuous as that of British longevity in Figure 40 it is often desirable to combine several months. Let us take the three consecutive birth months with the longest life—July, August, and September—and compare them with the three having the shortest span of life—December, January, and February. The difference amounts to only 0.54 year, or a little more than one-third as much as between the two single months of greatest extremes. Since the number of persons born in three months is much greater than in one month, the ratio between the actual difference and the probable difference is reduced merely to 1.8, but this means that there is 1 chance in only about 4 that the difference is accidental. It is commonly held that, unless the ratio between the actual and the probable differences rises as high as 4.0 (1 chance in 142), a relationship other than mere chance is not established. Because of this, and also because the ratio between the actual and probable differences falls so sharply when we use three months instead of one, we may dismiss the British data as inconclusive. This does not necessarily mean that there is no connection between month of birth and length of life in Britain. That can be determined only by a more extensive study of ordinary people of all ages. It is quite clear, however, that if there is any relation between length of life and month of birth it is far less important in Great Britain than in the United States or Italy. In Russia, on the contrary, we should expect it to be important.

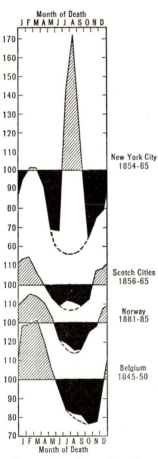

FIG. 41.—Deaths under Five Years of Age.

The most reasonable interpretation of this contrast between Britain and America seems to be that in Britain both the summers and the winters are so mild and healthful that it does not make much difference at what season people are born. One evidence of this is seen in Figure 41, where the death rate of children under 5 years of age in Scotch cities in 1856-1865 shows only a faint hint of a summer maximum whereas the similar curve for New York City rises tremendously. Similar data for England are not available, for the English keep their vital statistics on the basis of quarters of the year instead of months. The Nor-

wegian and Belgian curves in Figure 41, however, make it
clear that in the whole North Sea region the summers are
so mild that they had very little harmful effect upon children
even before the advent of modern hygiene. The winters on
the other hand, produce a similar increase in deaths in all
four of the regions of Figure 41, although in Scotland and
Norway, the two most oceanic countries, the effect is less than
in New York and Belgium.

The magnitude and significance of the difference in climate between New York and London are rarely appreciated. Set down in cold figures the contrast appears thus for
the years 1911 to 1920:

	January Temperature	July Temperature
London.................	39.9° F. (4.4° C.)	61.2° F. (16.3° C.)
New York..............	31.9 (−0.6)	72.8 (22.7)
Departure of New York from London..........	−8.0 (−5.0)	+11.6 (6.4)

The fact that New York is 8° F. colder than London in winter and nearly 12° warmer in summer may not sound very
important, but it is obviously connected with an astonishingly
great difference in health during the summer. Even now,
with our modern hygiene, this difference has not wholly disappeared. The reason for so great a difference is that in
both summer and winter the London temperatures approach
closely to what appear to be the optima for the respective
seasons. The facts are especially clear in summer. Taking
the year as a whole the area centering in London comes
close to having the most healthful of all climates for people
in our stage of civilization. In such a climate no season is
especially bad.

This does not indicate that the British are free from the
effects of the seasons. The seasonal swing is very clear in
respect to both births and deaths. In the case of births it is
of substantially the same character among Scotch infants
(left side, Figure 22, page 97) and among long-lived leaders
(*F*, Figure 83, page 349). Both curves show not only a

main maximum in February or March, but also a secondary cultural maximum in the autumn. Among leaders the cultural maximum is much smaller than among ordinary people, perhaps because leaders come mainly from social groups which are not subject to seasonal migration. For our present purpose the important fact is that both curves also show a general seasonal swing in harmony with the basic animal rhythm.

Let us now treat the American data of Table 5 in the same way that we have treated the British data, comparing the three-month periods which are associated respectively with the greatest and least length of life. The results appear

TABLE 6

LONGEVITY AND SEASON OF BIRTH

		Months			Difference between Maximum and Minimum		
A	B	C	D	E	F	G	H
Section in Fig. 40	Group of People	Maximum	Minimum	Actual	Probable	Ratio E/F	Ratio Table 5
I	Am. Leaders	Feb.-Apr.	May-July	0.88	0.21	4.2	(4.8)
II	Br. Leaders	July-Aug.-Sept.	Jan.-Feb.-Mar.	0.54	0.30	1.8	(3.3)
III	New England	Feb.-Apr.	July-Sept.	2.97	0.42	7.1	(7.5)
IV	New England	Feb.-Mar.	July-Sept.	3.98	0.92	4.3	(4.2)
V	Middle Atlantic	Feb.-Mar.-Apr.	June-July-Aug.	2.70	0.45	6.0	(7.5)
VI	South Atlantic	Jan.-Mar.	July-Sept.	3.77	0.50	7.5	(6.1)
VII	Ordinary Americans	Jan.-Apr.[1]	July-Aug.-Sept.	3.00	0.25	12.0	(9.0)

[1] January and April are almost identical, the figures being: January 49.6, February 50.3, March 50.8, and April 49.6. If all four months were used in our study of probable differences the ratio between the actual and probable differences in Column G would rise to 13.3.

in Table 6. The numbers in parentheses in Column H at the right-hand side of this table are repeated from the last column of Table 5. They show the ratio between the actual and probable differences when the single months associated with maximum and minimum longevity are used. When comparing the one-month ratios with the three-month ratios (Column G) we see that in Britain (No. II) there is a great drop from 3.3 to 1.8. In the American data, Nos. I, III, and V also drop, but not so low as to lose their significance; No. IV shows little change; No. VI rises about as much as the others fall; No. VII, which is the most significant, rises very notably. There a ratio of 12 between the actual and probable differences means that there is only 1 chance in billions upon billions that we are being misled by accident. Thus the same process which emphasizes the slightness of the relation between season of birth and length of life in Britain adds to the probability that there is a real and important relationship in America.

When all the data for America, Britain, and Italy are considered together, there scarcely seems room for doubt that season of birth is intimately related to length of life, and that this relationship varies in proportion to the degree to which the climate at one season or another departs from the optimum. Hence in California or New Zealand we should expect the length of life to vary relatively little according to month of birth, whereas in Japan it probably varies greatly. Data to test these last suppositions are not available, but the American data make it practically certain that in a climate like that of the United States, with a strong contrast of seasons, the people born from January to March or April tend to live distinctly longer than do those born from July to September.

Before we accept the preceding conclusion we may well examine a seeming inconsistency. In all the regions employed in Figure 40, January, February, and March are now and always have been a season of poor health. July, August, and September, on the contrary, are now a time of excellent health in the northern United States. Even in the Southern States and central Italy they are by no means so bad as the cooler months. Figure 39 (page 168) indicates that in earlier times, when the people of Figure 40 were born, the summer in America was not so good as now for children above two years of age, but was better than the winter. Thus, on the whole, great longevity is associated with birth at a season when the general conditions of health are poor. Why this anomaly? Why should the people born in a season of poor health have the longest lives? In answering these questions we must consider both season of birth and season of conception, together with the period of pregnancy. One possible hypothesis is that variations in longevity may be due to a selective process whereby soon after birth the weaker children are killed off more rapidly in some seasons than in others. Hence the survivors among the children born at the most unfavorable season will be a selected group possessing greater constitutional vigor than the survivors born at seasons when the death rate is lower. This hypothesis fails to fit the facts. In the eastern United States, until the last few decades, the summer was the time of by far the greatest mortality among infants, while the late winter came next in this respect. Therefore, if this selective hypothesis is correct, the curve of longevity according to season of birth ought to resemble the New York curve of deaths of children in Figure 41. Long life should be associated with many early deaths, but the opposite is actually the case.

Since our first hypothesis is untenable we may frame a modification of it to the effect that hot weather and its accompanying ailments are equally fatal to children of all constitutional types, whereas cold weather and its diseases pick out the weaklings. This might give a result in harmony with the observed data, but certain stubborn facts seem to point in the opposite direction. For example, the work of factory operatives in both the United States and Japan (Huntington, 1924, 1935; and Yagi, 1933) seems to be depressed for a much longer time after severe heat than after severe cold. Again the rate of reproduction in Japan, Italy, Florida, and other regions is greatly depressed by heat, whereas the depression associated with cold weather is much less severe. These facts suggest that hot weather produces more severe and lasting harm than cold weather, and therefore is more likely to be selective in its effect on children. No positive conclusion, however, seems warranted.

Another hypothesis is that variations in longevity among

persons born at different seasons are not due to selective action, but to the direct effect of the seasons and their diseases in earliest infancy. Can we suppose that the conditions which led to the midsummer peak of deaths in New York in Figure 41 not only killed many young infants, but weakened the survivors so much that they were permanently handicapped and therefore did not live so long as their brothers and sisters who were born in February? In order to make this hypothesis workable we must assume that cold weather not only does less harm than hot, but that it is actually beneficial to infants. This is not the case, however, at least so far as mortality is concerned. Figure 39 (page 168) shows that in New York City during the middle of the nineteenth century children of all ages experienced a distinct maximum of mortality during the late winter. It is hard to believe that the conditions which produced numerous deaths in February gave the surviving children unusual vigor without any process of selection. Yet such an assumption seems necessary if we are to explain the seasonal distribution of longevity on the basis of the harm done by summer diseases and heat to young infants. We may, of course, assume that cold weather and hot weather during the first month or two of life imprint permanent damage upon young infants and thus affect their longevity. In that case the curve of longevity ought to follow the general shape of the New York curve of deaths among young children as given in Figure 41, but with an inversion so that short life would correspond to many deaths during early childhood. The curves of longevity in Figure 40, however, fail to show any hint of a minimum in February. On the contrary, the maximum span of life belongs to persons born in February or March when the conditions of health are decidedly poor, although not so bad for children as in summer. Thus the curve of longevity departs widely from what would be expected on the basis of the immediate effect of the seasons on the health of young infants, unless we assume that cold weather in early infancy produces a direct and long-lasting stimulus, whereas hot weather produces equally lasting harm and leads to short life.

If we turn now to the time of conception for an explanation of the relation of longevity to season of birth another hypothesis presents certain claims to acceptance. According to this hypothesis the children born in February or March live long because they are conceived at the season when their parents are best fitted to produce vigorous offspring. The fitness of the parents varies, we may suppose, in harmony with the basic rhythm whereby animals breed at such a time that their young are born at the season most favorable for survival. Because the parents are vigorous in May and June, the resultant children, born in February and March, possess a constitutional vigor which stays by them throughout life. For this reason, so the hypothesis runs, the curve of longevity in Section VII of Figure 40 reaches a peak in March, corresponding to conceptions in June. It falls to a minimum from July to September, corresponding to conceptions from October to December, and rises again above the average only in December, corresponding to conceptions in March. In other words, the curve follows the form of the basic animal rhythm as we have repeatedly found it in countries where the summer is warm.

The choice of the best hypothesis cannot be made until we have examined two sets of facts which must be postponed till later pages. One set, in Chapter IX, deals with sex ratios and abortions. The other, in Chapter XIII, deals with a peculiar access of vigor which occurs among both men and women of reproductive age during the months when conception takes place most freely according to the animal rhythm. All this leads us to believe that the facts are best fitted by the hypothesis that season of birth is related to length of life primarily, although perhaps not wholly, through the condition of the parents and hence of the germ plasm at the time of conception. This by no means excludes the hypothesis of a permanent depressive effect when a very young infant experiences undue heat or disease regardless of any selection through death. The case is like that of climatic and cultural influences upon the number of births. Both types of influence seem to play a part, and the great task is to unravel them. In view of the evidence thus far given, however, and of that which will be presented later, it seems probable that what we may perhaps call a semi-inherited effect, due to the physical condition of the parents at the time of conception, is the primary factor in determining the relation of length of life to season of birth. Nevertheless the effect of the seasons, and especially of hot weather, upon the infant soon after birth and upon the mother during pregnancy appears to be another factor of no small importance. We shall not discuss pregnancy for two reasons. One is lack of physiological training, the other is that the available evidence seems to us to focus attention upon the period when the ova and spermatozoa are being prepared for conception.

Let us return now to the main problem of this chapter, namely, the question whether the climatic conditions associated with the birth or conception of children are really of importance in respect to longevity. We have examined one kind of evidence in America and another in Italy, and the two agree in indicating a high degree of importance. We have found, however, that in the almost ideal climate of the North Sea region the season of birth has little to do with length of life. In Australia still a third kind of evidence is available. Though it does not show anything as to season of birth, it does show that, when other conditions such as race and mode of life are eliminated, the climate in which people are born appears to have an intimate relation to their length of life. The pertinent data are given in Table 7. They were most kindly furnished me in manuscript in 1923 by the Commonwealth Statistician, C. H. Wickens, Esq., and were published in *West of the Pacific* (pages 363 ff.)

The table shows clearly that there is a marked difference in death rates and hence in length of life between persons *living* in Queensland, but not necessarily born there, and persons *born* in Queensland, regardless of where they happen

TABLE 7

DEATH RATES PER "STANDARD POPULATION" AT AGE 15–49 YEARS IN
VICTORIA, NEW SOUTH WALES, AND QUEENSLAND, ACCORDING
TO PLACES OF BIRTH AND RESIDENCE, 1920, 1921, 1922

| Birthplace | Residence | | | | | | Average | | |
| | Victoria | | New South Wales | | Queensland | | | | |
	Male	Female	Male	Female	Male	Female	Male	Female	Both sexes
Victoria............	4.38	4.01	3.60	3.38	4.28	3.72	4.09	3.70	3.90
England............	3.65	3.87	3.78	3.39	4.66	3.99	4.03	3.75	3.89
Scotland............	4.83	4.13	3.94	3.48	4.85	3.47	4.54	3.69	4.08
New South Wales...	4.47	4.27	3.76	3.57	4.84	4.03	4.36	3.96	4.16
Queensland.........	5.22	5.01	4.42	4.13	4.87	4.27	4.84	4.47	4.66

to live at the time of death. The numbers in the table show
the death rate among persons from 15 to 49 years of age in
three Australian states; namely, Victoria, which is the coolest
state aside from Tasmania; New South Wales, which lies so
far to the south that it is reasonably cool; and Queensland,
which lies to the north and has a quarter of its population
within the tropics. The death rate has been calculated according to a "standard population," so as to eliminate any
differences arising from the fact that there are more young
people in one section than in another. The residents of the
three states have been divided according to their birthplace,
the great majority of Australians being natives of one of the
three states, or else of England or Scotland.

The significant fact about the table is this: no matter
whether they reside in Victoria, New South Wales, or Queensland, and regardless of their sex, the people who are born
in Queensland have a higher death rate than those born in
the other two Australian states, or in England, or Scotland.
In other words, those born in the hot climate do not live so
long as the others. If we combine the four upper entries in
the last column, it appears that the residents of Australia
who were born in Victoria, England, Scotland, and New
South Wales have an average death rate of 4.01. On the

other hand, the death rate among the people born in Queensland, no matter where they reside, is 4.66, or approximately 15 per cent greater.

If this percentage prevailed at all ages, and if the average death rate were 16 per 1000 population, it would mean nearly 10 years less life for Queenslanders than for the others. The high death rate of Queenslanders in Victoria, or New South Wales, may be due to the fact that Queenslanders whose health is impaired migrate to those cooler states. But in that case the born Queenslanders who remain in Queensland ought to be stronger than the average, and their death rate should be correspondingly low. On the contrary, their death rate exceeds that of the Queenslanders born in any of the other four regions. In other words, taken as a whole the people whose *residence* is in Queensland have a lower death rate than those who were *born* there. A considerable percentage of the persons over 15 years of age who reside there were born elsewhere and have had the advantage of a childhood spent in a comparatively invigorating climate. Moreover, the Queenslanders as a whole represent recent and relatively difficult migration. Hence they have been through a somewhat drastic selective process which has weeded out the weaklings. Naturally, then, their death rate is normally low. A careful analysis of this death rate suggests that, although the people who go to Queensland are so highly selected that they reduce the general death rate to a low level, the hot climate renders their children less healthy and shorter-lived than are those born in the cooler climates of the more southerly parts of Australia or in the old country. Just at what age the climate exerts its greatest effect is not clear. The preceding pages suggest that the effect begins at the time of conception, but it presumably continues throughout life.

The Australian data are especially significant because, so far as I am aware, they represent the most exact available facts as to the relation between climate and longevity. Of course there are innumerable data as to the death rate in countries with many diverse types of climate The trouble, however, is that countries differ enormously in race, culture, and types of parasitic diseases. Therefore when their death rates are compared it is difficult to know how much of the difference is due to these factors and how much directly to climate. Among the people born in Queensland, however, other factors are almost eliminated. Whether the people born in Queensland stay there or migrate to other parts of Australia, they are of the same race as those around them, they are subject to the same diseases and the same sort of medical practice, and they live and work in much the same way. Aside from a very small number who live under extreme frontier conditions, the major difference lies in the fact that the Queenslanders were born in Queensland, whereas the people with whom they are compared were born in cooler climates. In this respect they are comparable with the Americans of Figure 40 who were born in one month as compared with another. They, too, differ only in the season at which they were born. Thus the data from Australia, America, Italy, and Britain are all in harmony with the hypothesis that climatic conditions at the time of conception (or birth?) play an important part in determining longevity. If the climate is extreme, the effect in reducing length of life is noteworthy; if it is mild and approaches the ideal, as in Britain, the effect is slight and may not be evident.

In concluding this chapter a few words may be said as to practical applications of our findings concerning climate and longevity. When the Australian figures were published, the Australian officials were not at all pleased. They had not realized what the data indicate, and did not approve of anything that seemed to be opposed to the dominant policy of urging white people to settle in tropical Australia. Hence, although the responsible officials admitted the accuracy of the data, they attempted at first to minimize their importance. Now, however, the government realizes that white people who are born and bred in a tropical climate cannot be as efficient as those who live where it is cooler. Hence the national policy toward the sparsely settled stretches of northern Australia has undergone a change. Elsewhere a similar new viewpoint toward practical problems of tropical colonization and even toward migration within countries such as the United States is now growing up.

The data of this chapter as to age and season have an important bearing upon personal as well as political and economic conduct. They indicate that a slight change in the season at which children are born would make a readily appreciable change not only in length of life, but in general health and vigor as well. When the entire 39,000 Americans of Figure 40 are taken together, the difference between the best and the worst months, as we have seen, amounts to 3.8 years. Since the average span of life among these people was approximately 49 years, this means a difference of nearly 8 per cent. Those born in the more favorable months must have suffered correspondingly less from the various ailments which gradually or suddenly, as the case may be, brought earlier death to those who were born in the wrong months. Of course, length of life depends on many other factors beside the weather. Our daily habits and occupations, the amount of travel in automobiles and airplanes, the kind of communities in which we live, and the inheritance with which we are endowed all enter into the matter. Pearl (1934) has shown that people who live to the age of 90 years or more spring from parents and grandparents who on an average lived about 11 years longer than the corresponding ancestors of the ordinary person who reaches the age of about 50. Part of this difference may be because Pearl's old people, unknown to him, were born in climatic environments and at seasons of the year more favorable than those of his younger group. Nevertheless, there can be no doubt that constitutional vigor is a major factor in determining length of life. Here, as in many other cases, we see that different factors may produce the same result. The fact that long life is hereditary does not in any way conflict with the conclusion that length of life varies according to season of birth and climate.

CHAPTER IX

SEX, SEASON AND CLIMATE

Few questions have a wider interest than those pertaining to sex. Scores of abandoned theories litter the path of investigation as to how sex is determined. The geneticists have discovered that, if both members of one particular pair of human chromosomes are alike when the parental cells unite in reproduction, a female is produced, but if the two members are different, the result is a male. This, however, sheds little light on the immediate problem of how sex can be controlled in any particular mating. In fact, many people feel that it definitely puts the control of sex beyond our reach. How can we dictate which of millions of spermatozoa shall fertilize the ova? Nevertheless, the relative numbers of the two sexes *do* vary, and there must be reasons for this. This book is concerned with these reasons, because the weather appears to be one of them.

The easiest way to express the relative numbers of the sexes is by means of a ratio showing how many males there are for every 100 females. A sex ratio of 100 denotes equality. All over the world boys are usually born in larger numbers than girls. Only in rare cases are girls as numerous as boys. In most civilized countries, the ratio at birth is about 105, but it varies considerably even in Europe. This, however, is a *secondary* ratio. The primary ratio is that which exists at the very beginning of pregnancy.

According to the laws of genetics, the number of male and female embryos must be equal unless some agency interferes with one sex more than the other. Among the 24 pairs of chromosomes which are the most vital part of every growing human cell, one pair is different in the two sexes. In the female it consists of two similar members, X and X; in the male there is only one X chromosome—the other is a smaller type known as Y. In the process of reproduction, each pair of chromosomes separates so that the actual reproductive cells contain only 24 chromosomes instead of 48. This leaves an X chromosome in every female cell, or ovum; but half the male cells, or spermatozoa, contain an X chromosome and half a Y chromosome. If the two types of spermatozoa behaved exactly alike, the laws of chance would cause half the fertilized ova to contain two X chromosomes, thus giving rise to females, and half, an X and a Y chromosome, thus producing males.

Inasmuch as the two sexes are not born in equal numbers there must be some alteration in this simple mechanism of inheritance. Any valid explanation of such an alteration must account not merely for the secondary sex ratio of 105 males per 100 females, but for the additional males lost in stillbirths and abortions. Among stillbirths the sex ratio often rises to 130, and among spontaneous abortions (miscarriages) to 200 or even 400. Inasmuch as far more males than females are thus lost, the primary sex ratio at the beginning of pregnancy must be at least 110 and more probably near 125.

The simplest hypothesis in explanation of the high primary sex ratio is that the spermatozoa which carry the Y chromosome are more vigorous than those that carry the X chromosome. Hence there are many more X–Y embryos (males) than X–X embryos (females). A possible modification of this is that the two types of spermatozoa may be equally vigorous, but after fertilization the female embryos may at first be very sensitive, and hence perish in large numbers at the very onset of pregnancy. This scarcely seems consistent with the fact that spontaneous abortions are not only especially numerous in the first three months of pregnancy, but have the highest sex ratio—the most males—at that time. Therefore the most probable form of this hypothesis is that X-bearing spermatozoa are less vigorous than those bearing the Y chromosome, and hence are more easily influenced by their environment. Nevertheless, when fertilization has once taken place the females with their two X chromosomes are more vigorous than the males with an X and a Y.

If we put this hypothesis in terms of survival through selection, it implies that for the preservation of the species strong females are more important than strong males. Therefore the type of human being that has survived is one in which the weaklings among potential females are weeded out even before conception, whereas male weaklings survive in much larger proportion. They are eliminated as abortions during pregnancy, or by death at birth or later, when the death rate among boys is systematically higher than among girls. Another view might be that among primitive people the dangers to which the male is subject necessitate the birth of more males than females, but this does not explain why the males have a high death rate even before birth. Perhaps males are of secondary importance, and their selection is taken care of after the selection of strong females has been assured. Whatever may be the truth as to these matters, the hypothesis of differential vigor in the two kinds of spermatozoa carries with it the implication that environmental conditions may have more effect upon those carrying the X chromosome than upon those carrying Y.

Many geneticists, not satisfied with the preceding hypothesis, hold another of a purely genetic type. According to the genetic hypothesis the X chromosome is the repository of certain genes which in one of their several forms are recessive and lethal. If such a gene meets a corresponding gene of the dominant, non-lethal type, no harm results. The dominant gene determines the character of the offspring, and the recessive gene merely lies low, so to speak, and waits for another chance. That chance can never come so long as the chromosome in question mates with a Y chromosome and produces a male. The Y chromosome, according to the hypothesis, always supplies a dominant gene to counteract the lethal one. But suppose that two X chromosomes which both carry the lethal gene come together, as is bound to happen sometimes. Then the double lethal dose makes life impossible, and the fertilized ovum soon perishes.

The facts which we shall present as to the relation of season of birth to the sex ratio seem to be fully in harmony with the first of the two hypotheses sketched above, but not with the second. Systematic seasonal variations in the sex ratio apparently occur because the condition of the human body fluctuates with the weather, and X chromosomes appear to be influenced by such fluctuations more easily than Y chromosomes. On the other hand, a gene that is lethal under one condition of environment must also be lethal under other conditions unless the genes are far more influenced by environment than geneticists have been willing to admit.

Figure 42 shows seasonal variations in the sex ratio among 11 mutually exclusive groups in 7 countries. Index numbers in parentheses indicate the number of births on which each curve is based and the weight which each receives in the summary curve (L). Each unit in these numbers indicates approximately 250,000 births. The final curve is based on about 52,000,000.

The curves of Figure 42 present three outstanding features: (1) a distinct period of low sex ratios in the spring; (2) a period of high ratios in the summer; and (3) a lack of any decided character from August onward. Either February or March has a sex ratio below the average in every one of the 12 curves; in 8, if we include the summary curve, both months have a ratio below the average. In the entire 12 curves there are 24 chances that at least one of these two months will be below the average. According to the laws of chance 12 of these chances should find the curves below the average and 12 above. As a matter of fact, 19 are below the average in February or March. On the other hand, June and July generally show sex ratios well above the average. Out of their 24 chances, they are above the average 18 times, and at the average once, whereas they are below it only 5 times.

In addition to this, the curves of Figure 42 which are

based on great numbers of people, that is, those of the rural and urban United States (*E* and *F*), together with Orthodox Russia (*I*) and Japan (*K*), are the ones which most clearly display a minimum sex ratio in February and March and a high ratio in June and July. The curves based on smaller

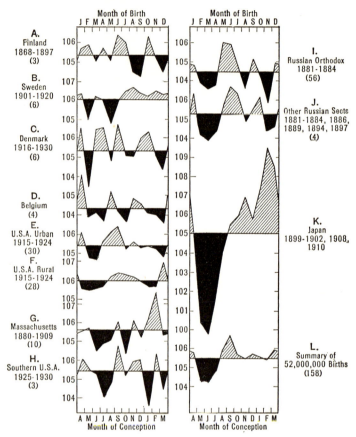

Fig. 42.—Sex Ratio at Birth.

numbers of people display a good deal of irregularity, which suggests that other conditions as well as the seasons are important. Nevertheless, when the curves based on smaller numbers of people are averaged together, the result is essentially the same as the curves for the 4 larger groups of people.

This can be seen in Figure 43, where *L*, the weighted summary curve for the 11 sections of Figure 42, appears in inverted form as *A*, while the unweighted inverted average of the minor groups is shown as *B*. This latter curve is inserted merely to show its parallelism to *A* and is not rightly placed in respect to the scale on the left.

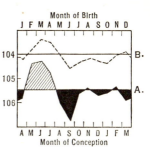

FIG. 43.—The Sex Ratio at Birth, Inverted.

The indefinite character of the fluctuations of the sex ratio during the second half of the year is significant because the same condition prevails in a great number of curves showing seasonal fluctuations in the *number* of births. Thus the curves for the sex ratio and for the number of births agree closely in three main respects, as is clear in Figure 43. There the high parts of the inverted summary curve indicate femininity, or an approach to equality in the numbers of the sexes. Putting the matter in this way we see that in general the seasonal fluctuations in the femininity of births and in the number of births agree in having (1) a pronounced maximum in February and March, (2) a pronounced minimum in June and July, and (3) a succeeding period which varies from place to place. This suggests that the swing of both femininity and the number of births from a low level in December or January to a maximum in February and March and then to a minimum in June or July is due to the basic animal rhythm. In other words, the basic animal rhythm of reproduction appears to manifest itself in the sex ratio as well as in the number of births. Many births and a close approach to equality in the numbers of the sexes go together.

But why does the sex ratio depart from the smooth curve of the basic animal rhythm in the second half of the year? The answer seems to be the same as in the case of the similar condition in the curves showing the number of births. Births from July to November represent conceptions from

October to February—that is, the part of the year when the number of conceptions is most influenced by the return of men who have been away from home. Many such migrants are young married men, at the height of their vigor. They return home in the best of health after their summer's work. Their physiological condition is presumably like that which prevails in the late spring or early summer, when children are conceived in greatest numbers and the proportion of girls is highest. Reproductive vigor, many births, and an approximation toward equality in the numbers of the two sexes go together.

In order to make this last point clear let us turn back to Figure 42 and examine the curves for Russia and Japan. These two countries are of unusual interest because in them the contrast between a good season and a bad season is especially prominent. In Russia, the winter is bad; in Japan, the summer. Also in Russia there used to be much seasonal migration; in Japan there is relatively little. The two Russian curves (*I* and *J*) are closely similar. This in itself is significant, for one curve is based on approximately 14,000,000 births among Orthodox Christians and the other on about 1,000,000 births among Moslems, Protestants, and other non-Orthodox Christians. Jewish births are omitted because of the defective registration of girls. The low sex ratio in March needs no further comment; it agrees perfectly with the maximum in the number of births as seen in Figures 1 (page 30), and 14 (page 65). This would be more evident if Figure 42 were inverted, as is Figure 43, and a low sex ratio were indicated by an upward bulge, thus suggesting favorable conditions. The great preponderance of boys indicated by the ruled shading of the Russian sections (*I* and *J*) of Figure 42 in May and June corresponds to conceptions in August and September. These are the months when the younger men are away from home in greatest numbers.

The Japanese curve (*K*), in Figure 42 is more impressive than that of Russia. This is presumably because the contrast between the excellent Japanese winter and the very trying summer and early fall is greater than the contrast between the favorable Russian summer and the unfavorable winter. It will be remembered that, in order to get children into school as early as possible, Japanese parents sometimes report that children really born in April or May were born in March. The Japanese value boys much more than girls. Therefore it seems highly probable that there is an especially strong tendency to report boys as having been born earlier than was actually the case. This would tend to give March a high sex ratio. Nevertheless, in Japan, far more than elsewhere, the sex ratio drops low among births in the spring. In March it actually falls to 99.8. In November, on the contrary, it rises about 10 per cent higher, to 109.5.

A range of practically 10 per cent from minimum to maximum is so great that one wonders whether there is some statistical error. Can it be that the more ignorant Japanese fail to report the births of girls during the early part of the year, and then, for fear of the law, report them toward the end? This is improbable because the minimum sex ratio comes in March instead of January, and the maximum in November, whereas the statistical error would bring it in December. Three other considerations also suggest that the Japanese curve is essentially correct. First, its minimum agrees very closely with those of other countries and with the basic animal rhythm. Second, the minimum sex ratio comes at the same time as the maximum birth rate. And third, the sex ratio of Japan is like the birth rate and death rate of that country in being subject to seasonal fluctuations more extreme than in almost any other country. This is in harmony with the extreme contrast between the delightful and invigorating cooler season, and the very depressing hot wet season.

The significance of the Japanese data can perhaps be better appreciated by reference to Figure 44 where Hokkaido, the most northerly province (Curves *A* and *B*), is compared with Kagoshima, the most southerly province (Curves *F* and *G*). The solid lines represent the sex ratio, but have been inverted so that a high level indicates a high degree of femininity, which usually means a close approach to equality in the numbers of the two sexes.   The dotted curves represent

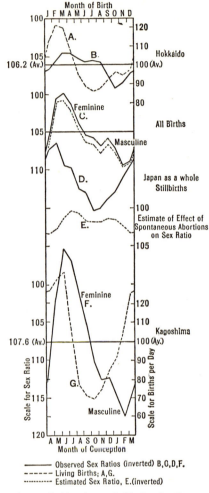

Fig. 44.—Sex Ratios and Number of Births in Japan, 1899–1903 and 1908–1910.

the number of births according to our usual method.   The first point to note about Figure 44 is that the range from maximum to minimum in the sex ratio, as well as in the number of births, declines from north to south. In Hokkaido (Curve *B*), where the summers are not especially trying, the difference between the sex ratio in October (conceptions in January) and in March and April (conceptions in June and July) amounts to 4.7 per cent, as may be seen from the inverted scale on the left. On the other hand, in Kagoshima (Curve *F*), with its terrible summers, the difference is 22.2 per cent. This contrast is even more surprising than the corresponding contrast in the seasonal distribution of births (Curves *A* and *G*). The essential point however, is that the curves for both the sex ratio and the number of births are flatter in the north than in the south.

The next noteworthy point in Figure 44 is that all three inverted curves for the sex ratio—not only *B* and *F,* but also *C,* which embraces the entire country—conform closely to the basic seasonal rhythm. In their inverted form they closely resemble the Belgian curve (Figure 1) with which we began our study of births, except that the amplitude from maximum to minimum is greater. Another point is that during the first half of the year, these inverted curves of sex ratios agree with the curves showing the total number of births (*A* and *G*), but continue to drop in the autumn after the others have begun to rise. The agreement during the first half of the year corresponds with what we find practically everywhere among both kinds of curves. It indicates that during the half of the year when the basic animal rhythm is dominant the number of births and the proportion of female births vary in harmony, the lowest sex ratio occurring when conception takes place at the season which is best for birth according to the animal rhythm.

The fact that during the second half of the year the curves showing number of births draw away from those of both the basic animal rhythm and the sex ratio affords interesting grounds for investigation. We shall return to it after we have studied other phases of the problem.

Meanwhile let us inquire whether the remarkable seasonal variation in the Japanese sex ratio can be explained on the basis of stillbirths and abortions, or must be ascribed to something occurring at the time of conception. Abortions, as we have said, have a very high sex ratio. Hence they tend to reduce the percentage of males. According to the Japanese definition stillbirths form 8 or 10 per cent of all births. This figure is much higher than among most Europeans, but not greatly different from that of American Negroes, namely, 8.5 among the urban type, and 6.9 among the rural. Even if the Japanese reckon as stillbirths some that would be counted as living births elsewhere, it is evident that an unusually large proportion of Japanese infants die either at birth or very shortly thereafter. This agrees with the very high rate of infant mortality which still prevails in Japan. The seasonal incidence of stillbirths is much the same as that of living births. When deaths are numerous, stillbirths are also numerous. Moreover, when stillbirths are expressed as percentages of total births, the percentages also vary almost in harmony with the deaths. In certain typical years, for instance, the percentage was 9.3 in December. It fell from this maximum to a minimum of 8.4 in April; rose again to 9.2 in July; and then fell to 8.6 in October. Thus the proportion of stillbirths rises in both winter and summer, but does not exactly follow the general mortality.

The seasonal variation in the sex ratio of stillbirths is illustrated in Curve D of Figure 44. It follows approximately the same course as the number of births (the dotted lines A and G) but departs decidedly from the course of the sex ratio among living births, C. Nevertheless, if all the stillborn children should live, the seasonal trend of the sex ratio among living births would be changed very little. The solid line of C would merely become the fine dotted line.

It is not easy to estimate the effect of spontaneous abortions upon the sex ratio because statistical data are almost non-existent. According to such authorities as Stander and Williams (1936), abortions do not depend upon the health of the mother at the time of their occurrence so closely as do stillbirths. This is because they are also influenced greatly by the condition of both parents at or before the time of conception, that is, during the period when the ova and spermatozoa are being formed. For the sake of argument, however, let us assume that abortions vary from season to season in the same proportion as deaths in general. In other words, let them vary in harmony with the health of the mother. This apparently gives them the maximum allowable weight in support of the hypothesis that the sex ratio depends mainly upon the frequency of abortions. In order to simplify the problem we will assume (1) that conceptions are equally numerous at all seasons, (2) that they are equally divided between the sexes, (3) that 20 per cent of all conceptions result in spontaneous abortions, (4) that the abortions are distributed throughout the months of pregnancy in accordance with the findings of Kopp (1934), and (5) that the sex ratio during successive months of gestation varies in accord with Table 8 which shows the ratios among the incomplete reports published by the United States Census.

TABLE 8

Sex Ratio Among Stillbirths (Abortions) in the Available Portions of the United States

Registration Area 1922–1933

Duration of Pregnancy	Sex Ratio	No. of Cases
Under two months.............	271	89
Two months..................	438	576
Three months................	375	2,769
Four months.................	202	7,288
Five months.................	143	14,372
Six months..................	124	21,029
Seven months................	115	26,961
Eight months................	127	31,253
Nine months.................	136	84,879
Ten months..................	135	3,353

Kopp's data show that among the spontaneous abortions reported as the result of careful questioning of 10,000 maternity cases in New York City 9 per cent occurred in the first month of pregnancy, 42 per cent in the second, 32 in the third, and only 17 from the fourth onward. In the first month, however, unreported abortions may have been more numerous than at any later time. Stander and Williams (1936) believe that this is the case. The embryos that thus escape are so undeveloped that the woman herself is not conscious of their loss. In the great majority of cases abortions that occur in the early months are not reported, as is evident in Table 8 which gives only the number of abortions reported to the Census Bureau. If Kopp's percentages apply to all of the limited number of states on which Table 8 is based, and if we draw the line between abortions and stillbirths at the end of the sixth month of pregnancy, those states alone must have had not less than 82,000 abortions in the second month of pregnancy and twice as many in the first four months. But even this large number is far below the reality, according to Stander and Williams.

The preceding assumptions probably give too much weight to abortions. They are purposely framed to err on that side, except where they depend upon actual statistics. Taking them, then, for what they are worth, the sex ratio of living births in Japan would vary from season to season as shown in Curve E of Figure 44 if abortions were the sole cause of variation. This curve, with its main maximum in April, bears a certain resemblance to the actual curve (C), with its maximum in March. Both curves have minor maxima in September. On the other hand, the estimated curve (E) is very much flatter than the other, and the two maxima are much more nearly equal. Moreover, the summer minimum in the estimated curve is relatively more important than in the real curve, while the winter minimum, which corresponds to high masculinity, is more pronounced in the actual curve. Of course the estimated curve is based on assumptions derived from other countries, and does not pretend to be exact. Inasmuch, however, as the assumptions give abortions more weight than they apparently deserve, we seem to be safe in saying that Curve E represents the maximum suppositious effect of spontaneous abortions upon seasonal fluctuations of the sex ratio. That effect is too small to account for the reality. Some other cause must be operative. Hence we conclude that although abortions, in conjunction with stillbirths, are unquestionably a factor in determining the sex ratio, other factors are still more important.

Among these other factors the chief place is presumably held by the condition of the reproductive cells of both parents at the time of fertilization. This in turn must depend upon the physiological fitness of the parents during the weeks immediately preceding conception. Our curves of birth show that such fitness is at a maximum in May or June in Japan, as well as in many other countries. Hence our final conclusion is that a certain type of weather not only sets the date at which children are conceived in greatest numbers, but also provides conditions such that female embryos have the maximum chance to be produced, or at least to survive; and the children resulting from such conceptions and born the following March tend to have a low sex ratio. From June onward the fitness of Japanese parents for reproduction apparently declines almost steadily until October if we judge by the reduction in the number of conceptions that result in living births (Curves *A* and *G*, using the lower scale of months). If we judge by the growingly masculine quality of the sex ratio (Curves *B*, *C*, and *F*), however, it declines until January or February, as shown on the scale at the bottom. We shall discuss the cause of this discrepancy after we have considered the relation of the sex ratio to various other factors.

The conditions in Japan seem to be typical of other countries, except that climatically Japan is more extreme than most countries, whereas from the standpoint of seasonal migrations it is quite moderate. It is interesting to note that in the sex ratios of Japan, just as in the total number of births in Belgium, we find no indication that the return of cool weather brings reproductive conditions as favorable as those accompanying the return of warm weather in the spring. The return of cold weather is, to be sure, accompanied by an increase in conceptions, as is also true in many other countries. Nevertheless, on the return to cooler weather after a hot summer the reproductive cells do not display the kind of vigor which leads to approximately equal numbers of the two sexes. The full nature of this relationship is by no means clear, but in general the sex ratio seems to conform to the basic animal rhythm more closely than does the number of births.

The geographical distribution of sex ratios confirms our conclusion as to the effect of the weather. Figure 45 illus-

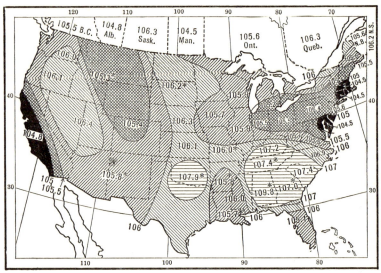

FIG. 45.—Sex Ratio at Birth, Rural Whites in the United States, 1924–1933.
* Based on less than 10 years.

trates the geographical distribution of sex ratios at birth among the rural whites in the United States. From 1923 to 1929 the United States Census defined "rural" as places with less than 10,000 inhabitants, and from 1930 onward as places with less than 2500, but the people included in this classification belong mainly to smaller and more truly rural places. The geographical distribution of sex ratios in these rural districts is very interesting. From the northern part of the Atlantic coast a heavily shaded area of relatively low

sex ratios extends westward to Illinois.   In California there
is another low area.   The South shows high ratios, as appears from the light shading, but Florida drops rather low.
A somewhat similar situation is seen in Figure 46 illustrat-
ing the distribution of sex ratios among Negroes.   In general, although with some exceptions, the sex ratios of whites
and Negroes are low or high respectively in the same parts of
the United States.

The resemblance of these two maps becomes still more significant when we compare them with maps of climatic energy,

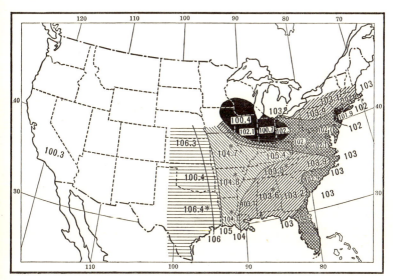

Fig. 46.—Sex Ratio at Birth Among Negroes in the United States, 1924–1933.

health, social progress, and various types of human activity.
All these maps are essentially alike.   The one for climatic
energy, or perhaps we should say climatic efficiency (Figure
47), shows to what extent the climate approaches the ideal for
human health and activity.   It is a purely climatic map based
on data discussed in *Civilization and Climate*.   Although by
no means identical with the map of the sex ratio among
whites, it agrees with it in the following major aspects: (1)
dark shading (equivalent to favorable climatic conditions

on one map and to a low sex ratio on the other) is found in the North from the Atlantic coast to Illinois; (2) light shading (equivalent to less favorable climatic conditions, and to a high sex ratio) prevails in the South; (3) the area of light shading extends into Nevada; (4) heavy shading occurs on the Pacific Coast (California); (5) dark shading characterizes the prairie provinces of Canada, though this is merely suggested in Figure 47 because the climatic map ends at the boundary of the United States.   To a considerable

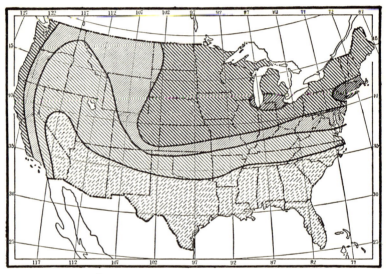

Fig. 47.—Climatic Efficiency in the United States on the Basis of Factory Work.

extent, although with distinct modifications, these same conditions are repeated in the map of Negro sex ratios, so far as that map goes.

The chief difference between the climatic map and the map of sex ratios among rural whites is that, on the map of sex ratios (Figure 45), the Rocky Mountain section is shaded heavily, whereas on the climatic map (Figure 47) it is shaded lightly.   This difference disappears, in part at least, when certain other factors are considered.   The most important of these is probably the size of families.   Figure 48 shows the net reproductive rate, which is essentially the same as the size of the family. The resemblance between this map and the one for the sex ratio among rural whites (Figure 45) is evident. Where the sex ratio is high, the reproductive rate is also high as a rule. The correlation coefficient between the two is 0.565 with a probable error of ±0.074. Inasmuch as the coefficient is 7.6 times as large as the probable error, there is only one chance in a hundred million or so that the agreement is accidental. A still closer agreement

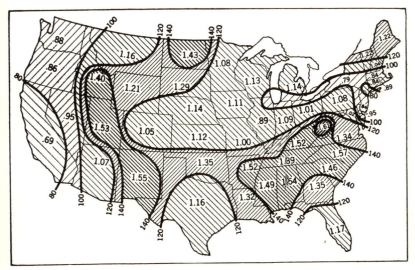

Fig. 48.—Net Rate of Reproduction in the United States.

would be found if allowance were made for the fact that the first children in a family tend to have a higher sex ratio than the later ones, as we shall see in a later chapter. But suppose that the small families of regions such as California and the strip from New England to Iowa should become as large as those in the South and in the Rocky Mountain area? The sex ratio of those regions would presumably fall even lower than now. This would increase the resemblance between the climatic map (Figure 47) and the map of sex ratios (Figure 45). A similar argument applies to the map of Negro sex ratios (Figure 46). Thus it seems clear that among both whites and Negroes the sex ratio varies in fairly close harmony with the degree to which the climate as a whole is invigorating, although other factors such as urbanization undoubtedly have considerable influence.

The condition of the Negroes is especially interesting. In Figure 46 we see that their sex ratio is low in a strip from New Jersey to Iowa, and also among the few Negroes in California. It is fairly low along the Atlantic coast from Virginia to Florida, but becomes high toward the center of the southern half of the country. Only there, in the Mississippi Valley and Texas, does it rise to approximately the same level as that of the whites. In the rest of the South, where the Negro ratio ranges from 103 to 104, it is from 2 to 4 per cent lower than the rural white ratio; in the North and Far West, where the Negro ratio is 103 or lower, it falls still more below the figure for whites. Thus we see among the Negroes three tendencies. First the Negro sex ratio tends to be lower than that of the whites. Second, it displays a tendency like that of the whites toward geographical variation in accordance with the degree to which the climate is healthful. Inasmuch as the families are smallest and hence have the highest percentage of first births in the most healthful regions, this tendency is even stronger than appears in Figure 46. The third tendency is toward a higher sex ratio as one goes away from the Atlantic coast, but this is true only in the South and not in the North. It can scarcely be due to intermarriage of whites and Negroes, for mulattoes appear to be as common in the north as in states like Texas, Oklahoma, and Kansas. Perhaps the pureblooded Negro thrives best in a relatively humid climate and hence has a lower sex ratio near the Atlantic coast. This is one of the many points that demand investigation. For the present, the main conclusion is that the geographical distribution of sex ratios among both whites and Negroes suggests that the ratio varies in harmony with the climate, being low where the climate is most conducive to health and high where the climate is less favorable. The seasonal and the geographical distribution of sex ratios lead to the same conclusion.

The intimate relationship between sex ratios and climate is confirmed by the conditions in Europe. Figure 49 shows the geographical distribution of European sex ratios. The ratios are lowest around the North Sea. They increase outward in all directions, but especially toward the east and

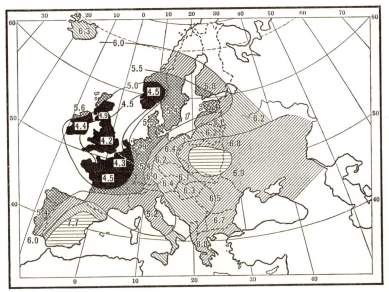

FIG. 49.—Excess of Males per 100 Females in Europe, 1926–1929 or Later.

south. If allowance is made for the size of families and the proportion of first-born children, the contrast between the sex ratios around the North Sea and those in countries like Russia, Bulgaria, and Spain becomes even more prominent. Those countries have large families, which presumably reduces the sex ratio. A similar situation is seen also in Australia, where the sex ratio is lowest in cool Tasmania and highest in warm Queensland. In its essential features the European map of sex ratios strongly resembles a map of climatic efficiency (Figure 50). Like the map of sex

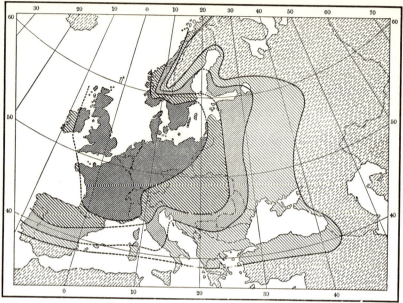

FIG. 50.—Climatic Efficiency in Europe.

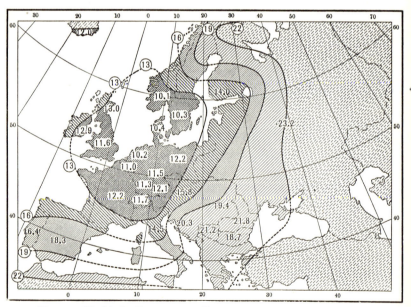

FIG. 51.—Health in Europe according to Standardized Death Rates.

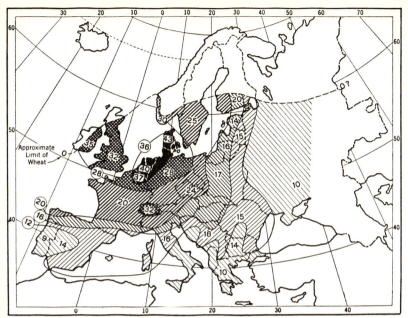

FIG. 52.—Annual European Yield of Wheat per Acre, Bushels, 1910–1929.

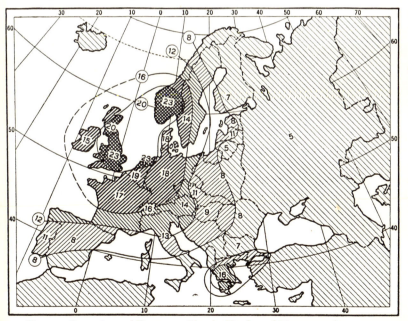

FIG. 53.—Percentage of European Men in Trade and Transporation, 1930.

ratios among Negroes in the United States, however, it shows a divergent feature in a comparatively low ratio along a warm coast. The low ratio in Portugal resembles the low American ratio in Florida not only among Negroes (Figure 47) but also among whites (Figure 46). Among Negroes the state of South Carolina also shows a low ratio. The European map of sex ratios resembles not only the corresponding map of climatic efficiency (Figure 50), but many others such as Figure 51 showing mortality or health. This in turn is closely similar not only to a map of the yield of wheat per acre (Figure 52), which is primarily a climatic map, but to others representing such conditions as the degree to which trade and transportation are developed (Figure 53) and many other conditions. Thus it appears that the sex ratio is one of many human characteristics whose geographic distribution is greatly influenced by differences in the climatic environment.

CHAPTER X

SEX RATIOS, RACE, AND BIRTH RANK

The conclusions of the preceding chapter as to the correlation between a low sex ratio and favorable conditions of weather and climate ought to be tested in every possible way. Let us make a further study of the extent to which differences of race may account for differences in the geographical distribution of sex ratios. Many authorities speak of race as an important factor in causing the sex ratio at birth to differ from one geographical region to another. Jastrzebski (1929), for example, cites several cases where racial groups living in supposedly similar environments differ considerably in the proportions of the two sexes at birth. A typical example is the statement that the Jews in Austria show a ratio of 109.1 males per 100 females, whereas the corresponding figure is 106.5 among the Italians of the Dalmatian coastlands, 106.0 among the Poles of Galicia, 105.6 among the Czechs of Bohemia and Moravia, and 103.7 among the Serbo-Croats in the uplands of Dalmatia.

Such figures are not convincing. In the first place, little reliance can be placed on the Jewish data as will shortly appear. In the second place, there is no evidence that the difference of 2.8, for instance, between the sex ratios of the Italians of the Dalmatian coast and the Serbo-Croats of the Dalmatian upland is racial. We are not even sure that the facts are correctly indicated. The Italian statistics as to sex ratios contain so notable an error at the end of the year that we have not tried to use them in this book. Jugoslavic statistics were imperfect even under Austrian rule. Moreover, some social groups fail to report girls as fully as boys. But even if the statistics were perfect, we cannot safely conclude that they indicate a racial difference, for we have already seen that pronounced geographic differences in the sex ratio are closely correlated with differences in climate. In later pages we shall also find that the sex ratio varies with birth rank, and hence with size of family, and also with economic status. Even if data for these conditions were available in the countries mentioned above, which is not the case, there is as much reason for attributing the difference in the sex ratios to diet, or mode of life, as to race.

The common practice of citing the Jews as an example of a race with a peculiarly high sex ratio at birth seems to be groundless. The apparently high Jewish ratios are due largely, if not wholly, to social or religious customs. In Russia, for instance, the sex ratios reported among Jewish infants are extremely high, but this means mainly, if not wholly, that the births of girls are not reported. During the years 1886, 1889, 1894, and 1897, for example, the average sex ratio among Jewish births in the province of Minsk was 175.7 according to the official figures, whereas among the Moslems of Kazan it was 105.0. For the years 1881 to 1884 in Russia as a whole the sex ratios at birth among certain main groups were as follows: Orthodox Christians, 104.6; Roman Catholics, 104.9; Protestants, 104.9; Moslems, 105.8; large cities, 108.2; small cities, 110.9; rural districts, 104.9. The Jewish ratio was about 150.0. The ratios of the other religions all cluster at approximately 105, even though racially the Moslems are distinct from the rest.

Any doubt on this matter seems to be set at rest by Table 9, showing the sex ratio at birth among Jews as reported in 13 Russian provinces where people of that persuasion were numerous in the nineteenth century.

It is irrational to suppose that most of the world's people, regardless of race, have almost the same sex ratio, but that the Jews of neighboring provinces differ biologically in such a fashion as to give ratios as low as 114 and as high as 180. Even within the limits of a single province the reported sex ratios of the Jews show a similar difference from one year to another. In 1881, 1882, and 1883 the Bessarabian Jews

TABLE 9

SEX RATIOS AS RECORDED AMONG RUSSIAN JEWS, 1881–1884

Province	Sex Ratio	Births	Province	Sex Ratio	Births
Ekaterinoslav...	113.8	9,051	Volhynia......	156.0	36,976
Chernigov......	125.2	11,876	Vilno.........	157.2	13,270
Kherson........	125.6	30,860	Moghilev......	159.4	14,470
Kovno.........	137.1	26,048	Minsk.........	164.2	23,819
Kiev..........	144.0	47,485	Grodno........	170.0	24,601
Podolia........	150.0	38,125	Vitebsk.......	180.2	14,178
Bessarabia......	153.8	15,883			

reported sex ratios of 167, 161, and 165. In 1884, however, when only half as many births were reported, presumably from the cities, the apparent ratio dropped to 107. The obvious fact is that religious and social customs deter the less-enlightened Jews from reporting the births of girls. Therefore the sex ratio of any group containing Jews must be viewed with suspicion until evidence is produced to show that the Jewish girls are being recorded as fully as the boys. It is mainly the presence of Jews, not the nature of the cities, which causes the large Russian cities cited above to have a sex ratio of 108.2 and the small ones, where Jews are more numerous, 110.9.

Even in so enlightened a city as New York the borough of Bronx shows a consistently higher sex ratio than the other boroughs year after year, as appears in Table 10. There the average sex ratios from 1916 to 1923 are compared with the percentage of Jews in 1920. Bronx is the borough not only where Jews are most numerous (38 per cent) and the sex ratio highest (107.0), but where Jews are most crowded together so that old customs brought over by recent immigrants persist most strongly. In Brooklyn there are many Jews (30 per cent of the population) but they are the Americanized type. They report the births of girls as carefully as those of boys. They are also comparatively prosperous. Hence the sex ratio of Brooklyn (104.9) is low—a trifle lower than in any other borough. In view of all this it seems im-

possible to entertain the idea that the real sex ratio of the
Jews differs materially from that of the people among whom
they live. Nevertheless, the apparent sex ratio of any city
may be influenced by the presence of Jews, especially if they
are kept in isolation. Moreover, if the Jews or any other
group have unusually small families, as we shall soon see,
their sex ratio at birth will be high.

TABLE 10

Sex Ratios at Birth in Boroughs of New York City as Reported
for 1916–1923

Borough	Sex Ratio	Percentage Jews, 1920
Bronx	107.0	38.0
Brooklyn	104.9	30.0
Manhattan	105.3	28.8
Queens	105.1	18.4
Richmond	105.1	14.7

This does not necessarily mean that there is no such thing
as racial differences in the sex ratio. Among tropical races
the ratio is almost universally lower than among Europeans.
For example, ratios for whites and colored respectively, as
reported by Jastrzebski (1929), are given in Table 11.

TABLE 11

Sex Ratios at Birth Among White versus Colored People,
After Jastrzebski

Locality	Authority	Ratio for Whites	Ratio for Colored
U. S. A.	Jastrzebski	105.7	100.0
Cape Colony	"	105.4	102.6
Colombia	"	105.0	100.0
New York	"	104.5	101.6
New Orleans	"	102.0	98.2
U. S. A. (1st births)	Little (1920)	115.5	93.6
Colombia	Nichols (1907)	106.2	103.0
Cuba	Heape (1909)	108.42	101.2

We do not trust all these figures, but they are impressive.
Let us try to discover whether the difference which they

seem to indicate between the races is innate or merely cultural. The United States furnishes perhaps the best means of testing the matter. There whites and Negroes live side by side, and can be compared state by state, even though their mode of life is not quite the same. In Figure 54 the states have been arranged according to the sex ratio of the Negroes, as indicated by the solid line. The sex ratio of the rural whites is shown in the dashed line, and that of the urban whites in the barred line.

In Figure 54 it is evident that on the whole the Negro

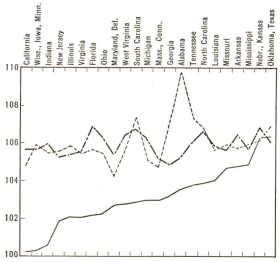

Fig. 54.—Sex Ratio at Birth in the United States, 1924-1933.

sex ratio is systematically lower than that of the whites. It is also more variable, but perhaps this is purely accidental. The minimum (100.3) occurs in California where there are few Negroes, and the maximum (106.4) in Oklahoma and Texas where the records are as yet too short to be conclusive. On the other hand, aside from the exceptional, and probably inaccurate case of Alamba (109.8), the rural whites vary only from 104.8 to 107.4. The urban whites vary much less, namely, from 105.7 to 107.0. The average difference between Negroes and whites is only about 2.0. For example, in 1926 the ratio among whites was 105.8 and among Negroes 103.9. The difference may be greater than this, however, because colored people probably fail more often than do whites to report the births of girls. This would make their reported ratio higher than the true ratio.

Other factors such as size of family and abortions must also be considered. First births, as we shall soon see, appear to have a different sex ratio from later births, and the percentage of first births among colored people is low because families are large. According to Little (1920), the first births among colored people have the very low sex ratio of 93.6 in contrast to 115.6 for whites. This seems almost incredible, but we have not been able to test it. The figure for whites, however, is consistent with that reported for first births elsewhere, for example, New Zealand 108.1; children in *Who's Who in America,* 111.2; and old American stock, 115 to 129. If the Negro sex ratio among first births is really below 100, this fact alone is enough to account for the differences shown by Figure 54 and Table 11 in the sex ratios of whites and Negroes. But before we can decide whether a low sex ratio among first births is a biological characteristic of Negroes, we must discover whether it is due to an excess of female conceptions, or to a great loss of males through abortion. It may arise from an innate reproductive superiority such that the X-bearing spermatozoa are rarely injured and few female embryos are lost at the inception of pregnancy. It may also arise from poor health resulting in excessive spontaneous abortion.

The only exact facts which I have been able to find as to abortions among Negroes are those of Titus (1925). In studying 274 patients in the Johns Hopkins Hospital at Baltimore he found that the total number of abortions reported by white women was 1.6 times as great as by colored. If more extensive investigations substantiate this finding, the low Negro sex ratio cannot be due to abortions. The small number of cases reported by Titus, however, scarcely warrants any generalization, nor is there any assurance that the

Negro women reported their abortions as fully as the whites. Moreover, stillbirths in the later months of pregnancy are twice as common among Negroes as among white women. From 1922 to 1928, for example, the stillbirths reported in the United States, chiefly in the North, amounted to 3.8 per 100 live births among urban whites, and 3.3 among rural whites, whereas they rose to 8.5 among urban Negroes and 6.9 among rural Negroes. If the stillbirths had a sex ratio of 133, which is not far from the average, their occurrence depressed the sex ratio among live births 0.6 per cent farther among Negroes than among whites. In the South where the death rate among Negroes is much higher than in the North, the effect may be correspondingly greater, but as to this there is no certainty.

It seems probable, then, that stillbirths alone account for not far from half of the difference between the sex ratios of whites and Negroes. It also seems probable that spontaneous abortions are more numerous among Negroes than among whites, even though the data of Titus point otherwise. If Titus is right, the explanation of the low sex ratio of the Negroes must apparently be that as a race their metabolism or their reproductive system is superior to that of whites. This would prove that in one case, at least, race does play a part in determining the sex ratio at birth. Even if this is true, however, it does not necessarily mean that there is an innate racial tendency toward a certain sex ratio. The racial trait may manifest itself through other conditions such as size of family, and this in turn may depend upon environmental causes.

Size of family is important for our present purpose because the sex ratio at birth varies according to birth rank, that is, according to whether a person is the first, second, third, or later child to be born to its mother. This subject has been little studied. In Australia a sex ratio of 105.2 is reported for first births in comparison with 105.0 for all others; in Budapest 105.1 against 104.9. In New Zealand, where special attention has been given to this matter, the following ratios are reported, and are almost certainly significant:

> 1919-1925, First births 107.8
> Other births 105.2
> 1925-1934, First births 106.1
> Other births 105.7

New Zealand also supplies more detailed information. Since 1919 the authorities have looked up the record of every child who is born as the fourth in a family where these children previously born to the same mother were still alive. Then they have calculated the sex ratios of the first-born, second-born, and so on. This procedure has the great advantage of eliminating social, economic, and biological differences. The first-born are exactly like the second-born, third-born, and fourth-born in parentage, economic status, social level, and every other respect aside from matters connected with birth rank. Their sex ratio, nevertheless, varies systematically, as appears in Column A of Table 12. It declines rapidly from the first to the second births and less rapidly to the third, and then begins to rise a little.

Other lines of investigation confirm this result. In about 2800 families recorded in *Who's Who in America* (Column B in Table 12) the sex ratio falls off just as in New Zealand, but more rapidly, from 111.2 among first children to 101.7 among third children. Then it rises with extreme rapidity to 142.7 among sixth or later children. Little confidence can be placed in this last figure since it is based on only 172 children. Otherwise, the agreement with Australia is close. The only trouble is that the number of families declines rapidly as the number of children diminishes, so that both heredity and environment change from one birth rank to another. In Column C of Table 12 we have obviated this difficulty by using only families with 4 or more children in two genealogical books. Here again the situation is the same as in New Zealand so far as the first 4 children are concerned, except that the variation in sex ratios according to birth rank is more extreme. Column D shows that among the smaller

TABLE 12

SEX RATIOS ACCORDING TO BIRTH RANK

Number of cases in parenthesis

Birth Rank	A New Zealand	B Who's Who in America	C New England I[1]	D New England II[2]	E Old I[3]	F Colonial Stock II[3]	G III[3]
1	108.1	111.2 (2778)	129.0 (1205)	115.5 (1319)	113.0 (3923)	116.6 (3122)	119.9 (3027)
2	105.4	104.2 (2130)	109.8 (1205)	116.2 (854)	113.7 (2751)	117.7 (3230)	117.0 (3020)
3	104.1	101.7 (1285)	103.5 (1205)	113.0 (412)	93.9 (1359)	106.3 (3122)	110.3 (3010)
4	104.4	113.4 (696)	124.5 (1205)	....	....	117.4 (3044)	116.4 (3040)
5	....	115.2 (220)	108.6 (893)	....	....	113.0 (1921)	115.8 (3024)
6 (or later)	....	142.2 (172)	97.1 (739)	....	....	100.4 (898)	107.8 (3028)
7	....	....	94.3 (478)	....	....	....	107.5 (2961)
8	....	....	105.9 (350)	....	....	....	121.9 (2206)
9	....	....	110.1 (227)	....	....	....	121.9 (1742)
10 (or later)	....	....	111.2 (283)	....	....	....	116.3 (2046)
All	105.5	107.2	111.0	113.8			

[1] I = All completed families with four or more children in Flanders and Huntington Genealogical Books.
[2] II = All completed families with one to three children in Flanders and Huntington Genealogical Books.
[3] Data compiled by C. L. Ziegler from many genealogical books, and divided into families with 1–3 children, 4–6 children, and 7 or more children.

families recorded in these same books the children born third in their families had the lowest sex ratio, although the ratios for all three birth ranks are very high.

A more conclusive investigation by Mr. Ziegler is based on many genealogical books. Figure 55 and columns E, F, and G, show the sex ratio according to birth rank in three types of families divided according to size. Solid lines indicate the part of each section based on an approximately uniform number of families and hence reliable for comparisons between one birth rank and another. Dotted lines indicate data based on a number of families smaller than is used for the first-born children, and hence of doubtful value. At

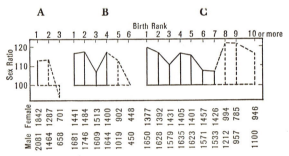

FIG. 55.—Sex Ratio According to Birth Rank among Old American Families Completed before 1885.

least two significant features are evident. First, the sex ratio of the first-born increases from 113.0 in small families with 1 to 3 children (A) to 116.6 in medium-sized ones with 4 to 6 children (B), and then to 119.9 in the large ones with 7 or more children (C). Second, in spite of considerable irregularity, all three types of families show a distinct tendency toward a lowering of the sex ratio among later births. This is especially clear in the solidly shaded portions of Section C where the first 7 children in large families are compared.

Before we point out the connection between these facts and the problem of sex ratios in relation to climate, weather, and race, let us inquire as to the conditions which favor a high sex ratio among first births. How much effect does the age of the mother have? Do abortion or stillbirth enter into the matter?   In considering the age of the mother, it is well to remember that small families include many mothers who married late, whereas practically all the mothers of the large families married young.   In New Zealand, as appears in Column B of Table 13, the sex ratio is practically identical among the children of mothers in the age group "under 20 years" and "20 to 24 years."   As the age of the mother increases, the ratio falls, except that there is a curious increase between the ages of 30 and 35.

TABLE 13

SEX RATIO OF FIRST BIRTHS ACCORDING TO AGE OF MOTHER IN NEW ZEALAND, 1910–1934, AND DEATH RATE OF INFANTS IN 8 CITIES OF THE UNITED STATES.

A	B	C	D	E
			Index Number of Deaths of Infants in 8 Cities Born at	
Age of Mother	Sex Ratio	No. of Births	Specified Ages of Mother (After Woodbury, 1925)	No. of Deaths
Under 20 yrs.	106.5	9,901	122.0	215
20–24 yrs.	106.6	48,853	98.3	753
25–29 yrs.	106.3	40,392	91.2	671
30–34 yrs.	109.0	17,005	94.2	443
35–39 yrs.	105.7	6,133	113.8	340
40 yrs. or more	101.9	1,672	122.9	131

The general decline in the sex ratio as the mother's age increases agrees with Figure 55.   When their first children were born the mothers of Section C in the figure, where the sex ratio of first-born children is 119.9, must have averaged between 20 and 25 years of age; those of Section B, where the sex ratio is 116.6, must have been older; and those of A, where the sex ratio of the first-born is 113.0, must have averaged still older, although probably under 30 years.   A more potent factor in the low sex ratio of the small families, however, is found in the fact that the mothers of the small families were almost certainly more subject to abortions than were the others.   Spontaneous abortions are everywhere one

of the great causes of small families, and they tend to produce a low sex ratio.

Another interesting fact is that in all three sections of
Figure 55, just as in all columns of Table 12, the sex ratio
reaches at least a minor minimum with the third child.
This apparently corresponds to the slight decline in the sex
ratio of first-born children which is indicated in New Zealand (Table 13) as one goes from mothers aged 20-24 years
to those aged 25 to 29 years. On an average the third
child is probably born when the mother is in this latter age
group, 25 to 29. Then, with the fourth child of all our
examples where there is such a child (Columns A, B, and C
of Table 12, and Sections B and C of Figure 43), the sex
ratio again rises. In Column B of Table 12 and Section C
of Figure 55 the sex ratio of the fifth child rises still more.
The majority of the fourth and fifth children in all these
families were presumably born when their mothers were not
far from 30-35 years of age. Therefore their high sex ratio
agrees in a mild way with that which is found in New Zealand among children who were the first-born of mothers at
the same age (Column B of Table 13). Finally, in Section
C of Figure 55 and in Columns C and G of Table 12, the sex
ratio tends to decline after the fourth child. Then with the
eighth child the ratio rises once more.

These confusing fluctuations in the sex ratio from one
birth rank to another apparently can be explained on the
basis of two distinct types of relationship. One type consists
of changes in the facility with which the X chromosomes as
compared with the Y chromosomes reach the ova. The other
consists of changes in the amount of abortion. Both changes
presumably take place in response to changes in the age of
the mother, but it is possible that the age of the father also
enters into the matter. As for the chromosome changes, the
hypothesis is that first children of mothers of all ages tend
to have a high sex ratio at the time of conception, because
the chemical conditions of the genital tract are not favorable
to the X-bearing spermatozoa. Of course the primary sex

ratio may be altered later by abortions and stillbirths. With second and third children, unless there is some weakness in the mother, the sex ratio apparently declines after the first birth, and again after the second, because the reproductive tract of the mother assumes a condition which makes it easier for the X chromosomes to reach and fertilize the ova. Then, as the mothers grow older, a reversal presumably takes place, the conditions become less favorable for the X chromosomes, and the percentage of ova fertilized by Y chromosomes and hence becoming males increases. All this, taken by itself, would lead to a high sex ratio with first births, a low ratio with third births, and then a steadily increasing ratio among later births.

The type of result that might be expected according to this hypothesis is actually found in the data for *Who's Who* in Column B of Table 12. The extremely high ratio of 142 there given for sixth and later births is probably accidental, but ratios of 113 and 115 for fourth and fifth children are reasonable. They are ratios which might be expected if abortions did not enter into the matter, as explained in the next paragraph.

The effect of abortions and stillbirths upon the sex ratio of different birth ranks is illustrated in Table 14. Column B shows that according to Kopp's (1934) study of 10,000 maternity cases the percentage of pregnancies terminated by spontaneous abortions rises steadily from the first pregnancy onward to the eighth. It probably would continue to rise with later pregnancies, were it not that the few of Kopp's cases who had 10 or more children were presumably women of unusual vigor. If data for them were available separately, we should doubtless find that their percentage of abortions begins very low and rises steadily to 10, which is the figure for the tenth or later pregnancies in Column B. According to Woodbury (1925), stillbirths (Column D, Table 14) follow essentially the same course as spontaneous abortions, except that they are numerous with first births and fall to a low level with second births. From only 2.5 per cent among second births the number of stillbirths rises to 5.5 among births occurring tenth or later.

The last column in Table 14 shows what the sex ratio would be if we assume (1) that it is 110 at the very beginning of pregnancy; (2) that it averages 300 among abortions up to the end of the sixth month of pregnancy and 133 among still births thereafter, as the available data indicate to be approximately the case; and (3) that the percent-

TABLE 14

PREGNANCIES TERMINATED BY SPONTANEOUS ABORTIONS PER KOPP; AND STILLBIRTHS AS PERCENTAGE OF ALL BIRTHS, PER WOODBURY, ACCORDING TO RANK

Rank of Pregnancy (Column B) or of Birth (Column D)	A No. of Pregnancies per Kopp (1934)	B Percentage Terminated by Spontaneous Abortions	C Births per Woodbury (1925)	D Percentage of Stillbirths	E Estimated Sex Ratio
1	9583	6	6491	4.0	106.7
2	8101	7	5080	2.5	106.3
3	6271	9	3423	2.8	106.3
4	4593	9	2555	2.9	106.3
5	3242	9	1830	3.4	106.2
6	2273	12	1310	3.6	103.7
7	1579	11	968	4.9	104.0
8	1071	13	707	4.2	103.1
9	709	12	480	3.9	103.6
10 and later	1563	10	927	5.5	104.4

ages of abortions and stillbirths follow the courses indicated by Kopp and Woodbury in Columns B and D, Table 14. The estimated sex ratios are only approximations, but with any other reasonable set of assumptions the general relationship between early and late births would be the same. According to Column E the sex ratio resulting from abortions and stillbirths alone declines a little from the first to the second birth (106.7 to 106.3). It remains almost stationary through the fifth birth (or pregnancy), and then declines rapidly. Thus up to the third birth the changes in the frequency of abortion re-enforce the conditions which favor the X chromosomes, and the two conditions together give a low sex ratio among third children. Thereafter, however, the two tendencies work in opposite directions. At first the X chromosomes are dominant and raise the sex ratio, but afterward abortions and stillbirths play the leading rôle, and the ratio declines.

In the light of these two tendencies let us see how Table 12 and Figure 55 are interpreted. In Column D of the table and Section *A* of the figure we are dealing with families of only 3 children. Inasmuch as these families belong to a period when there was little limitation of births, their small size must be due mainly to late marriage, poor health, or death of at least one partner, but death generally indicates poor health. Such health presumably has the same effect as increased age not only in making it more difficult for the X chromosomes to fertilize the ova, but also in causing abortions. Therefore, as we have already indicated, the relatively low sex ratio of all the births in the two smaller types of families in Figure 55 may reasonably be attributed to abortions. Even in the smallest New England families (Column D of Table 12) the sex ratio is lower than in the first and second births illustrated in Figure 55.

Carrying the matter further, we can perhaps explain the very slight increase in the sex ratio from the first to the second child in our two groups of families numbering only 1 to 3 children. It may be due to the normal increase in the sex ratio which appears to occur because the X chromosomes find greater difficulty in fertilizing the ova as the age of the mother increases beyond the optimum. We do not stress this, however, for the increase is so small that it may be accidental. In the same way, in the absence of any exact data as to the age and health of the parents of these small families, we do not know whether to ascribe the relatively low sex ratio among third births to increased abortions or to some other cause. We suspect, however, that abortions are the cause. We are presumably dealing here with mothers who, on the average, are past 30 years of age, and in many cases cease to have children because they are subject to abortions. It must be remembered that only a small percentage of the mothers in this particular group had even as many as 3 children, and we do not know anything about the qualities of this percentage in comparison with those of the larger percentage whose families comprise only 1 child.

In Table 12 and Figure 55 the second and third children among all groups which have as many as 4 children show a declining sex ratio. According to the hypothesis now before us, this is because the physiological condition of the mothers becomes increasingly favorable to the X chromosomes which produce females. With the fourth child, however, the average woman has presumably passed the period of life most favorable for childbearing, and increasing difficulty for the X chromosomes leads to a larger proportion of males. With later children an increase of spontaneous abortion appears to overbalance the tendency toward an increase in male conceptions which we have suspected in connection with fourth and fifth children. Abortions and stillbirths remove not only the extra males due to this tendency, but some of the other males as well.

It must be clearly understood that the only case in which the facts as to children beyond the fourth are unequivocal is the part of Section C, Figure 55, drawn in solid lines. There alone are we free from complications due to the fact that the number of families changes when we get beyond the fourth child. In the part of Section C pertaining to the first 7 children an increasing rate of abortions and a changing rate of masculine conceptions apparently combine to form a rather complex curve. The contrast between this curve and the data for *Who's Who in America* (Column B, Table 12) appears to be due to the social status of the group in *Who's Who*. The continued rise of the sex ratio among the later children of that group suggests that the few mothers who had 6 or more children experienced practically no tendency toward increased abortions because of increased age. Probably they were not only physically strong, but unusually well nourished and cared for because of their social status. In addition to this the tendency toward masculine conceptions may have increased rapidly among these women because in this favored group they take too little exercise and live a very sedentary life, but this is pure surmise.

In dealing with the sex ratio and abortions according to birth rank we have indirectly been studying the question of age at which women are best fitted for motherhood. Further light is thrown on this by Column D of Table 13 (page 225). There data collected by Woodbury (1925) in 8 American cities show that the death rate among infants reaches a pronounced minimum when the mothers are 25 to 29 years of age. A rate of 91 deaths per 1000 births among children born to mothers aged 25 to 29 years is very different from a rate of 122 among those born to mothers aged under 20 or over 40. Much of this difference, however, may be due to the fact that among the less privileged and less healthy classes of society the proportion of both unusually young and unusually old mothers is high. Hence there is no knowing how far the contrast found by Woodbury is economic and how far physiological. Nevertheless social differences probably do not account for the whole of it.

A study of families of the nobility in Germany eliminates this social factor. Ploetz (1922) tabulated the children of such families according to birth rank. His data, as given in Table 15 (Column B), show that although the vitality of the children born in any rank from first to ninth varies but little, the second, third, and fourth children have a weighted mortality of 25.6 per cent during the first 5 years of life as compared with 26.4 among first births and a steadily rising percentage among births from the fourth onward. This culminates in 34.4 per cent among children who are born tenth to nineteenth in their families.

A study of old New England families gives a similar, but more conclusive, result, as appears in Figure 56. There the lower section shows the deaths per 1000 births up to and

TABLE 15

PERCENTAGE OF CHILDREN DYING IN CHILDHOOD IN GERMANY AND THE UNITED STATES

	Germany per Ploetz[1]		United States (See Figure 56)							
	A	B	Families of 4 to 6			Families of 7 or more			Flanders[2] Family	
			C	D		E	F		G	H
Birth Rank	No. of Births	Percentage of Deaths under 5 Years of Age	No. of Births	Percentage of Deaths		No. of Births	Percentage of Deaths		No. of Births	Percentage of Deaths Under 5 Years
				Under 2 Years	Under 21 Years		Under 2 Years	Under 21 Years		
1	614	26.4	2808	6.3	14.1	2756	7.1	15.9	1749	13.1
2	539	24.9	2917	6.7	15.0	2746	6.9	15.3	1392	10.9
3	455	26.4	2804	6.4	14.1	2735	7.2	13.9	1188	7.9
4	386	25.6	2782	6.1	13.0	2767	6.0	13.7	754	9.8
5	311	26.0	1745	5.7	12.8	2747	7.5	14.7	575	10.2
6	249	26.1	830	5.4	11.3	2747	7.8	14.4	417	11.3
7	463	26.3	....	....	....	2697	7.1	13.8	311	11.6
8	....	....	....	....	....	2009	6.0	14.2	224	10.7
9	....	....	....	....	....	1615	4.8	11.5	145	11.8
10 or more	302	34.4	....	....	....	1879	8.1	14.5	186	14.5
	3319	26.7								

[1] From *World Almanac*, 1922.
[2] Average of male and female death rates, and total number of births.

including the age of 20 among children and young people recorded in American genealogical books.   The two upper sections show the average length of life among persons of this

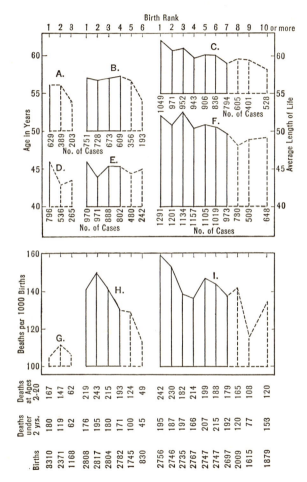

Fig. 56.—Longevity and Youthful Death Rate among Old American Families.

same kind who survived at the age of 2 years (middle section), or at the age of 20 (upper section).   In each section the left-hand diagram illustrates families of 1 to 3 children; the middle diagram is for families of 4 to 6; and the other for those with 7 or more. The last are the most important because up to the seventh child the same families are concerned in each birth rank. So far as heredity and economic status are involved there is essential uniformity throughout the 7 birth ranks that are shown by solid lines. In the middle diagrams, for families of 4 to 6, there is uniformity only in the first 4 birth ranks, which again are shown by solid lines. In the small families the number of cases varies with each birth rank.

In interpreting Figure 56 it must be remembered that the data as to age are much more reliable than those as to deaths. Our information as to date of death is, indeed, much less abundant among poor and inconspicuous people than among those who are more prominent. This makes little difference for our present purpose, however, because at the time when the persons used in this tabulation were born the size of families was practically the same in all classes. On the other hand, when we consider the *number* of deaths we are faced with very serious errors. Many families in which all the children died are recorded in the genealogical books as childless. The proportion of such families of course increases greatly as one goes from the large to the small families. One reason for this is that the chances that all the children will die vary inversely as the number of children. If there is only 1 child, and other things are equal, the chances that it will die are approximately the same as that any child in a 7-child family will die, but they are 7-fold greater than that death will overtake *all* the children in the larger family. Moreover, other things are not equal. In the days of unrestricted families the size of the family was closely correlated with the physical vigor of the parents, regardless of whether their vigor was due to age, constitution, or mode of life. Hence in families where there were few children the death rate was relatively high because many of the parents were not strong. In addition to this, a first child dying very young is more likely to be omitted from the record than a later child, because the brothers and sisters who often supply the records are less likely to know about the earlier death than about the later one.

Let us begin with the death rate, diagrams *G, H,* and *I.* A very low death rate is suggested by diagram *G* for families of 1 to 3 children. In all three birth ranks this is probably due to deficient records. The higher level of the second child may be more nearly correct. The low level of the third child is probably due to the fact that the number of families on which it is based is only 686 in comparison with 993 for the second child and 1911 for the first. The parents who had 3 children may have been more vigorous than those that stopped with 2 or 1. Therefore their children may have had a lower death rate. If this were true, however, one would expect the death rate in the larger families to be still lower, but such is not the case. It may be that the small families, even in the nineteenth century, belonged mainly to the upper social levels where the death rate is normally low.

Diagram *H,* showing the mortality in infancy and childhood in families of 4 to 6 children, is more reliable than diagram *G.* We suspect that a good many deaths of first-born children are omitted, and that this is the reason why the death rate of the first-born appears to be lower than that of the second-born. From the second to the fourth children we are dealing in all cases with the same families except that here, as in all data based on genealogical books, a death has now and then failed to be recorded in the books through accident. The death rate declines steadily from the second to the fourth child. This is continued with the fifth child, but as there were only about 1700 fifth children in this group, in contrast to 2800 in each of the earlier birth ranks, the parents of the fifth children may have been a stronger group than the others. This is still more the case with the sixth children, but the continued and strong decline in the death rate is interesting.

The most significant part of the lower section of Figure 56 is Diagram *I.* There the record is comparatively good, because the members of such families are numerous and long-lived, as we shall soon see, and hence likely to supply better information than members of smaller and less long-lived families. Among the 7 earlier birth ranks, which are based on essentially the same families, the death rate declines decidedly but irregularly as the birth rank becomes greater. This continues with the later children, although there is some irregularity as the number of children per family increases and the number of available families becomes less.

The general conclusion to be drawn from these data seems clear. In large families the death rate during infancy and childhood is greatest among the first-born. It diminishes rapidly until about the fourth child, but thereafter the difference between one birth rank and the next becomes less and less. The high death rate among first-born is probably due partly to the difficulties of childbirth, which diminish with progressive births. The later children also fare better because of the growing skill of the parents and the assistance of the older children in taking care of their brothers and sisters. Their better health does not appear to be due to any tendency toward greater vigor on the part of the later children, as we shall now see.

The upper two sections of Figure 56 leave no doubt that, when the size of families is not restricted, the members of large families live longer than those of small ones. No matter whether we consider length of life among persons who survive beyond the age of 2 years or 20, those in the large families live longer. The difference is considerable. It is certainly no small matter that at the age of 2 among the people born in the first half of the last century the boys belonging to families of only 1 to 3 children were destined to live on an average to the age of 46.8 years and the women to 43.4; whereas the boys belonging to families of 7 or more were destined to live longer by 6.2 years and the girls by 4.1.

So far as longevity is concerned, the general tendency is for the oldest child to be the most long-lived. This is clear in the diagrams for the small families (*A* and *D*) and for the large families (*C* and *F*). The same condition appears to be true for the families of medium size, but by no means to so great an extent. If we omit the dotted portions of diagrams *B* and *E*, it appears that in families of 4 to 6 children the length of life varies only a little among the first four birth ranks. The case becomes clearer when we note that in both of these diagrams a decrease in length of life appears with the fifth child. Nevertheless, the regularity of diagrams *B* and *E*, and also of *H*, suggests that families of 4 to 6 children are more normal and better balanced than either the larger or smaller families. Diagram *C*, however, is also very regular. It seems to indicate almost beyond question, that in very large families length of life declines almost steadily from the oldest to the youngest child.

Putting together the facts as to child mortality and length of life, we conclude that, when the size of families is not restricted, the mortality up to the age of 20 is greatest among first-born children, and declines quite steadily among those born later. If people survive until they are adults, however, the further years of life that can be expected are most numerous among the first-born, and decline steadily among those born later. This seeming contradiction is presumably due to the combined action of several conditions. First, a high death rate would be expected among first-born children because the dangers of childbirth and the accidents or ill health arising from lack of parental experience are greatest with them, and decline thereafter. Second, long life would be expected among the earlier children because the vigor of the parents, especially of the mothers, begins to decline after the age of about 30. Third, high mortality in childhood among those in the earlier birth ranks presumably exerts a selective effect, so that the survivors display a degree of constitutional vigor proportional to the number of weaklings who die before reaching maturity. Thus a high death rate in youth among the first-born and a steadily declining death rate among later births do not seem to be inconsistent either with unusual vigor among the first-born who survive to maturity, or with progressively lower vigor among adults of later birth rank.

We must now inquire what all this means as to the relation of sex ratios to racial traits and climate. Since sex ratios vary according to birth rank, the size of families must always be taken into account in appraising their importance. A population composed primarily of small families is bound to have a high sex ratio simply because it has a high percentage of first-born children. This does not make much difference so far as the seasonal distribution of sex ratios is concerned. It makes a great difference geographically, however, as we have already seen. Regions such as western Europe, the northeastern United States, and the Pacific coast of America have low sex ratios and also a high proportion of small families. Therefore, as was said in the last chapter, their sex ratios must be reduced still more in order that they may fairly be compared with those of regions such as Russia, Italy, and the agricultural sections of the United States where the families are large. When this is done, we find more reason than ever to be impressed by the contrast between the low sex ratios of the most progressive parts of the world, where the climate and diet are especially healthful, and the high ratios of the less progressive parts with their less favorable climate and diet. We seem forced to conclude that a low sex ratio among the population as a whole in regions such as Europe or the United States is an indication of good physical environment and of physiological conditions such that the X chromosomes are less handicapped than in regions with a less favorable environment.

This at once raises the question of the Negroes. What does their low sex ratio indicate? The answer depends partly on the extent to which Negro women continue childbearing until late in the reproductive period, and suffer from abortions and stillbirths. In the parts of the United States where Negroes are numerous they certainly have much poorer health than the whites, and their women tend more strongly than the whites to continue having children well on toward the end of the reproductive period. These two conditions together seem to indicate that, in spite of the facts quoted from Titus in the last chapter, the percentage of abortions must be higher than among whites. We have already seen that even in the North, where Negroes have comparatively good health, their proportion of stillbirths is more than twice that of whites. Therefore it seems probable that their percentage of abortions is correspondingly high.

If this is true, and if the number of pregnancies per woman is decidedly higher than among whites, as appears to be the case, the low sex ratio among Negro births may be due wholly to the same conditions which cause poor health. Only if those conditions arise from innate racial traits can we say that the low sex ratio is likewise due to such traits. Even then the racial character may find its primary expression in the degree of social progress whereby health and size of family are regulated, rather than in any innate biological quality which directly causes a low sex ratio. Therefore the question of whether Negroes are biologically different from whites in respect to the sex ratio still remains open. Nevertheless, this chapter seems to lead to at least one conclusion which is of considerable interest. A low sex ratio at the beginning of pregnancy appears to be an indication of a favorable environment. The clearest evidence of such a ratio is now found in regions where the general health is good and the families are of relatively small size. Under such conditions conceptions are rare among older mothers, and the danger of abortion is diminished. Therefore, a low primary sex ratio due to good health has the best chance to manifest itself as a low secondary ratio at birth. Nevertheless, a low sex ratio at birth may be an unfavorable sign if it occurs where the size of families is subject to little restriction, and where abortions are common among the later births. On the whole, however, among the advanced peoples of the world a high primary sex ratio at conception and a high secondary ratio at birth both appear to be signs of weakness. We shall test this conclusion further.

CHAPTER XI

SEX RATIOS AND CULTURAL ENVIRONMENT

The two preceding chapters have led us to conclude that the sex ratio at *conception*—the primary ratio—varies according to weather, season, climate, diet, birth rank, age of the mother, and possibly race. Favorable conditions of climate, season, and diet, and a fairly early but not the earliest stage in the reproductive period of the mother, seem to bring the numbers of the two sexes toward an equality, thus lowering the sex ratio. The ratio at *birth*, however—the secondary ratio—depends not only upon the numbers of the two sexes that are conceived, but also upon the numbers that are lost during pregnancy. The losses depend upon abortions and stillbirths, both of which tend to lower the sex ratio because they are predominantly masculine. It therefore seems advisable to give still further study to the conditions that cause abortions and stillbirths. The first question that confronts us is whether their relation to economic and social status is consistent with our conclusions concerning the relation of the sex ratio to climate.

Winston (1931) has advanced the view that a high sex ratio is an indication of favorable economic conditions. He apparently holds that such a ratio can arise only when there are few losses through abortion. Therefore he says that such a ratio must indicate good health and comfortable economic conditions. Taking the three volumes of Virkus's *Compendium of American Genealogy,* he divided 5466 completed familes into groups according to the number of children, with the result shown in Table 16. These ratios seem high, but we have seen that other genealogical records give similar ratios. Family records probably show a systematic tendency to record the birth of boys more carefully than

TABLE 16

SEX RATIO AT BIRTH AMONG OLD AMERICAN FAMILIES ACCORDING TO
NUMBER OF CHILDREN BORN PER FAMILY, AFTER WINSTON

Children per Family	Number of Families	Sex Ratio
1	1166	117.1
2	1463	121.3
3	1223	112.8
4	820	110.3
5 or more	794	106.2
Total	5466	112.0

those of girls. But even though Winston's ratios are high, the change in them from the small families to the large is significant. Aside from an irregularity in the 2-child families, the sex ratio declines steadily from 117.1 in families with 1 child to 106.2 in those with 5. Winston concludes that this is due to differences in the quality of large and small families. In support of this he states that small families predominate among people belonging to the higher social and economic levels. Hence the mothers have better health and are better cared for than those in the lower social levels. This is supposed to reduce the number of spontaneous abortions and stillbirths and thus give a sex ratio higher than that of the supposedly poorer relatives who have large families.

This reasoning needs to be examined carefully. The general relation of favorable conditions to the sex ratio has often been discussed. For example, Heape (1907) long ago pointed out that his experiments on canaries and his studies of the sex ratio in Cuba indicate that when basal metabolism is high the conditions for reproduction are favorable. Hence female embryos tend to develop in greater numbers than when metabolic activity is diminished. This means that among people who are well fed and in good health the primary sex ratio at the beginning of pregnancy should not be so high as in less-favored groups. Winston apparently holds that, even if this is true, abortions and stillbirths are so rare among the most-favored and best-nourished classes that the primary sex ratio, which appears always to be high, remains almost unchanged until birth. Thus two opposing tendencies appear to be in conflict. At the inception of life, that is, at the time of conception, the most favorable conditions of nutrition and health apparently tend toward femininity because they favor the development of female ova in numbers almost equal to those of male ova. During pregnancy, however, these same conditions tend toward masculinity because they prevent stillbirths, and are not accompanied by any appreciable number of abortions.

Let us see what bearing this has on Winston's hypothesis that among old American families the small families have a high sex ratio because they belong to the upper classes and hence suffer little from abortions and stillbirths. We note first that small families are often a sign of poor health. This was especially true in the old days before the size of families was limited. Physical defects, chronic illness, or death are even now the main reasons which limit families to only 1 child. Most parents want at least 2 children, and feel that they can afford that number. Large families, on the contrary, are usually a sign of physical vigor. Therefore it is extremely doubtful whether either spontaneous abortions or stillbirths really are more common in large families than in small, provided that mothers of similar age are compared. The probability is all the other way.

In the second place, obstetricians such as Lee (1933) say that abortions are more frequent in the city than in the country, and among the upper than the lower classes. City people and the upper classes are the ones who now most often have small families. This does not help us much, however, for we are not sure how far such statements distinguish between spontaneous and induced abortions. Moreover, it must be remembered that in the period when the families used by Winston were born there was much less difference than now in the size of families among the various social classes. So far as abortions are concerned, the only exact data which I have found are those of Malins (1903), who compared 2000 comparatively poor out-patients in London maternity hospitals with 2000 of his own prosperous patients. He obtained the results shown in Table 17. These figures

TABLE 17

ABORTIONS ACCORDING TO SOCIAL STATUS (MALINS)

	Under-Privileged	Privileged
Children per woman..............	3.84	2.22
Abortions per woman.............	0.72	0.42
Abortions per 100 children.........	18.85	19.23
Abortions per 100 pregnancies......	15.86	16.13

date from a period before induced abortion had begun its recent rapid increase, and apply almost wholly to spontaneous abortions. They show that in proportion to the number of children abortions were more numerous among the privileged than among the under-privileged classes, but the difference was only 2 per cent. This is by no means enough to account for the large differences found by Winston in Table 16. If abortions terminate 20 per cent of all pregnancies, and if the sex ratio of all abortions is 300, a difference of 2 per cent in abortions would make a difference of only about 0.3 in the sex ratio. Moreover, even this 2 per cent may be doubtful, for the women of the upper classes perhaps reported their "miscarriages" more fully than did the others. Not only would their greater intelligence lead to this, but having little more than half as many miscarriages to report, they would be more likely to remember them all.

With stillbirths the case is quite different. Up to about the sixth or seventh month of pregnancy, according to Stander and Williams (1936) and others, abortions do not show such close conformity with health as would be expected. The unborn children of under-nourished mothers are often very well nourished. It is only toward the end of pregnancy and at birth that the mother's poor health becomes the dominant factor in causing the loss of foetuses that have once been well started. Before that time defective germ plasm seems to be the main cause of such losses. In late pregnancy, however, stillbirths become especially numerous among under-privileged groups and among people in poor health. The fact that they follow the general seasonal course of deaths in the community as a whole (Figure 11) shows their intimate dependence on the health of the mother.

Among stillbirths the difference between the health of the upper and lower classes is very evident. Winston cites the case of Halle in Germany, where stillbirths formed 2.1 per cent of all births among the upper classes, and 5.0 per cent among laborers. In Holland, among the rich, a percentage of 2.5 was found, and among the poor, 3.2. Such differences, however, are far too small to account for the differences which Table 16 shows between the sex ratios of families of different sizes. If the sex ratio of stillbirths be taken as 133, the difference between 2 per cent and 5 per cent of stillbirths would change the sex ratio by only 0.4. Hence we seem forced to suspect that even if the average social station of the small families in the *Compendium of American Genealogy* is somewhat higher than that of the large families, any consequent ill health of mothers during pregnancy is not the main cause of the difference in the sex ratio.

This suspicion is in harmony with the abundant evidence presented by Lee (1933), Stander and Williams (1936), and others that in both man and animals the father is often responsible for abortions. His spermatozoa may be defective because of general debility, undue sexual activity, alcoholic poisoning, syphilis, and many other causes. Streeter, in a study of data reported by J. L. Huntington, concluded that the essential cause of 81 out of 104 abortions was defective germ plasm. Defects may be due to either parent. They probably have a maximum effect at or soon after the time of conception, but they continue to be influential for a long time. Stander and Williams (1936) say that 20 per cent of all pregnancies probably end in spontaneous abortions. They cite Mall to the effect that 7 out of 20 aborted embryos are pathological to a high degree, and 1 is actually a monster. The other 12 are called normal, but many, especially the younger ones, show hints of departures from the normal, suggesting that if their growth continued, they too would become monsters. Hence Stander and Williams conclude that about 12 per cent of all pregnancies end in abortions of pathological ova. It would seem, they say, "that abortion is nature's method of discarding most of the unsuccessful products of conception." It is clear from the context that they have the father as well as the mother in mind when saying this. Only when pregnancy is well advanced, they say, does the health of the mother become the major factor in determining the loss of embryos. Late abortions and stillbirths would have to rise to extraordinary proportions if poor health on the part of the mother were to cause the loss of enough male embryos to offset the earlier losses of females, and thus give a low sex ratio.

Returning once more to the hypothesis that high sex ratios indicate economic comfort, another objection is that practically all the people in Virkus's *Compendium of American Genealogy* belong to a relatively high level of society, as Winston himself emphasizes. Therefore the economic and social contrast between his large and small families is far less than between the two groups studied by Malins. Moreover, the children reported in *Who's Who in America* show a sex ratio of only 107.2 when all birth ranks are averaged together, in contrast to 112.0 for all those in the *Compendium of American Genealogy*. But the people in *Who's Who* come overwhelmingly from a social level even more favored than that of Winston's 5000 families. This is directly opposed to the hypothesis that groups which are favored in economic position and health have a high sex ratio because of few abortions and stillbirths. The difference between the two groups is probably due almost wholly to the greater accuracy of the data in *Who's Who*.

In searching for an explanation of Winston's interesting data as to a high sex ratio in small families and a decline in the ratio as the size of the family increases, we must not overlook what we have found as to the relation of birth rank to sex ratios. Even if no other factors played a part, we should expect families of 1 child to show a high sex ratio because they consist entirely of first births. Moreover, the rapid decline in the sex ratio among second and third births is in itself sufficient to explain a considerable part of the contrasts found by Winston between small and large families. We have seen also that in New Zealand, at least, the first births among women aged 30 to 34 show a high sex ratio. One-child families contain a high percentage in which marriage is delayed and the first birth does not occur until the mother has reached the age of 30.

From all these lines of evidence it seems that the high sex ratios found by Winston in families of 1 or 2 children indicate unfavorable rather than favorable conditions. The unfavorable conditions include (1) a high proportion of first births; (2) a high percentage of late marriages; (3) a high proportion of families which are limited by poor health on the part of the father as well as the mother. The weakness of the mother, to be sure, means many abortions which would tend toward a low sex ratio. That of the father, however, means weak spermatozoa, and therefore unusually great handicaps for the weaker type of spermatozoa which carry the X chromosome and produce females. On the other hand, in spite of Malins' British data, when women of the same age and the same duration of marriage are compared, the more privileged classes probably suffer less than the underprivileged from abortions. This is certainly true in respect to stillbirths. The small size of such losses is clearly a factor in raising the sex ratio of the privileged classes, and would tend toward a high sex ratio in Winston's small families, if they were really especially privileged. The important point, however, is that any effect produced in this way appears to be of decidedly less magnitude than the contrary effect arising from the high proportion of first-born children, late marriages, and poor health among the parents of small families.

A correct understanding of the sex ratio is so important that we may well analyze the matter still further. Table 18 summarizes the main lines of evidence on which Winston bases the conclusion that losses during pregnancy are much more important than conditions at the time of conception in determining the sex ratio at birth. The table presents averages of data which are cited as evidence that the sex ratio at birth is higher among favored than among unfavored groups.

The obvious fact about this table is that the sex ratio in each case is higher in the group which Winston considers the more favored. It would be absurd to doubt that abortions and stillbirths lower the sex ratio, but the real question is the extent of their effect compared with that of other factors. The first contrast in Table 18 is between whites

TABLE 18

SEX RATIOS AT BIRTH UNDER FAVORABLE AND UNFAVORABLE CONDITIONS, MAINLY U. S. DATA 1918–1927 AFTER WINSTON

Basis of Comparison	Favored Group		Less Favored Group		Excess of Favored over Unfavored
1. U. S. whites vs. Negroes....	White urban	106.1	Negro urban	102.4	3.7
2. U. S. whites vs. Negroes....	White rural	106.2	Negro rural	104.0	2.2
3. U. S. urban vs. rural........	Rural white	106.2	Urban white	106.1	0.1
4. U. S. urban vs. rural........	Rural Negro	104.0	Urban Negro	102.4	1.6
5. U. S. native vs. foreign parentage.................	Native white	106.2	Foreign white	105.3	0.9
6. Urban vs. rural outside U. S..	Rural	103.9	Urban	102.9	1.0
7. Legitimacy U. S., 1923–7....	Legitimate	106.1	Illegitimate	105.0	1.1

with a high sex ratio and colored people with a low ratio. This is a widespread contrast, but are abortions its cause? We have seen that the sex ratios of both whites and Negroes tend to become low instead of high under conditions where health is best and where abortions and stillbirths play the smallest part. Then, too, in the United States as a whole, the percentage of first births is higher among whites than among colored people, for the whites restrict their families far more. This alone must account for much of the difference in the sex ratios of the two races. The frequency of abortions and stillbirths among the older Negro women presumably accounts largely for the rest of the difference unless a genuine racial element is involved.

The next contrast in Table 18 is between rural and urban, the rural condition being counted by Winston as the more favorable, and hence as the reason for the higher sex ratio. Figure 54 (page 219) shows that there is no uniformity in the relation between rural and urban sex ratios among the whites of the United States. Only about half of the states or groups of states there given show the rural ratio as the higher. The slightly lower urban rate for the country as a whole is presumably due to the fact that the large cities are located mainly in areas which have low sex ratios because of their geographical location. Apparently this more than counteracts the effect of a high proportion of first births which lead to masculinity.

The next contrast in Table 18 (No. 5) is between white children of native and foreign parentage in the United States. The foreign whites have the lower ratio. This is what we should expect because their families are larger than those of the native whites and hence the proportion of first births is low. We know of no evidence that spontaneous abortions are especially numerous among them. We should expect the contrary because immigrants as a rule are vigorous. The constitutional weaklings are left in the old country. The final contrast in Table 18 is between legitimate and illegitimate births, the legitimate having the higher sex ratio. Abundant data from many countries show that generally, although by no means universally, this is the case. This may be because of a high proportion of spontaneous abortions and stillbirths among the illegitimate, but some account should be taken of the fact that illegitimacy is often the result of physical vigor and fitness for reproduction. In other words, other things being equal, people whose metabolism is perfect are more subject to the urges which produce illegitimacy than are those with poorer metabolism. But good metabolism apparently tends to lower the sex ratio.

Further light on the origin of differences in sex ratios is shed by a study of changes in the sex ratio from one period to another. If we are right as to the variation of the sex ratio according to the birth rank of the children and the age of the mother, the recent restriction of families and postponement of childbirth must have raised the sex ratio in all progressive countries. Improved conditions of health ought apparently to work in the same direction by reducing the number of abortions and stillbirths with their high percentage of males. But they appear also to work in the opposite direction by improving the general conditions of metabolism, thereby promoting equality in the conceptions of the sexes. Thus two opposing tendencies are at work.

Both of these tendencies were interrupted more or less by the World War. Figure 57 shows changes in the sex ratio of 18 regions for more than half a century. Each curve is tied by vertical lines to the horizontal line representing a sex ratio of 105. Thus one can tell at a glance not only how much the ratio in any given region has varied, but whether the ratio is high or low compared with other countries. Most of the curves, when viewed as a whole, are higher on the right than on the left, which means that since 1880 the general tendency has been toward greater masculinity. This is in harmony with what we should expect from (1) improved health, provided this results in fewer abortions and stillbirths; (2) the modern decrease in the size of families and consequent increase in the proportion of first births with their high masculinity; and (3) the modern tendency toward postponing first births for some time after marriage, thus causing the mother to be older than formerly and hence more likely to give birth to boys.

On the other hand, the recent high sex ratios disagree with what we should expect from improved health so far as this results in better metabolism and thereby favors a low primary sex ratio at the time of conception. It should be noted, however, that previous to the World War the sex ratio showed a downward tendency in many countries—France, England, Scotland, Austria, the Netherlands, Denmark, and Switzerland, as well as Italy and Japan. This may be due to

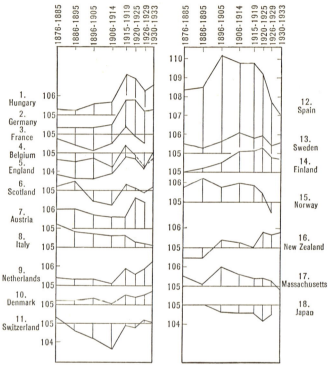

FIG. 57.—Secular Changes in Sex Ratio at Birth.

improvements in health, and hence in metabolism, before the recent great decline in the birth rate set in.

Five curves in Figure 57 show a general downward trend not only in early years, but after the World War. In Italy (Curve 8), Spain (12), Norway (15), Massachusetts (17), and Japan (18), the sex ratio is declining rather than increasing. This is in harmony with what we should expect from improved metabolism, due to better diet, hygiene, and medi-

cal practice, provided the effect of such conditions is not
neutralized by other factors such as limitation of families and
postponement of childbirth. In Italy, Spain, and Japan,
these other factors are not important, for there has been little
change in marital customs and size of families until very
recent years. Nor have the death rate and the general mode
of life changed so much as in many other countries. Therefore, an important rise in the sex ratio is not to be expected.
Moreover, in both Italy and Spain there is reason to doubt
the accuracy of the statistical data on which the curve is
based.

In Italy, as we have seen, the people have shown a strong
tendency to omit or delay the record of the birth of boys,
hoping thereby to postpone the time of military service.
This has been especially true in the south. Moreover, it
is increasingly evident in the statistics until within the last
few years. Only recently, under the influence of such men
as Professor Gini, who has contributed much to our knowledge of sex ratios, has it begun to be corrected. Thus the
steady decline in the Italian curve may be due in part to a
growing tendency of parents to postpone and sometimes to
forget the registration of births in order to postpone the
military service of their sons. Part may also be due to a
general improvement in nutrition and mode of life. A
similar situation may prevail to a slight degree in Japan, but
the departure of the Japanese curve from a horizontal line is
very slight. Such a lack of departure is what would be expected in a country where both the death rate, the birth rate,
and the mode of life have changed so little.

In Spain the apparently high sex ratio up to the World
War is probably due largely to failure to record the birth of
girls. The extent of this failure is much greater than is
commonly supposed, as we saw in studying the Jews. The
sudden drop in the sex ratio of Spain since the war is probably due to increased care in recording the births of girls
as well as boys. The Norwegian curve resembles that of
Spain, although less extreme. There, too, in the remoter vil-

lages there may have been carelessness in recording the birth of girls. The correction of this in recent years would cause the curve to swing downward. The other possibility is that changes in diet and mode of life have improved the metabolic conditions and thereby lowered the sex ratio more rapidly than changes in marriage customs and birth rates have raised it. This last supposition seems to be the only tenable one in the case of Massachusetts, for that state has unusually accurate vital statistics. It is possible that such drastic changes as the introduction of the automobile and the enormous recent increase in recreation may have a bearing on the sex ratio.

Let us turn back again to the 13 curves of Figure 57 that rise higher with the course of time. How far does this rise indicate that the modern restriction and postponement of births are having a widespread tendency to raise the sex ratio at birth? Does it mean that advances in medicine and hygiene create a favorable environment which prevents abortion and thus permits the survival of male foetuses that would previously have seen the light as abortions or stillbirths? Does it mean that males are being born in greater proportions than formerly because of the greater percentage of first births and the greater age of the average mother at the birth of her first child?

One of the most pronounced features of Figure 57 runs directly counter to the hypothesis that a favorable environment promotes a high sex ratio. This is the sudden tendency toward a high ratio during the World War, and the distinct decline thereafter in the countries most affected by the war. The upper 8 curves on the left pertain to countries which were actively engaged in the war. For 5 of them, Hungary, Germany, France, Belgium, and England, the curves are almost alike. They show relatively little change in the sex ratio previous to the war, a sudden rise during the war, and thereafter a decline which has been reversed since 1929. The general level from 1930 to 1933 was distinctly above that of pre-war times. Scotland shows the same conditions as the other war countries during and after the war, although in earlier times the ratio fell to an unusual degree.   In Austria, for some reason which we do not understand, the sex ratio jumped suddenly after the war, but not while it was in progress.   It is true that Austria has been under special stress, but not more so than some other countries, and the number of births from 1925 to 1929 was not much different from before the war.   The Italian curve as we have said, may owe its peculiar aspect to a persistent statistical error.   On the whole, however, the war countries show a sudden increase in the sex ratio during the war.

Below the war curves of Figure 57 are 3 others (Nos. 9-11) belonging to Switzerland, the Netherlands, and Denmark. These small countries did not fight during the World War, but were under great stress.   All show the same general features, namely, a decline in the sex ratio before the war, a rise like that of the combatants during the war, a slight drop in the next 5 years, and then once more a slight rise. In other words, these countries repeat the conditions of the war countries, but on a less extreme scale.   Turning to the right-hand side of Figure 57 we may omit Spain because it is probably inaccurate, and Norway because we do not understand it.   This leaves 5 curves.   Two of these, Sweden (13) and Finland (14), represent countries which were under stress during the World War, but were not so hard hit as Holland, Denmark, and Switzerland.   They both show a general rise in the sex ratio with a peak from 1920 to 1925. This rise is what one would expect, both from improvements in health and the consequent decline in spontaneous abortions and stillbirths, and from the progressive increase in the proportion of first births and in the age of mothers at the time of first births. During recent years both countries also show a slight tendency back toward the old conditions.

Lower down on the right of Figure 57 we have 3 countries —New Zealand (16), the United States (Massachusetts) (17), and Japan (18)—which took part in the World War, but were so far away that they did not suffer the kind of privation that occurred in Europe. We have already suggested that improvements in diet, hygiene, and metabolism may have been a probable cause of the downward tendency in Massachusetts and Japan. The important point here is that these countries show no appreciable effect of the war. Thus the extent to which the countries of Figure 57 show a peak during the World War is in fairly close harmony with the degree to which they suffered.

New Zealand seems at first sight to contradict the last statement, for it shows a marked drop in the sex ratio during the war. As a matter of fact, such a drop confirms our suspicion that the high sex ratio in western Europe during the war is the result of adverse conditions of metabolism. The New Zealand curve behaves just as one would expect. During the World War that remote country did not suffer from lack of food, or from any of the immediate horrors of war. Its young men, however, were away in large numbers for a long time. Hence a great many marriages were postponed and first births declined in number. This would naturally lower the sex ratio. When the young men returned home many marriages took place, first births became numerous, and the sex ratio jumped to a high level. A low sex ratio in New Zealand during the war is by no means inconsistent with the idea that the high ratio in the war-ridden countries of Europe arose mainly from an unfavorable physiological situation engendered by malnutrition, anxiety, and other unhealthful conditions. The absence of the young men there, as well as in New Zealand, must have reduced the sex ratio somewhat, but the privations of war apparently more than balanced this and caused the ratio to rise.

The evidence presented in the last three chapters seems to agree in suggesting that a low sex ratio generally indicates favorable conditions, but may have an opposite significance. The conclusion is the same no matter whether we consider climate, weather, birth rank, the age of the mother, racial differences, size of families, economic condition, or war. The primary determinant of the sex ratio appears to be the health of the parents. If their health were perfect the numbers of the two sexes would apparently be equal. At the time of conception the spermatozoa that bear the X and Y chromosomes would have equal chances of reaching the ova. At a later stage, during pregnancy there would be no losses through abortion and stillbirth. The degree to which reproductive efficiency departs from this ideal depends partly upon weather and climate. The more nearly these approach the conditions that are indicated as most favorable by other lines of investigation, the more nearly the two sexes are conceived and born in equal numbers. Taking the world as a whole, the geographical distribution of sex ratios seems to depend on climate more than upon any other single factor. Diet, however, appears to be an important modifying factor. A good diet with the right amount of vitamin E acts like a good climate to keep the sex ratio near 100.

Even if the weather, the climate, and the diet were perfect, the sex ratio would vary for several other reasons. One of these is the age of the mother and the consequent degree of difficulty experienced by the X chromosomes in reaching the ova. Before the female reproductive organs have reached their most effective condition, the difficulty appears to be great. The sex ratio which thus results is high and remains high even at birth because of the comparatively small number of abortions which terminate first pregnancies. Many stillbirths at the end of first pregnancies, however, oppose these two tendencies but are not sufficient to give a low sex ratio. With second and third births, the difficulties of the X chromosomes apparently decline, abortions do not increase much, and stillbirths fall to a low level. Hence the sex ratio is low among second, third, and even fourth births. Thereafter the increasing age of the mother seems to cause greater difficulty for the X chromosomes, and the sex ratio rises. This last tendency, however, is in turn opposed by an increasing frequency of both abortions and stillbirths as mothers advance in age. Thus the sex ratio of births beyond the sixth or seventh tends to be low except among people who are unusually well fed and cared for.

Economic conditions and war also play an important part in determining the sex ratio. Poor economic conditions apparently mean a high primary ratio at the time of conception, because they are accompanied by poor health which means difficulty for the X chromosomes. But these same poor economic conditions give rise to a tendency toward a lowering of the sex ratio at birth by reason of the more numerous abortions and stillbirths which accompany them. War acts in the same way. It disturbs reproduction not only by taking away the young men, but also by poor food, hardship, and mental strain. The rise in the sex ratio during the World War was presumably due mainly to failure of the X chromosomes at the time of conception, for it does not seem probable that abortions and stillbirths were diminished by the hardships of that period. Other factors, such as seasonal migrations, also influence the sex ratio, and there are doubtless many more that we have not even mentioned.

In concluding this chapter let us go back to the seasonal variations in the sex ratio with which we began. In Figure 42 (page 196) the most conspicuous curve is that of Japan. Therefore let us attempt a final explanation of it in the light of the fuller knowledge which we have gained in the last three chapters. Japan, it will be remembered, is very extreme in the seasonal range not only of its sex ratio but also of births and deaths. May and June are the culmination of several months of almost ideal weather. By that time, also, the deficiencies of the rice diet that prevails in winter have been considerably alleviated by the addition of green vegetables. The weather and diet together are such that in June the health of the Japanese is at its best (Figure 20, page 85). For that reason, and because the late spring or early summer is the optimum season according to the basic animal rhythm of reproduction, we should expect both a large number of conceptions and a low primary sex ratio. It will be recalled, however, that the rate of stillbirths, and presumably of abortions, is very high in Japan, and is at a maximum during the summer. The weather from July to September is very exhausting, especially to women. Embryos conceived in May and June are then at the stage of development when they normally perish in greatest number through abortion. Curve K of Figure 42 (page 196) makes it clear that the secondary sex ratio at birth among the Japanese children conceived in June and born in March falls to only 99.8. This extremely low ratio seems to find a full and satisfactory explanation as the joint result of (1) an unusually high percentage of female conceptions in June because of the highly favorable conditions during the preceding month or two, and (2) an unusual number of male abortions from July to September because of the very unfavorable weather.

Turning now to high sex ratios, we should expect the primary ratio in Japan to be high among conceptions a month or two after the climax of poor health arising from the hot, moist summer. The maximum would presumably occur among the embryos arising from reproductive cells which began to mature when people were weakest. September is the worst month, and the reproductive cells which then developed would presumably take part in conception during October or November. These in turn would lead to births in July and August, and, sure enough, Curve K in Figure 42 shows a maximum in August. The winter diet of Japan, however, is very poor, and is presumably lacking in the reproductive vitamin E, as well as in other respects. Therefore the worst conditions for conception probably occur somewhat later than would be expected on the basis of the weather alone. This may bring them in January and February, when cool or cold weather adds another depressing effect. This would lead to a high percentage of males among the conceptions at that time. The dangerous early months of pregnancy for these conceptions, however, coincide with the period of especially favorable weather and good health from March to June. Thus abortions would presumably be at a minimum among embryos in which males already greatly predominated. Hence from October to December the births resulting from conceptions from January to March would have a high sex ratio not only because few females were conceived, but also because few males were lost. This agrees with what we find in Curve K of Figure 42 (page 196), where the main maximum of masculinity occurs among births in November and December. Putting climate, diet, health, and abortions together in this way we find a satisfactory explanation of seasonal fluctuations of the sex ratio which would otherwise be extremely puzzling. Climate, weather, and diet thus fall into reasonable positions as important factors which co-operate in a highly complex fashion with other factors such as the age of the mother and the general economic status. It would be a mistake to magnify the climatic factor unduly, but in studying sex ratios, as in many other problems, it would be an equally grave mistake to overlook it.

CHAPTER XII

SURVIVAL AND INHERITANCE

In previous chapters we have concluded that a great body
of facts can be explained only on the hypothesis that the
human species inherits a highly complex adjustment to season
and climate. We have also been led to inquire whether
this inherited adjustment is so strong that its primitive form
remains evident even when migration to a new climate renders the original adjustment no longer the most favorable.
In order to get light on this problem we shall present three
diverse sets of data. The first deals with variations in the
number of spermatozoa from season to season. The second
shows how far the different parts of the world agree in their
seasonal distribution of conceptions. The third investigates
the death rate at various ages, and sheds light not only upon
the conditions of weather under which infants survive, but
also upon the peculiar quality of people's climatic responses
during the period of reproduction. All three lines of evidence indicate that human beings are more sensitive to
weather and climate than has commonly been supposed.
They also seem to point to a very deep-seated type of inheritance which causes certain specific climatic conditions to be
favorable for widely different types of people, but which is
slowly modified when people migrate into new climates.

It is highly desirable to investigate seasonal changes in
human reproduction by means of other criteria in addition
to the birth rate. By taking samples of semen from the same
individual at frequent and regular intervals during a period
of 2 years, Belding (1937) has discovered that there seem to
be seasonal fluctuations in the number of spermatozoa
(Figure 58). He finds that the spermatozoa are most numerous in December (births in February), decline to a mini-

mum in March (births in June), rise to a second maximum in May (August), and then fall to a main minimum in August (November). Comparing this curve of reproductive vigor with the number of conceptions in Massachusetts from 1915 to 1934, he concludes that there is a real relation between the two. The seasonal swing in the birth rate appears to be the direct result of a physiological swing whereby the number of spermatozoa ebbs and flows with the seasons. Belding recognizes the danger of generalizing from a single short record. Nevertheless, his results are significant, both because they represent a first attempt at a new line of investigation and because they agree with the results which have been obtained by other methods.

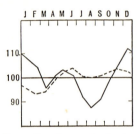

FIG. 58. — Seasonal Variation in Number of Spermatozoa and in Conceptions. After Belding.

Although the curve of spermatozoa in Figure 58 differs considerably from that of conceptions, there is a certain resemblance. It seems quite probable that if data for thousands of men were available the curve of spermatozoa would agree with that of conceptions. If this should prove to be the case, it would lead to two important conclusions. The first is that, although geographical and other variations in the birth rate for the year as a whole depend largely upon cultural habits, variations in the birth rate from season to season are strongly influenced by changes in the number and presumably the vigor of germ cells produced in the male. There is some evidence of corresponding variation in the maturation of ova in the female, but a study of this would carry us too far into the field of physiology. The second conclusion would be that the seasonal swing in reproductive vigor is not the same as the corresponding swing in health. The lowest point in the curve of spermatozoa comes in August, at a time when health, under our modern conditions, is at its best.

Our next problem resolves itself into two questions. First, to what extent are the weather conditions which promote conceptions the same in different parts of the world? We have already discussed this somewhat, but we shall here summarize all the available data in a single series of graphs. In the second place, how far does the seasonal distribution of births depend upon the weather at the time of conception as compared with the time of birth? Inasmuch as temperature appears to be by far the most important element of the weather, we shall confine ourselves to it. Our first step in answering both questions is to select seasonal curves of births from as wide a geographical range as possible in order to represent all types of climate. Confining ourselves to the data illustrated graphically in this book, we find 84 available curves of the seasonal distribution of births. Their geographical distribution is as follows:

Northwestern Europe (France to Finland) 12
Central Europe (Italy to Germany) 9
Russia 13
United States and Canada 26*
Japan 6
Australia 6
South Africa and temperate South America 7
Egypt, India, Mexico, and Central America 5

* These 26 include two curves from New York State, one being urban and thus mainly representing New York City, and the other rural so that it mainly represents the upper part of the state. By mistake, two different curves for the state of Mississippi were included in our tabulations. As this was not discovered until Figure 59 was ready for the printer, it has not been corrected, and the number of curves is stated in the text as 84, although the number of regions is only 83. This makes no appreciable difference in our results.

Where several curves from the same region are available, the latest has generally been chosen, although in a few cases a combination of two has been used because the maximum was especially clear in one and the minimum in the other. Since there are 84 curves, the number of months on which they are based is 1008 (84 x 12).

The curves having been selected, the next step was to tabulate the 1008 months according to their mean temperature. The result is illustrated in the upper diagram in

Figure 59. An average temperature of 17° C. (17.0–17.9) is there seen to be characteristic of 64 months. This does not mean 64 regions, for in some places such a temperature prevails for two months in midsummer, and in others during

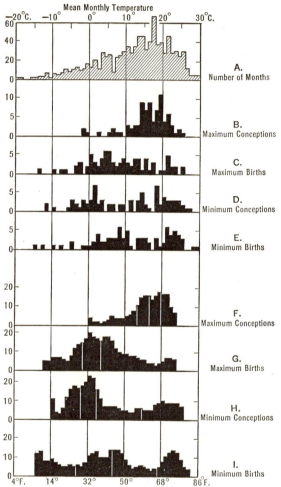

Fɪɢ. 59.—Summary of Relation between Births and Temperature.

one month when the temperature is rising and one month when it is falling. The highest mean temperature, 29° C. (84° F.), was experienced 5 times, and the lowest, −19° C. (−10° F.), only once.

In order to see how the mean temperature is related to births we next make the tabulations illustrated in the other sections of Figure 59. The first (*B*) shows the number of regions in which conceptions were at a maximum during months with any given temperature. This occurred twice, for example, in months with a mean temperature of −1° C. (−1.0 to −1.9) but never during the 86 months when the temperature was below that level. It occurred most frequently (11 times) when the temperature averaged 19° C. (66° F.). In warmer weather the maximum of births occurred only once during the 31 months when the temperature averaged 25° C. (77° F.) and never during the 27 months with still higher temperatures.

Diagram *C* for the temperature when births were at a maximum shows much less concentration at one particular level than does Curve *B*. The 86 months with temperatures averaging below −1° C., for example, include 9 in which the number of births was at a maximum for the region in question. Such a maximum occurred most frequently at temperatures of 4° and 5° C. (6 times each).

Turning to the minimum of reproduction, we find that the tendency toward concentration in any one season is less than with the maximum. In Curve *D*, showing the number of months when the minimum number of conceptions occurred with any given temperature, there is great irregularity, and it is hard to determine at what temperature the greatest concentration occurs. The same is more or less true of Curve *E*, representing the relation of months of minimum births to temperature.

Taken as a whole, the data of Sections *B* to *E* in Figure 59 suggest the following conclusions: (1) the maximum number of conceptions tends to occur at temperatures from 14° to 20° C.; (2) the maximum of births is more likely to occur at temperatures of 0° to 6°, and (3) the minimum of both conceptions and births occurs without much reference to the weather.

In order to make sure whether these conclusions are warranted, it is necessary to express the data of Sections C to E as percentages of Section A. This prevents any one type of climate from exerting an undue influence, and thus enables us to determine whether the high level of B, for example, at temperatures of 14° to 20° is anything more than a reflection of the fact that months with those temperatures happen to be numerous in our 84 regions. It is also desirable to get rid of the irregularities which are almost inevitable when a number no larger than 1008 is divided among so great a range of temperatures. Accordingly, before expressing Sections B to E as percentages of Section A, the data of all 5 sections were smoothed by the formula:

$$\frac{a+2b+3c+2d+e}{9} = c'$$

This enables us to draw Sections F to I where we get a true picture of the degree to which the maxima and minima of births and conceptions tend to be concentrated in months with any given temperature. In order to bring out the facts more clearly each section has been divided into quartiles by means of white bars. Thus one sees at a glance not only the degree to which there is concentration in any given range of temperature, but the median temperature above and below which the number of cases is the same.

Sections F to I of Figure 59 indicate at once that the maximum of conceptions tends to be concentrated within a few degrees of temperature. The method employed in their construction shows what would happen if months with each degree of temperature within the entire range shown in Figure 66 (–19° to 29° C.) were equally numerous. In 62 per cent of all cases the month with the maximum of conceptions would have a temperature of 14° to 21.9° C. (57.2 to 71.6° F.) even if cold and hot months were as well represented as months of medium temperature. This percentage would presumably be increased if we could make allowance for the fact that in hot regions, such as Panama, Salvador, and Bengal, there are no months cooler than 22°. It seems highly probable that, if these places experienced cooler weather, the maximum of conceptions would come at that time, for as things now are, it occurs at the lowest possible temperatures. Still another point to consider is that cultural agencies such as migration, fasts, and seasons of marriage tend to blur the effect of the weather. If their effect, as well as that of the regions where the temperature is always high, could be eliminated, Section F of Figure 59 would presumably show a distinct peak at a temperature between 14° and 21° C. (57° and 68° F.).

Even more significant, perhaps, is the fact that the median temperature at which the maximum of conceptions occurs is 16.6° C. (62° F.). This should be compared with the optimum temperature as determined in other ways. Among thousands of factory operatives whose work was measured during a series of years, I found that the most rapid and accurate work was done when the mean temperature for day and night averaged 60° F. Other studies of work and fatigue in the United States, England, and Japan give approximately the same result. (Huntington, 1924, 1935; Yagi, 1933). Millions of deaths in many countries show that the death rate is lowest and health is best when the mean temperature is about 63° F. Common experience indicates that we feel most comfortable in temperatures ranging from about 66° to 72° F., according to the relative humidity of the air. Such temperatures occur during the working hours of the day when the mean temperature for day and night together is about 63°. Carefully controlled laboratory experiments in rooms where the atmospheric conditions can be exactly regulated confirm our common experience (Yaglou, 1928). Studies of the relation of temperature to recovery after operations point to a similar importance of a mean daily temperature between 60° and 65° F. (16° to 18° C.) (Huntington, 1920). Thus a great body of evidence indicates that such temperatures are best for the great majority of people in many diverse parts of the earth. They stimulate conception, especially when the temperature is rising rather than falling;

they provide the maximum feeling of comfort; they stimulate people to the most rapid and accurate work; and they are accompanied by the best health, fewest illnesses, and lowest death rate.

The temperatures most frequently associated with the maximum of births are lower than those associated with the maximum of conceptions, as is evident in Section G. In comparing Section G and the others of its kind (F to I) with one another, the fact that the total shaded area is greater in some sections than in others must be disregarded. This is an accidental and inconsequential result of reducing the data of Sections B to E to percentages of A. Each section represents the same number of months. The essential points to be noted are: first, the relative heights of the different parts of each section individually; second, the number of degrees of temperature over which each section spreads; third, the number of degrees of temperature occupied by each quartile as indicated by the white lines; and fourth, the location of the median as indicated by the central white line.

Looking at the matter in this way we see that the maximum of births, as distinguished from that of conceptions, tends to be concentrated in months with temperatures ranging from $-2°$ C. to $7°$ C. ($28.4°$ to $44.6°$ F.), with a peak at zero. The concentration, however, is by no means so pronounced as in the case of conceptions. This is evident when one notes that Section G extends over a much greater range of temperature than does F, its left-hand end being $12°$ C. below the corresponding part of C. Another evidence of this same thing is that the two middle quartiles of G extend over $11.5°$ C., whereas those of F. extend over only $6.6°$ C. The same fact becomes still more impressive when we note that three-quarters of all the maximum months of conception have a mean temperature of $13°$ to $22°$ C., whereas in order to include three-quarters of the months of maximum births we must include temperatures from $-5°$ to $16°$, a total of $21°$ in contrast to only $9°$. It seems quite clear that the weather, or at least the temperature, at the time of conception has a great deal of influence upon the number of births.

In Section *H* of Figure 59 the minimum of conception shows a distinct tendency to occur at low temperatures, or else in less-pronounced fashion at high temperatures. We also note that the minimum of conceptions occurs under as great a range of temperature as does the maximum of births. Perhaps the most noteworthy feature of Section *H* is its comparative uniformity from a temperature of 4° C. upward. The final section of Figure 59 (*I*) suggests that the season at which the minimum number of births occurs has no appreciable relation to temperature. It covers a much wider range of temperature than any of the three sections above it— 42° on the Centigrade scale in contrast to only 24° in Section *F*. Moreover, it rises to three almost equal peaks, no one of which appears to have any special significance.

The upshot of the whole matter seems to be that the weather influences the seasonal distribution of births mainly because there is a strong tendency for the maximum of conceptions to occur when the mean temperature is not greatly above or below 62° F. (17° C.) and a much less distinct tendency for the minimum to occur at temperatures below 37° F. (3° C.). This distribution of conceptions must inevitably cause some concentration of births at special temperatures, especially maximum births at temperatures somewhat above freezing. Such concentration, however, is far less conspicuous than the corresponding concentration of maximum conceptions. It appears to be systematic only in the way that the chips which fall from the chisel of the wood-turner are systematically piled up on the floor.

This raises an interesting question. Does the maximum of conceptions coincide with the optimum temperature for health because health is best at that time, or is health best because that is the time most favorable for conception? There is a real and important distinction between these two alternatives. According to the first alternative, some unknown set of conditions has caused mankind in general to be so constituted that health is best when the temperature for day and night together averages about 63° F. (17° C), or perhaps it is better to say 60° to 70° in order to cover a wide range of regions. Therefore, conceptions are especially numerous when the temperature rises to that level. According to the other alternative, conceptions which occurred among primitive people when the temperature averaged about 63° F. resulted in children who were especially likely to survive because they were born at the time of year most favorable for abundant food and for resistance to the dangers of diseases incident to the seasons. Therefore, human types which were stimulated to conceive prolifically when the temperature averaged 63° had a stronger tendency to survive than the types which conceived most prolifically at some other temperature. Thus, little by little, a process of selection worked in such a way that human types which felt especially vigorous when the temperature rose to an average of 63° in the spring survived and became dominant, while those which were most vigorous at other temperatures were gradually eliminated. According to this second alternative, the necessities of the infant have fixed upon man a definite optimum of temperature.

The first alternative, it will be remembered, supposes that some unknown condition has imposed upon mankind, as upon other animals, a certain definite optimum in respect to temperatures. When that optimum occurs, reproduction becomes active. The second alternative supposes that among human beings, and likewise among animals, the optimum temperature is that which prevails at the time when conception will lead to birth at the season best fitted to insure the survival of the young. In other words, the primitive type from which modern races of men are mainly derived is supposed to have lived for a long time in some special type of climate. In that climate the infants who were conceived when the average temperature rose to between 60° and 70° F. had a better chance of survival than any others. Therefore, the parents who were stimulated to reproductive activity by such temperatures were able to bring up more children than were the parents who were stimulated by other temperatures. This process, going on for generation after generation, is supposed to have fixed in the human race a very definite optimum of climate. It seems to us that this view is more reasonable than the other.

This conclusion can be tested by certain old data on deaths in Belgium. In order to discover the exact nature of the response of young children to the seasons, I searched for data as to the deaths of infants in each calendar month and at every age from 1 month upward. The only tables of this kind which I was able to find were those of Belgium from 1844 to 1850. Fortunately, the tables present every evidence of being of high quality statistically. They pertain to one of the most healthful climates in any part of the world, and to a country which we have already selected for special study because of its good statistics. Less complete tables dealing with deaths in each calendar month by years of age were published in Scotland, New York City, and other places at about the same time as the Belgian statistics, but they do not give data according to both calendar months and months of life. The Belgium data show the number of deaths during January, February, and so forth among infants aged 1 month, 2 months, and so on up to the end of the first year of life, and then among those aged 12 to 15 months, 16 to 18, and so forth for periods of 3 months during the second year. Thereafter, up to 10 years of age, the data are for single years of life and then for 5-year periods.

It may seem strange that such exact and highly detailed tables were published so long ago, whereas in recent times no data whatever for deaths by both age and month are published in most countries. The reason is that a century ago, when vital statistics began to be published, the diagnosis of disease was very imperfect. It was evident to everyone, however, that deaths varied greatly from season to season. Therefore, the vital statisticians centered their interest upon the meteorological relationships of death. Evidence of a similar emphasis upon physical environment is afforded by numerous books on medical climatology, mineral springs, and health resorts which were published during the first half of the nineteenth century. This early interest in the influence of the physical environment was almost extinguished by the discoveries of Darwin. At any rate, his illuminating work, followed by that of Pasteur and others, switched the center of medical interest to specific diseases, parasitic infections, and physiological processes. Correct diagnosis became the main object of the physician. Hence, modern mortality tables show the number of deaths from several hundred specific diseases in great detail. The tables are as elaborate as those of old Belgium showing the deaths according to the seasons, but none, so far as I am aware, tabulate the deaths according to both age and month.

The Belgian figures for deaths by months, sex, and age are so interesting and suggestive that the data for the 6 years 1844 to 1845 and 1847 to 1850, which are the only ones to which I have had access, are fully illustrated in Figures 60 and 66. It is almost impossible to grasp their significance unless they are expressed in graphic form. In Figure 60, as in Figures 62, 64, and 65, the average number of deaths per day in any given month for males and females combined is represented by 200. Hence 100 represents the normal number of deaths that would occur in each sex if the two sexes were equal in numbers and if the death rate were uniform at all seasons. Solid lines indicate the actual deaths of males expressed as percentages of this normal; dotted lines represent deaths of females. Solid black shading indicates that there were more deaths of males than of females, and has been inserted where the solid, or male, line lies above the dotted, or female, line. Shading by means of horizontal lines indicates that the deaths of females were more numerous than those of males. Diagonal lines indicate periods during which the deaths of both males and females were below the average. This last type of shading is added simply to make the diagram easier to read.

The most surprising feature of these Belgian diagrams is the way in which the form of the seasonal curve varies from age to age. If Belgium is typical of the human species as a whole, and we believe that it is, the response of human beings to the seasons varies greatly according to age. This is so important that we may well examine the whole series of curves in order to determine the nature of the change from age to age. We believe that these changes are probably typical of many other countries and periods because the relation between deaths and the seasons which prevailed in Belgium a century ago was essentially the same as that which now prevails both there and in many other countries.

The upper left-hand pair of curves in Figure 60 represents stillborn infants—that is, deaths at the time of birth. There is a regular but moderate swing from an index number of about 114 in February to approximately 92 in July. In the winter when cold weather causes the general death rate to be highest, stillbirths are also at a maximum, and females predominate among them. In summer, when a close approach to the optimum temperature is associated with the lowest general death rate and the health of the mother is best, there are few stillbirths, and boys predominate among them.

The remaining sections of Figure 60, aside from the section showing stillbirths, are very interesting because of the way in which the response to the weather changes according to the age of the infants. The section for deaths during the first month of life shows that the seasons have much more effect upon the health of living infants during the first month of life than upon stillbirths. Throughout January, February, and March, the deaths among such infants stand at the high level of 136, according to our index numbers. Then they fall rapidly, and in July number about 78. Thereafter they once more increase. The seasons of maximum and minimum are the same as among stillbirths, but the effect of cold weather is prolonged, and the contrast between the seasons is increased almost threefold. It is evident that in old Bel-

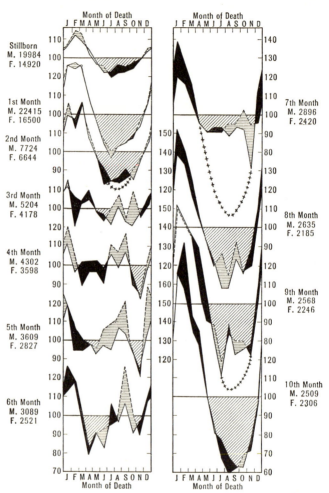

Fig. 60.—Deaths by Month and Sex in Belgium, 1844–1850. Ages 1–10 months unsmoothed.

gium cold weather was very unfavorable to infants during the first months of life, and warm weather very favorable. In this first month of life the deaths of the two sexes were practically equal in number, as is indicated by the way in which the solid and dotted lines coincide.

In the second month of life the response of the Belgium children to the weather is somewhat different from what it

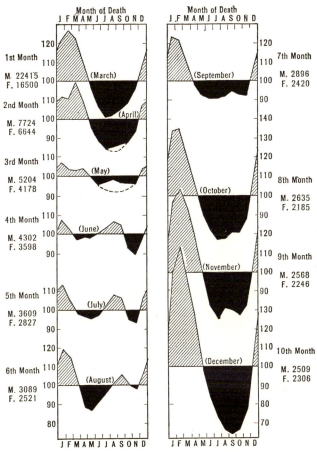

Fig. 61.—Deaths by Month and Sex in Belgium, 1844–1850. Ages 1–10 months smoothed.

was in the first month. January, February, and March are still the months of greatest mortality, but the number of deaths is proportionately not so great, for the effect of cold weather is not quite so bad as it was earlier. This is more clearly evident in Figure 61, where the two sexes have been combined and the resulting curves have been smoothed by the formula $\dfrac{a+2b+c}{4} = b'$. Inasmuch as stillbirths are omitted in Figure 61, its upper curve corresponds to the second pair of curves in Figure 60. It must be remembered that the total number of deaths is only about one-third as great in the second month of life as in the first, as is evident from the numbers beside the various curves. Our diagrams make no attempt to show this. In Figure 61, as in most of our diagrams, the number 100 means the average number of deaths per day during the year as a whole at the particular age in question, regardless of whether deaths were few or many.

The most notable difference between the first and the second months as illustrated in Figures 60 and 61 is that the period of few deaths in summer lasts longer—June to October—among the infants who are in the second month of life than among those in the first month. Even in November the death rate is still below the average for the year. One would expect the death rate to follow the line of little crosses in Figure 60, or the dotted line in Figure 61, thus giving a curve resembling that of the first month and of later months such as the tenth. The departure from what would be expected is slight and would not be important were it not that it seems to be a forerunner of a much greater departure in succeeding months.

The way in which both curves for the third month in Figure 60 waver up and down, but never get far from the line marked 100, appears to indicate a biological change as infants grow older. The differences between the death rates at one season and another in this third month of life are so small that February, July, and October all have minima of about equal depth, while January, April, August, and October all show approximately equal maxima. The true state of affairs can best be judged from Figure 61, where the two sexes have been combined and the resulting curve has been smoothed, thus getting rid of minor irregularities due to the shortness of available records. There we see that the response of infants to the seasons during the third month of life differs from the response during the two preceding months mainly because the great swing from a high winter maximum to a low summer minimum almost disappears.

Two new features also appear in the death rates of infants at this time. The first is a tendency toward a maximum of deaths in summer as well as in winter. In the unsmoothed curves of Figure 60 this is clearly evident, and in the smoothed curve of Figure 61 it leaves a wide space between the dotted line and the shading. The other new feature is an excess of deaths of girls in comparison with boys during the summer, as appears from the areas shaded with horizontal lines in Figure 60.

The three features of the death rate which have just been mentioned as characteristic of the third month of life do not appear to be accidental, for they are foreshadowed in the second month and repeated in later months. They reach a maximum development at some time from the third to the fifth month, and then disappear gradually. Two of them, namely, the small amplitude of the mortality curve from season to season, and the double maximum in both winter and summer, can be seen most readily from Figure 61. To begin with the variation from season to season, note that the smoothed curve of deaths during the first month of life makes a very regular swing from a maximum in February to a minimum in July, and back again. The second month tries, as it were, to do likewise, but meets with a slight interruption in both winter and summer. In the third month of life, the winter maximum and the summer minimum of deaths have both been reduced to small proportions. In fact, the sharp peak displayed in February by the curve of deaths during the first month of life has been replaced by a slight hollow, while the pronounced minimum in July is replaced by a slight bend in the opposite direction. Thus, the curve as a whole becomes relatively flat.

Going on to later months, we see that among the 4-month infants the winter peak has been still further reduced, and has been surpassed in size by a rapidly increasing summer peak culminating in August. The curve still remains quite flat. Among 5-month infants, the winter begins to increase once more, but the August peak still retains its size, and the curve is still quite flat. With infants in their sixth month, however, the winter maximum again becomes dominant, the August maximum (now in September) loses ground, and the contrast between the unfavorable winter and the favorable spring begins to assume something of its early importance, although by no means equal to the contrast between February and July among infants during their first months of life.

From the seventh month onward the changes which became apparent among children 6 months of age become steadily more pronounced. Among infants in their tenth month, the maximum of deaths has returned to February and is very pronounced. The summer maximum, on the other hand, has completely disappeared in Figure 61 and is indicated by merely a hint in Figure 60. Thus, in their tenth month of life infants show a perfect curve of deaths whose only essential difference from that of the 1-month-olds is its much greater extremes and the location of the summer minimum in September instead of July. Of course, the number of deaths in the tenth month is only about one-eighth as great as in the first, but the point that we are now interested in is the relative difference between the deaths at one season and another. Among deaths during the first month of life, the range in the smoothed curves is from 81 in July to 126 in February—45 points; during the third month of life the weather has so little effect that the difference between the maximum and minimum in Figure 61 falls to 11; in the tenth month, on the contrary, this rises to the enormous figure of 98. Although infants at the end of their first year of life have a far lower death rate than those at the beginning, their sensitiveness to variations in the weather has greatly increased.

The relative number of deaths of the two sexes is still a third condition which changes systematically as the Belgian infants grow older. In spite of the irregularity of Figure 60, the black shading shows that on the whole more boys than girls die during the winter and spring, and even during the fall, especially from the age of 6 months onward. Nevertheless, during the summer, especially from the third to the eighth months, the deaths of girls rise considerably above those of boys, as appears from the areas that are shaded horizontally in Figure 60. This looks as if digestive troubles and heat were more fatal to infant girls than to boys, but why this should be so we do not know.

Before attempting to explain the systematic way in which increasing age is correlated with variations in the seasonal distribution of deaths among young infants, let us examine Figure 62 to see what happens after the tenth month of life. The first two sections of Figure 62 show that during the eleventh and twelfth months of life the seasonal fluctuations in the death rate are approximately as great as in the tenth month. The only difference is that the maximum of deaths passes from February to March, while the minimum is retarded until October among children in the twelfth month of life. The next section tells us that during the first quarter of the second year of life (the thirteenth to the fifteenth months) the range from maximum to minimum diminishes appreciably, and both the maximum and minimum occur a little later than among younger infants. In the next stage of life (the sixteenth to the eighteenth months) the maximum number of deaths still occurs in March or April, and the minimum in October or November, but the range from maximum to minimum diminishes to not much more than half its previous amount. This is a repetition of what happened a year earlier in the life of the child. The flattening of the mortality curves during the second year is not so great as in the first, but it is of the same general type and occurs approximately 12 months later. If data for individual months of life from the sixteenth to the eighteenth were

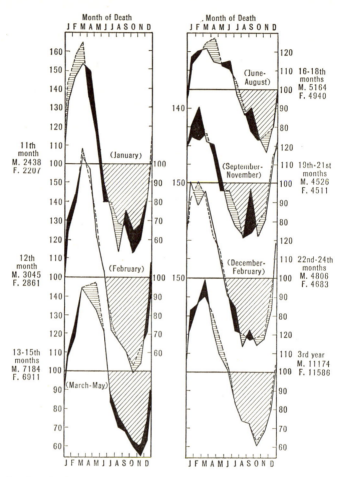

Fig. 62.—Deaths by Month and Sex in Belgium, 1844–1850. Ages 11 months to 3 years unsmoothed.

available, we might find that one of them gives a curve of death which is flatter than the average of the three, as given in Figure 62.

Be that as it may, the fact remains that among children 16

to 18 months of age the smoothed seasonal curve of deaths
ranges from 77 in October to 122 in March, or a total difference of 45, whereas the corresponding curve for the 3
preceding months ranges from 61 in September to 152 in
February, or a total difference of 91. Six months later, however, among children aged 22 to 24 months, the range has
risen again, for the difference between a minimum of 64
in September and a maximum of 145 in February amounts
to 81. Thus, the flattening of the seasonal curve of deaths
which occurs among Belgian children from the third to the
sixth month recurs a year later. Not only this, but the summer peak among children aged 3 to 7 months has a slight
counterpart in a similar peak among children aged 19 to 21
months. Inasmuch as the counterpart is separated from the
original by 13 or 14 months, instead of 12, and occurs among
boys rather than girls, we are in doubt as to how much
weight to attach to it. There can be little doubt, however,
as to the reality of the flattening of the curve of deaths from
the third to the sixth months of life and again a year later.
No matter what the season of birth may have been, these Belgian children were able to resist the influence of the weather
to an unusual degree when they were 3 to 6 months old,
and again when they had lived another year and were 14
to 18 months old.

Having seen the nature of the variation in the seasonal
incidence of deaths during successive months of infancy, we
next inquire what effect this has upon survival. Does it
promote the survival of any one type of infant rather than of
another? In order to test this let us compare the actual death
rate of Belgian infants born in the various calendar months
with the rate that would have prevailed among those same
infants if the seasonal distribution of deaths in every month
of the first year of life had been the same as the average for
all children under 5 years of age. In order to get the actual
death rate, we start with the number of deaths recorded for
each calendar month among infants under 1 month of age.
To the January deaths of this sort, for example, we add the

February deaths of children in the second month of life, the March deaths of those in the third month, and so on to the end of the first year. We thus find how many children who were born in January died within 12 months. Other months are treated in the same way. The result is Curve *A* at the bottom of Figure 63, which shows the percentage of deaths during the first year among children born in each calendar month.

Curve *B* is the same as *A* except that it covers the deaths

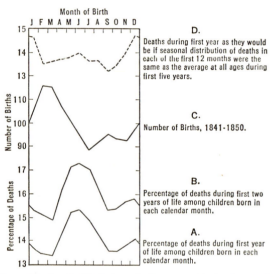

Month of Birth
J F M A M J J A S O N D

D.
Deaths during first year as they would be if seasonal distribution of deaths in each of the first 12 months were the same as the average at all ages during first five years.

C.
Number of Births, 1841-1850.

B.
Percentage of deaths during first two years of life among children born in each calendar month.

A.
Percentage of deaths during first year of life among children born in each calendar month.

Fig. 63.—Effect of Infantile Variations in Power to Resist Seasonal Handicaps in Belgium.

during the first 2 years of life. Compare these with Curve *C*, showing the number of children born each month. It is obvious that in general the chances of survival among these Belgian children varied directly as the number of births. Among children born in February and March, at the time of maximum births according to the basic animal rhythm, the percentage of deaths is very low; among those born in July, when births are least numerous, the death rate was very high. This may be in part because the infants born at the peak of the animal rhythm are stronger than the others, as we have seen from the greater length of life as shown in previous chapters. But it is also because of the peculiar changes in the seasonal distribution of births from one month to another during early infancy.

If the seasonal distribution of deaths were the same in all the early months of life, and if it agreed with the average distribution of all deaths under 5 years of age, the deaths during the first year of life among children born in the various calendar months would vary as in Curve *D*. A comparison of this with Curves *C* and *A* makes it evident that the peculiar flattening of the seasonal curves from the third to the sixth months of life has a distinct tendency toward the survival of infants who are born in harmony with the basic animal rhythm. In a country with hot summers this condition would presumably be much more important than in one like Belgium where the summer temperature closely approaches the optimum. In a warm climate the months of life from the third to the fifth or sixth are the time when children born in February or March are especially exposed to the great dangers arising from heat and especially from the accompanying digestive diseases. The names of the months attached to the various diagrams in Figures 61 and 62 make it easy to see how the flattening of the curves is related to the welfare of infants born in March at the height of the basic animal rhythm. Among primitive people the dangers of summer are very great. In many cases a quarter, a third, or even half the children die during the first year of life. Under such circumstances any condition which favors one special group more than another becomes of special importance and is likely to become established as an hereditary factor. The flatness of the Belgian curves from the third to the sixth months of life suggests that man has become endowed with an hereditary trait of this sort so that infants born according to the basic animal rhythm are less susceptible than others to the great danger of hot weather.

Let us now pass on to the years beyond infancy and see what more we can learn from the seasonal distribution of deaths in old Belgium. The period from the third to the fifteenth year, as illustrated in the final section of Figure 62 and in Figure 64, need not detain us long. All the curves

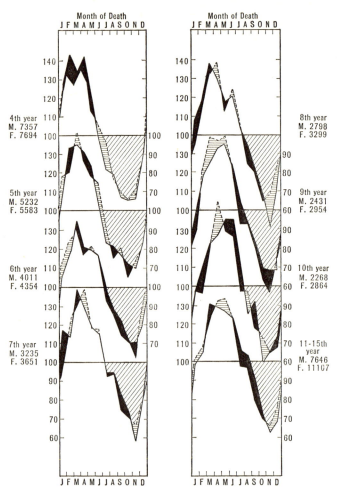

FIG. 64.—Deaths by Month and Sex in Belgium, 1844–1850. Ages 4–15 years unsmoothed.

are of essentially the same form, and their range, when smoothed to eliminate minor irregularities, is essentially the same. The only important change is that as the children grow older both the maximum and the minimum of deaths occur later in the year. The maximum moves from March in the third year to April in the tenth. The minimum changes from October to November. The systematic way in which this occurs suggests that it is significant. It probably means that during these childhood years of most perfect health it takes a long time for disease to become fatal. Hence both the maximum and the minimum of deaths are long delayed.

The mortality curves of Belgium during the reproductive ages show special characteristics which are quite as interesting as those during infancy. In Figure 65 the mortality of both sexes at ages 16 to 20 reaches a maximum during April. This agrees essentially with the conditions in earlier years, as shown in Figure 64. Nevertheless, the range between maximum and minimum at ages 16 to 20 is considerably less than at ages 8 to 10. In other words, at the onset of puberty people seem to become endowed with a new ability to resist the normal seasonal fluctuations in health. The next section of Figure 65 shows that at the ages of 21 to 25, after the reproductive functions are well established, not only does the contrast in the mortality of the worst and the best seasons diminish still further, but the peak of mortality in the late winter or early spring is cut off. We should normally expect it to follow approximately the course of the line of little crosses. Essentially the same situation continues until the age of about 45 when the reproductive period is coming to an end. It is especially noticeable at ages 36 to 40, as may be judged by comparison of the actual mortality with the line of crosses.

In strong contrast to this the seasonal decline in mortality during the summer and the low minimum in October or November remain essentially the same from the beginning to the end of the reproductive period. In fact they remain the same as in childhood, as is evident from a comparison with Figure 64. It is evident therefore that we are dealing with a condition which is peculiar to the reproductive season of the year as well as to the reproductive ages of life. As the end of the reproductive period approaches, the flattening of the main peak of the mortality curves begins to disappear. It is still visible at ages 46 to 50, but beyond 50 it practically

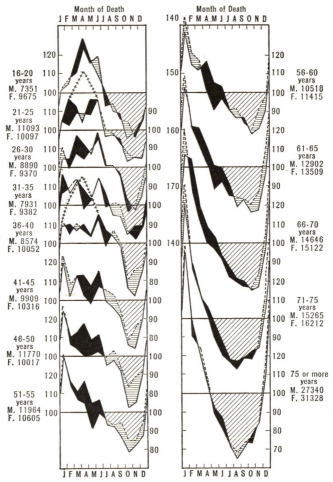

FIG. 65.—Deaths by Month and Sex in Belgium, 1844–1850. Ages from 16 years upward unsmoothed.

disappears. Thereafter, little by little, the mortality curves swing back to a very sharp peak in January and a low minimum in August, with a great contrast between the seasons.

The main features of the change in mortality from puberty to old age can be studied in Figure 66 more easily than in Figure 65. In Figure 66 the two sexes are combined and the curves are smoothed according to our usual method. Beginning with ages 16 to 20 we see a curve which is essen-

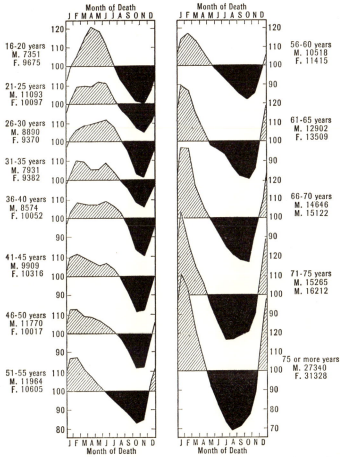

Fig. 66.—Deaths by Month and Sex in Belgium, 1844-1850. Ages 16 years upward smoothed.

tially the same as that of infants in the first month of life except that the maximum of deaths comes in April instead of February, and the minimum in November instead of July. This suggests that at the ages of 16 to 20, when health is almost at its best, the few deaths that occur are largely due to ailments which last a long time. Young people who become sick in winter may not die till April. In similar fashion the good effect of summer lasts far into the fall. Among infants, on the contrary, the period of illness lasts only a few days. Hence deaths are at a maximum soon after the worst of the cold weather, and at a minimum soon after the optimum temperature in summer.

At ages 21 to 25 and again at 26 to 30 Figure 66 shows a truncation of the maximum, but no significant change in the minimum. At ages 31 to 35 and 36 to 40 a well-developed minor minimum replaces the maximum of younger days, but the main minimum still remains unchanged. At ages 41 to 45 and 46 to 50 the minor minimum has begun to fade away and a maximum in February, like that of young children, has begun to appear once more. In the next curve for ages 51 to 55, the peculiar features of the reproductive period disappear entirely, except that the contrast between the seasons still remains relatively slight compared with either the end of the first year of life (Figure 61), or with childhood (Figure 62). From the age of 55 onward, however, the contrast between the seasons increases. At the same time the maximum mortality tends to be more sharply concentrated in the coldest weather (January at ages above 70), and the minimum tends to swing back to the warmest weather (July or August at ages above 70). In old age the effect of the seasons is almost the same as in the tenth month of life, except that the response of old people to the weather is even more prompt than that of the children.

One of the most significant facts about the Belgian curves of mortality is their obvious alteration during the period of reproduction. During the childbearing ages the harmful effect of cold weather is to a considerable degree mitigated. This mitigation applies to both sexes, but is much more pronounced among women. This is evident in Figure 67 where the mortality of each sex at ages 21 to 45 in Belgium is shown separately. In order to bring out the facts more clearly the scale is twice that of Figure 66. The solid line shows the deaths of males and the dash line that of females. The line of crosses at the top of the male line shows what would be expected if the mortality rose smoothly to a maximum as it does below the age of 20 and above 50. The line of little circles shows the corresponding curve of expectation among females. The contrast between the curves of expectation and the actual curves makes it obvious that some systematic and effective agency begins to operate upon both men and women in the late winter and spring. Among women it begins in February and continues until May. Its maximum influence appears to come in April. Its effect is to reduce the deaths in that month by approximately 8 per cent below what would be expected. The real reduction is even greater than this, for more children are born in February and March than at other times

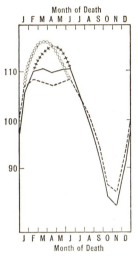

Fig. 67.—Belgium Deaths, 1844-1850. Ages 21-45. Unweighed averages of age groups.

of the year. Therefore, if there were no special health-giving factor the deaths among women in childbirth would raise the female death rate at that time above that of men. For this reason we have allowed the line of circles in Figure 67 to rise higher than the line of crosses.

The limitation of this reduction in the death rate to a special season seems to be important. In Belgium (Figure 21, page 95), February and March are the months of maximum births. May and June are therefore the months of most numerous conceptions. Figure 67 shows the maximum reduction of deaths in April between the maxima of births and conceptions. Several possible explanations of this may be mentioned. First, the reduction as a whole may represent an adaptation to climate whereby women, and to a less extent men, acquire an unexpected power to resist disease during a period which includes the maxima of both births and conceptions according to the basic animal rhythm. Another possibility is that the maximum reduction among women occurs in March and in April because that is the time when the ova which will be fertilized in May or June are passing through an especially critical stage in their early development. No one knows how long it requires for an ovum to develop before it is ripe for fertilization, but the general supposition is that at least 1 month and perhaps 3 are necessary. The less-pronounced reduction in deaths among men may mean simply that to a certain degree the male inherits an adaptation which is needed only by the female. Or possibly the male death rate is held down because the chances of infection by respiratory and other diseases are reduced by the fact that the women have relatively good health. A more probable explanation is that good health for a month or two immediately before the procreation of young is as important in the male as in the female. We do not know how long it takes for the spermatozoa to develop, but the time required is probably less than for the ova to mature in the female. If this is true, and if the vigor of the offspring is especially influenced by the conditions of health at the time when the spermatozoa first begin to develop, the period of a month or so before fertilization is especially important in the male as well as the female. On this basis the offspring would have the maximum vigor if the males had some special advantage in health perhaps a month before conception and the females perhaps 2 months. In Figure 67 the lines of crosses and dots, although hypothetical, suggest that something of this kind occurs. The crosses representing males are at a maximum distance above the actual curves about 1 month before the maximum of conceptions, while the dots, representing females, occupy a similar position about 2 months before that time.

It has been said above that the peculiar Belgian adaptations to the seasons are presumably characteristic of people in general. Data for testing this among infants are not available, but the mortality of New York City two or three generations ago is in full harmony with the Belgian figures as far as adults are concerned. In Figure 39 (page 168) the death rate of both sexes at ages 2 to 5 and 5 to 10 shows a strong maximum in the late winter and spring, a minimum in June which disappears among boys 5 to 10 years old, a minor maximum in August, and a deep minimum in October. Among people 10 to 20 years old the part of the curves from August onward does not change greatly and the June minimum is about the same as among children of 2 to 5 years. The winter maximum, however, is reduced in size; among boys it becomes lower than the August maximum. When the reproductive period is fully reached among people 20 to 40 years of age this reduction in the winter maximum becomes very pronounced. In both sexes, the deaths from February to April are much less numerous than in August. Moreover, the whole curve is flattened. Among persons aged 40 to 60 years this same condition still prevails, although among men it is disappearing. When old age arrives, however, it disappears, and among people over 60 years of age the winter maximum is once more the high part of the curve. In other words, here, just as in Belgium, both the season and the age when special vigor is needed for reproduction are marked by a pronounced lowering of the death rate in comparison with what would be expected from the experience of children and old people.

Further evidence along this same line is found in Strandgaard's study of seasonal variation in the weight of tuberculous patients in Denmark, as quoted by Madsen (1930), and in L. Brown's similar study in America (Huntington, 1924). In both cases the average weekly gain in weight (151 grammes in Denmark) is at a minimum in February or March and rises to a maximum in September (316 grammes). Curiously enough, however, in Denmark March and April show an unexpectedly high level (193 and 180), but May (157) drops back almost to the February level. A slight hint of this rise is seen in America in May. Moreover, the general death rate in Denmark reaches a maximum in both February and April but in March it declines a little. The great majority of tuberculous patients are in the reproductive ages of life. Therefore, it appears that people at those ages experience an access of vigor which enables sufferers from tuberculosis to make an unexpected gain in weight. This same vigor apparently holds the general death rate down somewhat in March.

As yet we are only on the threshold in our knowledge of this whole matter, and our interpretation may be wrong in detail. Nevertheless, there seems to be solid ground for believing that the peculiar truncation of the mortality curves of both men and women throughout the reproductive period during the months when the basic animal rhythm of reproduction is at its height represents a deep-seated adaptation to seasonal fluctuations of the weather. The same thing appears to be true of the peculiar way in which young infants show varying degrees of resistance to the weather according to their age. The concordance of these two sets of conditions is in itself remarkable. It is still more remarkable to find how closely these conditions harmonize with previous conclusions as to the basic animal rhythm and the relative vigor of children born at its height. The fact that the same general hypothesis of a close innate dependence of health, vigor, and reproduction upon climate and weather seems to explain all of these diverse phenomena adds weight to the hypothesis.

CHAPTER XIII

LEADERSHIP, BIRTH RANK, AND SEASON OF BIRTH

The main result of this book thus far has been the conclusion that several important factors show a closely related seasonal distribution which seems to be set in motion by the weather. The weather appears to initiate fluctuations in births, longevity, and sex ratios. It does this apparently through its influence upon the vigor of the parents, as well as in more direct ways. Fluctuations in these same conditions according to birth rank and economic condition also suggest that the effect of environment upon physical vigor ranks with heredity and training as one of the three great factors in determining human capacity. In the next few chapters we shall test our previous conclusions by what we may call eminence, leadership, success, or even genius. Whatever the name may be, the thing that we want to investigate is the qualities which make a man stand out above his fellows. We want to find out how far such success depends on physical vigor in comparison with innate genetic qualities on the one hand, and training and opportunity on the other.

In previous chapters our studies of birth rank have been so interesting that we shall begin with that subject before examining the seasonal distribution of the births of successful people. Mr. Ziegler has picked out from genealogical books some 1210 persons whose records indicate achievement and character above that of the average in *Who's Who*. He has tabulated them according to both birth rank and size of family. This gives a fairly clear picture of the extent to which the leadership of America has come from families of various sizes, and from persons of various birth ranks within these families. Table 19A shows the number of leaders falling in each birth rank and each size of family. Column A, on the right, gives the totals for families of each size. Col-

TABLE 19A

EMINENCE COMPARED WITH BIRTH RANK AND SIZE OF FAMILY

I. Number of Cases

Size of Family	Birth Rank															A Total	B Number of Families
	1	2	3	4	5	6	7	8	9	10	11	12	13	14	15		
1	46															46	971
2	59	33														92	1,104
3	73	35	32													140	1,107
4	53	42	47	28												170	946
5	43	34	22	24	18											141	769
6	27	15	24	21	20	19										126	126
7	25	18	18	22	14	14	23									134	588
8	12	7	12	8	14	12	14	14								93	510
9	13	15	6	10	11	7	10	8	10							90	438
10	12	7	8	5	7	9	10	8	11	6						83	296
11	3	4	5	3	1	6	2	6	3	1	3					37	234
12	6	3	3	4	2	0	2	4	2	1	0	3				30	109
13	4	2	0	2	0	0	3	0	1	3	0	0	3			18	66
14	0	0	2	0	0	0	0	1	1	0	1	0	0	0		5	31
15	0	0	0	0	0	0	0	0	1	1	0	0	1	1	1	5	16*
Total	376	215	179	127	87	67	64	41	29	12	4	3	4	1	1	1,210	

* Estimate

umn B shows the normal number of families of each size according to several good genealogical books which serve as an average sample. Table 19B is like 19A except that index numbers are used. They are obtained by dividing the numbers of leaders in Table 19A by the corresponding number of families in Column B, and then multiplying by 1000 to avoid fractions. Their absolute size has no significance. The only thing that counts is their relative size. Column C contains index figures for families of each size when all birth ranks are included.

Before examining the index numbers further a word of caution is needed. The number of small families in Column

TABLE 19B

EMINENCE COMPARED WITH BIRTH RANK AND SIZE OF FAMILY

II. Index Numbers

Size of Family	Birth Rank												C
	1	2	3	4	5	6	7	8	9	10	11	12 or more	All
1	47	....	....	....	....	....	....	....	....	....	....	......	47
2	53	30	....	....	....	....	....	....	....	....	....	......	42
3	66	32	29	....	....	....	....	....	....	....	....	......	42
4	56	44	50	30	....	....	....	....	....	....	....	......	45
5	56	44	29	31	23	....	....	....	....	....	....	......	37
6	40	23	36	31	30	28	....	....	....	....	....	......	31
7	43	31	31	37	24	24	39	....	....	....	....	......	32
8	24	14	24	16	27	24	27	27	....	....	....	......	23
9	30	34	14	23	25	16	23	18	23	....	....	......	23
10	41	24	27	17	24	30	34	27	37	20	....	......	28
11 ⎫	....	....	....	....	....	....	....	....	....	....	....	......	14
12 ⎪	....	....	....	....	....	....	....	....	....	....	....	......	23
13 ⎬	29	20	22	20	7	13	15	24	18	13	9	23	21
14 ⎪	....	....	....	....	....	....	....	....	....	....	....	......	12
15 ⎭	....	....	....	....	....	....	....	....	....	....	....	......	21

B is undoubtedly understated. The reason is that if all the children of a family die in childhood, or even in early maturity, the family may be recorded as childless in the genealogical books. The greatest opportunity for such error is of course in 1-child families. There is twice as much chance that all the children will die in a 1-child family as in a 2-child family, and 3 times as much as in a 3-child family. Therefore the numbers in Column B ought to be considerably larger in the 1-child group, somewhat larger in the 2-child group, larger by a small amount in the 3-child group, and so on. If we make allowance for this, all the index figures for small families in Table 19B become smaller, and those for the 1-child and 2-child families should probably be considerably smaller. In families of 4 or more, however, the error becomes negligible.

Let us now examine Column C. If we make allowance for the omission of small families as described above, the index numbers for the 1- and 2-child families in Column C would probably be smaller than those for the 3-child families. In that case the average degree of leadership probably reaches a maximum with the 4-child families. The number of cases is too small to give certainty. It is quite clear, however, that leadership decreases considerably in the larger families. This presumably means that, although the limitation of families had not gone very far when the leaders here studied were born, the people from whom such leaders mainly came were less likely than others to have families of more than 7 children. This agrees with *After Three Centuries,* (Huntington, 1935), where the leaders in a single line of Puritan descent came mainly from families of moderate size, both the small ones and the large being deficient in leadership.

Another phase of the matter is seen when the index numbers for individual birth ranks are examined in Table 19B. The index number for the first child increases from 47 in the 1-child families to 66 in those of 3. The contrast would be considerably greater if allowance were made for the small families which are omitted in the books because all the children died young. From the 4-child to the 7-child families a fairly high level of achievement continues among the firstborn, but thereafter a sharp drop ensues.

An examination of the various birth ranks in families of any given size shows the advantage of the first child very clearly. In the 2-child families, for example, the index of leadership is 59 for the first child and only 33 for the second. This cannot be a matter of inheritance. It must be either because the older of the two children is better trained and has greater opportunities, or because the second child is physically weaker than the first. Both suppositions probably contain some truth, but it seems as if the influence of health must be the greater of the two. It is generally conceded that children get a better training in a reasonably large family than where there are only 1 or 2 children. Nevertheless, families of every size up to and including 5 show at least 50 per cent more leadership among the oldest members than among the youngest. This is a very pronounced difference. It is at a maximum in the small families and diminishes in the larger ones.

When first-born leaders are compared with last-born, they outnumber them according to the ratios of Column F in Table 20. The decline from an average ratio of 2.0 in families of 2 to 4 children to 1.25 in those of 7 or more is

TABLE 20

EMINENCE OF FIRST-BORN COMPARED WITH LAST-BORN

A	B	C	D	E	F	G	H
	Eminent Number of			Ratio of First-born to			
Size of Family	First-born	Inter-mediate	Last-born	Inter-mediate	Last-born	Last-born, per Ellis	Last-born, per Ellis and Huntington
2	59	0	33	....	1.8	1.3	1.7
3	73	35	32	2.1	2.3	1.4	2.1
4	53	89	28	1.2	1.9	3.3	2.2
5	43	80	18	1.6	2.4	1.4	2.2
6	27	80	19	1.4	1.4	1.3	1.4
7 and 8	37	153	37	1.3	1.0	1.9	1.2
9 to 15	38	204	26	1.6	1.5	1.0	1.4

impressive. The last child in a small family formerly suffered such a handicap that his first-born brother was twice as likely to become eminent. In large families, however, the contrast between the first-born and last-born diminishes.

Children between the first and the last are apparently less handicapped than the last-born, as appears from the fact that the ratios in Column E are smaller than in F. Nevertheless, they are handicapped compared with the first child as appears from the fact that all the ratios in Column E are above 1.0.

Many features of Table 20 seem to illustrate the effect of the health of the mother, and perhaps of the father, upon the vigor of the child at conception and birth. In the old days many families were limited to 1 child because the mother died at the birth of that child or at the birth of a later one which also died. Many others were limited to 2 because the mother was not well at the time of the second birth. If she did not die at that time, she perhaps died at the stillbirth of a third child which is not recorded in the genealogies, or else because of her weakness she had no more living children, even though she herself continued to live. Thus in the small families the last child, whatever its rank, frequently was born weak because its mother was not well and was near the end of her childbearing career. Such weakness, we suspect, is the main reason why the last child, and to a less degree those that intervene between the first and the last, are less able than the first to achieve leadership. On the other hand, the table shows that in the big families, where the mother's strength enabled her to keep on bearing children for a long time, the intermediate children achieved leadership in more nearly the same proportion as the others. Even the last child had almost as much chance to achieve leadership as the first in the families of 7 or 8. This seems to mean that, when the mother's strength is maintained, the vigor of the children is approximately the same regardless of their birth rank.

Several independent bits of evidence should be considered in this connection. For example, in his *Study of British Genius,* Havelock Ellis finds that British leadership pre-eminently comes from first-born children. We have calculated the ratio between first-born and last-born among the 309 persons for whom he supplies data, and find that they agree in general with our ratios, but are much more irregular (Column G of Table 20). Ellis, however, does not note the increasing equality of the birth ranks as one goes from small to large families. He also concludes that intermediate children are less likely to succeed than are last-born as well as first-born. Our more abundant data, however, indicate that in small families the chances of conspicuous success among intermediate children are also intermediate. In the larger families, however, the intermediate children do not rise so high as either the oldest or the youngest child. It seems as if this must be a matter of training and opportunity. In the last column of Table 20 Ellis's data and ours are combined. Even so, the data are not sufficiently abundant, but they at least leave little doubt that first-born children are more likely to win fame than those born later, but this difference becomes slight in large families.

Another point to consider in estimating the importance of physical vigor as an aid to eminence is the fact that leaders in all countries appear to live to a great age on an average. It is true that a man must usually live to full maturity in order to achieve leadership, but very few men add much to their reputations after the age of 60 or even 45. Nevertheless the people in the *Dictionary of American Biography* live on an average to an age of more than 69 years, and those in the *British Dictionary of National Biography* live to about 71. Several people have shown that approximately this same length of life has prevailed among great leaders at all stages of history. Such longevity is an indication of constitutional vigor. Still another line of evidence is found in the fact that practically no great leaders have come from tropical countries. Akhenaton and the other most famous ancient Egyptians were born in latitudes 26° to 30°, as was Gautama, the founder of Buddhism. Mohammed was probably born in about latitude 24°, but on a relatively cool upland. The Mexican dictator, Diaz, was born in Oaxaca in latitude 17°, but his birthplace, too, was on a high, cool plateau. Search as one will, it is almost impossible to discover great leaders who were born in tropical climates other than cool highlands, and only a very few even there. It is customary to say that this is because of the low status of tropical civilization, but back of this low status lies lack of energy not only in tropical people as a whole but in the gifted men who might have become famous if they had possessed greater physical energy.

For our present purpose another line of evidence is much

more important than such disputed points. In Figure 56 (page 233) we saw clear evidence that even in families of 7 or more children the first-born who survive beyond childhood live about 3 years longer than their brothers and sisters who are born sixth or seventh. Such length of life appears to be a constitutional trait. If it is also the reason why first-born children display greater leadership than others, it cannot be the result of selection through infant mortality. Our index numbers for leadership are based on the number of births, not the number of survivors beyond infancy. Thus we seem forced to conclude that physical vigor is one of the main elements in leadership. Innate ability is certainly necessary and may be set down as the first great requisite. Training and opportunity together form a second great factor. But leadership, success, eminence, or whatever we call it, likewise requires physical vigor, and this is the third great factor. Of course, a superlative combination of the first two factors may produce striking results, especially in such matters as poetry where the inspiration of the moment is of supreme importance. But in most lines of effort great success is almost impossible without prolonged and strenuous work. In professional life and in business the most successful men are almost invariably harder workers than their less successful rivals. They have an inner drive which makes them work when there is no necessity of doing so. This inner drive appears to be greatly helped by physical vitality and endurance.

For decades or even generations there has been a widespread idea that men of genius are more likely to be born in February than in any other month. In America the fact that Washington was born on February 22 and Lincoln on February 12 has doubtless had something to do with this. Among the 31 presidents of the United States, no less than 26, or nearly 4 per month, were born in the 7 cooler months from October to April, and only 5, or 1 per month, in the warmer months from May to September. Among the 67

known birthdays of persons in the Hall of Fame at New
York University, 27 or about 40 per cent occur in February,
March, and April.

Several tabulations of world geniuses indicate a similar
tendency. Cattell (1903), Ireland (1925), Gini (1912), Kassel (1929), Pintner (1933), and Petersen (1936) are some
of the writers who have discussed the fact that eminent people tend to be born in cool weather, especially from January
to March. The group of geniuses most commonly used is
Cattell's list of 1000 greatest names of all time, among whom
the birthdays of 271 are known. The seasonal distribution
of these births is shown in Curve *A* of Figure 68. Three
other groups of leaders are added for comparison, namely, *B*,
the 1226 Americans included in the fourteenth edition of the
Encyclopædia Britannica (tabulated by Mr. Ziegler); *C*, 1374
scientists who are starred as outstanding leaders in *American
Men of Science* (tabulated by Pintner); and *D*, 1078 leading
American women of the nineteenth century who are mentioned in *A Woman of the Century* (tabulated by Mr. Ziegler). These four curves have been smoothed by our usual
formula to eliminate the minor irregularities which are inevitable with small numbers of cases. All have a strongly
developed maximum in January, February, or March, an
equally distinct minimum in June, and a minor maximum
in August, September, or October.

Do the four curves show a winter maximum merely because births in general are most numerous at that time?
So far as the three American curves are concerned a negative
answer is given by the lowest curve of Figure 68. This represents nearly 5000 ordinary Americans of old American
stock whose birthdays were culled haphazard by Mr. Ziegler
from genealogical records. They were born mainly from
1750 to 1885 at approximately the same time as the distinguished Americans of the three preceding groups. They
represent the type from which distinguished Americans have
mainly sprung. Moreover, their seasonal curve of births is

essentially the same as that of old Massachusetts (Figure 24, page 100) and Michigan (Figure 25, page 102.* It therefore seems probable that the births of distinguished Americans

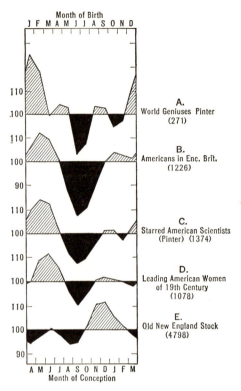

FIG. 68.—Season of Birth among Persons with Varying Degrees of Eminence.

show a seasonal distribution quite different from that of ordinary people.

Table 21 shows the degree of confidence that might be placed in this conclusion if it depended wholly on Figure 68. For the general reader the significant part of the table is lines I and J. They show that among the 271 geniuses of all time there is 1 chance in 23 that some accident may have caused the maximum to reach the observed level, and an

* Here and in later references it should be noted that the curves in Figure 25 are plotted according to month of conception, not birth.

TABLE 21

DEGREE OF RELIABILITY OF FIGURE 68*

In every set of data enough cases have been added to the short months to make them equivalent to months of 31 days.

	Curve A Geniuses	Curve B Amer. in Enc. Brit.	Curve C Starred Scientists	Curve D Am. Women 19th Cent.	Curve E Old New England	A to D Combined
A. Av. no. of cases per month	23.0	104.3	116.7	91.6	407.0	335.6
B. Standard deviation	4.6	9.8	10.3	9.2	19.3	17.5
C. Deviation of maximum	8.0	31.0	21.3	16.4	47.0	55.7
D. Deviation of minimum	8.0	29.3	20.6	16.6	26.0	68.7
E. Ratio C/B	1.74	3.16	2.06	1.80	2.44	3.18
F. Ratio D/B	1.74	2.99	2.00	1.76	1.35	3.93
G. Ratio C/B using periods of 3 months instead of 1	1.61	2.48	3.08	2.10	3.68	4.16
H. Ratio D/B using periods of 3 months instead of 1	1.46	3.69	2.56	1.70	2.14	4.53
I. Probability that maximum is accidental, 1 in	23	1267	53	27	136	1360
J. Probability that minimum is accidental, 1 in	23	716	43	24	10	23800

* It should be noted that the use of *unsmoothed* data causes the figures in this table to be different from what one would expect from inspection of Figure 68

equal chance that the minimum may have fallen equally far below the average. But the chances that both these things would happen in the same curve, and that the slopes connecting the maximum and minimum would be as regular as they are, fall to far less than 1 in 23. Using the unsmoothed data from which Curve *B* has been constructed, the chances that the well-developed maximum of births in February among the 1126 Americans in the *Encyclopædia Britannica* is due to sheer accident are only 1 in 1267, and the similar chances for the minimum are 1 in 716. But here, just as before, the chances that so high a maximum and so low a minimum would occur in the same curve, and that they would be smoothly connected by transitional steps, are far less than the chances that a certain maximum or minimum would occur. In fact, the chances that Curve *B* is due to mere accidents fall to only 1 in tens or hundreds of thousands. Among the starred scientists (*C*) the corresponding chances for the maximum and minimum are 1 in 53 and 43 respectively; in Curve *D*, among the women of the nineteenth century, they are somewhat larger, being one in 27 and 24.

When the four groups of Figure 68 are put together, as in the last column of Table 21, the chances of accidentally getting the observed maximum and minimum fall to only 1 in 1360 and 23,800 respectively. If we use periods of 3 months instead of 1 month, the actual number of births is such that there is only 1 chance in hundreds of thousands that either the maximum or the minimum is the result of accident. To go a step further, there is only 1 chance in millions that four diverse sets of data, such as form the basis of *A* to *D*, would accidentally give four curves showing the systematic qualities actually observed. Inasmuch as *E* for old New Englanders agrees essentially with the curves for entire states, we may feel confident that its form is even less likely than that of Curves *A* to *D* to be the result of mere chance. Therefore, we may feel fairly confident that eminent people really do show a seasonal distribution of births different from that of the population as a whole, and substantially like that of Curves *A* to *D*. We shall soon be better able to judge how important this is.

Having satisfied ourselves that Curves *A* to *D* are reasonably reliable and portray genuine tendencies, we may inquire what else they show. One point to notice is that, the greater the degree of distinction, the greater is the tendency away from the ordinary seasonal distribution of births, and toward a maximum of births early in the year. Thus Curve *A* for world geniuses shows a very high maximum squarely in January, corresponding to conceptions in April. Its amplitude, that is, its range from maximum to minimum, amounts to 50 on a scale where 100 is the average. The Americans of Curve *B*, a group less distinguished than the people of Curve *A*, have their maximum in February, with an amplitude of 40 between maximum and minimum. The starred scientists (*C*), only about 7 per cent of whom are distinguished enough to find a place in the *Britannica,* also have their maximum in February. In March, however, their curve is almost as high as in February, and its amplitude is only 32. The women's curve (*D*), belonging to a still less distinguished group, has its maximum in March, and the amplitude is only 22. Finally the curve for ordinary old Americans (*E*) is like that of the women in having its earlier maximum—a very insignificant one—in March. The range from this to the June level is only 7. The total amplitude of the whole curve, to be sure, is 18, but even this is less than the amplitude of any other curve in Figure 68.

This résumé of the curves of Figure 68 brings out two features. One is a steady tendency for the maximum to occur later in the season as we go from the greatest geniuses to other leaders and then down to ordinary people. The other is for the amplitude of the curves to decrease as we go from the more to the less competent. The differences in amplitude between Curves *A* and *E* may be due in part at least to the small number of cases (271) on which *A* is based in contrast to the much larger number (4798) in *E*. No such explanation is possible for the other three curves, for they are all based on approximately the same number of cases. If we judge by them alone, the most distinguished people show a tendency toward birth in cold weather and toward an unusually great contrast in the number of births in winter and summer.

Another interesting feature of Figure 68 is the minor maximum of births in August, September, or October. It is visible in each section of that figure, and becomes of major importance in Curve E. We may omit Curve A, however, because it pertains to only a few people who were born in many lands and at many periods. Among the other curves we note that in Curve B for Americans in the *Encyclopædia Britannica* this late summer or early autumn maximum is so insignificant that no black shading follows it. In Curves C and D it becomes more distinct, and in E it is very prominent. Thus in a general way it increases in importance as we go from the most to the least distinguished groups. In a previous chapter we interpreted this maximum as due partly, but not wholly, to seasonal migration, which in former days caused the winter, especially December, to be a time when many husbands who had been at work elsewhere during the summer came home for a few weeks or months. If this is correct, Figure 68 suggests that the families where such migration takes place are not the kind where distinguished people are born in large proportions.

Let us now test these tentative conclusions by means of the *Dictionary of American Biography*. That book it will be remembered is the official publication of the Learned Societies of America and is the standard source of information as to eminent Americans. Using only those persons who were born in America, Mr. Ziegler has tabulated them according to the amount of space which they receive in the book.* Although space is only a rough measure of distinction, we may feel quite certain that, on an average, when hundreds of people are taken into account, those receiving much space

---

* Volumes 19 and 20 had not appeared when the present study was made.

excel the others in distinction and presumably in ability. Accordingly Figure 69 shows four groups of American leaders divided according to their degree of distinction, the most distinguished being at the top.

In general we see in Figure 69 a repetition of the same phenomena as in Figure 68. Curves *A* to *D* show a maximum in January or February and a minimum in June or July. This is followed by a second maximum later in the season, except in Curve *D*. The range from maximum to minimum diminishes steadily from the most distinguished (*A*) to the least distinguished (*D*).* Part of this difference is presumably due to the larger number of cases in the less distinguished groups. Nevertheless, Curve *A* for 298 persons with 5 columns or more of space in the *Dictionary of American Biography* does not rest on a

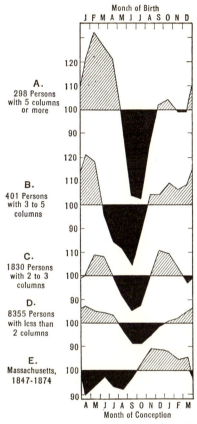

Month of Birth
J F M A M J J A S O N D

A.
298 Persons
with 5 columns
or more

B.
401 Persons
with 3 to 5
columns

C.
1830 Persons
with 2 to 3
columns

D.
8355 Persons
with less than
2 columns

E.
Massachusetts,
1847-1874

A M J J A S O N D J F M
Month of Conception

Fig. 69.—Seasonal Distribution of Births Among Eminent Americans in the *Dictionary of American Biography*.

very different foundation from Curve *B* based on 401 persons with 3 to 5 columns. Moreover, an amplitude of 26 between the maximum and minimum for the 1830 persons with 2 to 3 columns (*C*) is identical with what we found for the 1374 starred scientists in Figure 68. The degree of eminence in the

---

* In Curve *A* the chances of accidentally attaining the observed maximum and minimum are 1 in 32 and 160 respectively. For Curve *D* the corresponding numbers are 174 and 128.

two cases is approximately the same. On the whole, the amplitude of the curves appears to be more closely related to the degree of eminence than to the number of cases. In Europe, Japan, and elsewhere we have already seen many curves which are based on hundreds of thousands of cases, but show amplitudes like those of Figures 68 and 69. Hence we conclude that there is a genuine tendency for the amplitude of the seasonal curves of birth to increase with the degree of distinction. In other words, the greater the degree of distinction, the more chance there is that people will be born in February, or at least in the winter, rather than in summer. Among the 300 most distinguished Americans the relative number of births per month is about 132 in February (conceptions in May) in contrast to only 64 in June and July (conceptions in September and November).

Let us see how far Figures 69 and 68 agree in two important features. One is the change in the date of the maximum as one goes from the more to the less distinguished groups. This is not so regular in Figure 69 as in 68. Curve A, though high in January, is still higher in February, but the number of cases is so small that a few more might easily shift the maximum. Curve B, with its maximum in January, and C with a maximum divided between February and March agree with Figure 68. So does Curve E for people in general. The maximum comes later as the degree of distinction becomes less. Curve D, however, for persons with only 1 or 2 columns shows a maximum in January, and is thus out of step with the others. Perhaps this is due to the large proportion of southerners included in this group, especially generals and politicians. We have already seen that in the southern United States the maximum of births tends to occur more nearly in midwinter than in the North, and we shall soon see that this applies to intellectual people even more than to the rank and file. As Figure 69 now stands, however, it shows nothing more than a hint of a tendency for the maximum of births to occur earlier among more distinguished persons than among others of less distinction.

The other feature in which we may compare Figures 68 and 69 is the increase in the autumn maximum as one goes from the more to the less distinguished groups. Among the people with more than 5 columns (Group *A* in Figure 69) the September maximum is inconspicuous. In *B* the ruled area above the base line is large, but the actual drop of the curve in November is slight. In *C* the drop is conspicuous. Thus from *A* to *C* the autumn maximum increases. Among the large group of persons with the 2 columns of space (*D*), however, the autumn maximum fails to appear. This may be due once more to the high percentage of southerners. In that part of the country not only do the births of leaders fall off during the summer to a greater degree than farther north, but practically none of the white people have had the habit of going away to work during the summer. Therefore there is no large group of husbands to return home during the winter. If allowance is made for this, the agreement between Figures 68 and 69 in respect to the autumn maximum is fairly close. This agreement becomes more conspicuous when we include Curve *E* representing ordinary people of every sort in Massachusetts. Taking both the earlier and the later maximum into account there appears to be a real difference between the eminent people and the rank and file; and the difference is most marked in winter.

At this point we may well inquire still further as to the reliability of curves based on limited numbers of people. A mere calculation of the probability that a given departure from the average will occur is by no means enough. The essential feature of the present study is not merely the amplitude of the curves, but the number and season of the maxima and minima. The important thing is the degree to which one curve agrees with another, or varies from it according to some systematic relationship. Moreover, there is abundant evidence that among special groups, such as the very eminent, the characteristic seasonal distribution of births becomes manifest with a far smaller number of individuals than among average people.

Figure 70 illustrates a test of the matter by means of *Who's Who in New England* (1915). Some of the people in that book are really eminent, but the great majority are merely local leaders. The left-hand side of Figure 70 illustrates

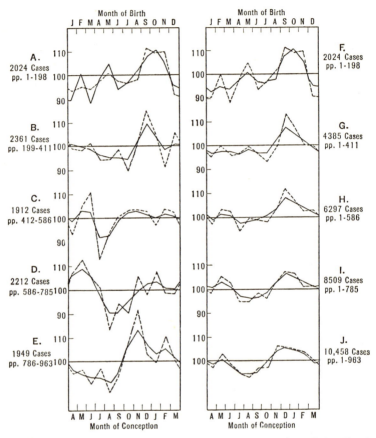

Fɪɢ. 70.—Seasonal Distribution of Births among Persons in *Who's Who in New England*. Unsmoothed curves, dotted; smoothed curves, solid.

what happens when we divide the book into five approximately equal sections, each containing about 2000 names. Confining our attention to the solid lines, which have been smoothed by our usual formula, we see that each of the left-hand curves shows a maximum in August, September, or October. This agrees with the early curves for Massachusetts and Michigan, as is evident in Figure 25 (page 102), provided we make allowance for the fact that there the curves are plotted according to the date of conception rather than birth. In other respects the five curves on the left of Figure 70 by no means agree so well. All, to be sure, show a summer minimum, but this ranges from April to July, and in Curve *A* is inconspicuous. A winter maximum appears in February in Curves *C* and *D*, and there is a hint of it in January in Curve *B*, but the other curves do not show it in their smoothed form. In view of such differences it seems obvious that a seasonal curve of births based on 2000 people is not truthworthy unless its indications are confirmed by other data.

Now let us see what happens to the curves on the left of Figure 70 when we increase the number of cases by adding successive increments of about 2000. The right-hand side of the figure shows what happens. Curve *F* is the same as Curve *A*; *G* represents *A* with the addition of *B*. In *H* the data of *C* have been added to those of *A* and *B*, and so until *J* represents all the 10,000 persons in *Who's Who in New England*. Curve *J*, however, does not differ significantly from Curve *I* based on 8000 people or from *H* based on 6000. Therefore we may feel confident that further additions would make no appreciable change. It is worth noting, however, that if Curves *C* and *E* had chanced to change places in the arrangement of *Who's Who in New England*, the winter maximum would not have appeared in our summary curves on the right until Curve *I*. Hence we conclude that for ordinary people at least 10,000 cases are needed before we can rely upon the results. This is important because several students have drawn sweeping conclusions on the basis of no more than a single curve based on less than 1000 cases. It must not be inferred from this, however, that small bodies of data are without value. The main feature of Figure 70, the maximum in late summer or early fall, is evident in every one of the curves. Moreover, if several curves based on a few data all agree, the probability that they can be trusted is high.

The difficulty of obtaining reliable results unless large numbers of cases are available is still further illustrated in Figure 71. There a part of the people in *Who's Who in New England* were tabulated according to their year of birth. The others were not so tabulated because the desirability of this was not realized until the work was well under way. The small group of 600 who were born before 1840 shows a

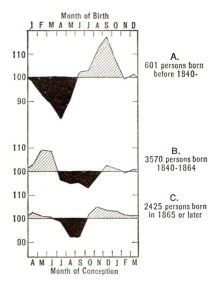

Fig. 71.—*Who's Who in New England,* Arranged by Date of Birth.

minimum of births in April and a maximum in September. This is somewhat like the earliest curves for Massachusetts and Michigan (Figure 25, page 102) except that in this smoothed curve there is no hint of a winter or spring maximum. The next curve, for 3570 persons born from 1840 to 1864, assumes what we have come to consider the standard form, with a maximum in February and March, a minimum in July, and a minor maximum in September. It almost duplicates many of our European curves; for example, early

Belgium, France, and Spain (Figure 22, page 97), or south Sweden, Germany, and north Italy (Figure 23, page 99). Among the 2425 New Englanders born from 1865 onward the curve of births bears some resemblance to that for the preceding period, but the maxima and minima come a little earlier, and the maximum in the second half of the year is higher than the one in the first half. The diversity of these curves emphasizes three points: (1) the seasonal distribution of births may change with the lapse of time; (2) in order to get reliable results there is need either of a large body of data or of a number of similar curves based on smaller bodies of data; and (3) curves for ordinary people based on a small number of cases show much greater irregularity than the curves for highly exceptional people.

The full significance of a seasonal curve of births pertaining to any special group of people can be appreciated only by comparison with the population as a whole in the same region. This obvious truth has led some students into error because they have not realized that there are great variations even in a single country, as we have seen in Figures 24 (page 100) and 30 (page 116). In order to facilitate the necessary comparisons and at the same time avoid this error we have endeavored to choose appropriate curves of large bodies of people for comparison with our special curves. Thus the curve of births in Massachusetts from 1847 to 1874 has been inserted at the bottom of Figure 69. This is legitimate, not only because the Massachusetts records are the best in America for that early date, but because that state is fairly typical of the part of the United States where the majority of the persons in the *Dictionary of American Biography* were born. In Figure 69 the reference curve at the bottom is based on approximately 5000 persons of old New England stock most of whom were born in New England and New York, but some in other states farther west. Although this group is somewhat small as a basis of comparison, it was chosen because it represents the same kind of people from whom most of the other Americans in Figure 69 have sprung, and because its seasonal curve agrees quite well with those of early Massachusetts and Michigan.

In Figure 72 another method has been tried. Instead of introducing a curve to serve as a standard, each curve has been shown not only in its original form (the dotted lines), but as it would be (the solid lines) if the index figures of

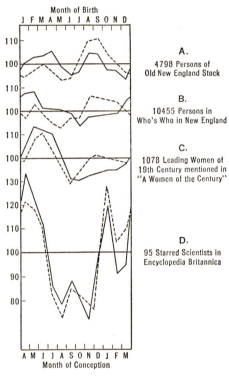

A.
4798 Persons of
Old New England Stock

B.
10455 Persons in
Who's Who in New England

C.
1078 Leading Women of
19th Century mentioned in
"A Women of the Century"

D.
95 Starred Scientists in
Encyclopedia Britannica

Fig. 72.—Index Numbers of Births per Month Expressed as Percentages of the Corresponding Index Numbers for Massachusetts, 1847–1889.

births for each month were expressed as percentages of the corresponding index figures for old Massachusetts. In other words, when a solid line is above the horizontal line marked "100," the number of births in the group in question is relatively high compared with births in general, as represented by Massachusetts. The effect of this in every case is to increase the importance of the winter or spring maximum, and to eliminate or reduce the autumn maximum. Curves *A* and *C,* for old New England stock and for women of the nineteenth century, are repeated from Figure 69, and Curve *B* for *Who's Who in New England* from Figure 79.

Curve *D* is new. It is introduced to show how small a number of persons is necessary to give a typical seasonal curve of births if we have a group which is very sensitive to seasonal influences. We have already seen that the tendency to be born in the winter increases as people become more distinguished. The 95 persons on whom Curve *D* is based are American scientists who not only are starred in *American Men of Science,* but also are included in the *Encyclopædia Britannica.* They were tabulated in order to discover how much duplication there is in Curves *B* and *C* of Figure 68 which represent respectively Americans in the *Britannica* and starred scientists. The results proved so interesting that their curve is reproduced. Like the curves for world geniuses (*A,* Figure 68) and the world's most famous women (*H,* Figure 75), it shows that among sufficiently eminent people even a very small group presents a highly characteristic seasonal curve of births. Taking periods of 3 months as the unit there is 1 chance in 12 that either the maximum or the minimum may have occurred accidentally, but the chances of thus getting a curve which agrees so closely with other curves of eminent people and which disagrees so radically with the curves for people in general are nowhere near so great.

After this interlude as to methods, let us return to our main problem. The seasonal distribution of births among leaders varies from region to region in the same way as among people in general, but to a greater degree. This is evident in Figure 73 where the people in *Who's Who in America* and in *American Men of Science* are grouped according to the location of their places of birth. Neither set of people can be called famous or even eminent as a whole, but both stand far above the average in general ability. The *Who's*

Who people apparently rank higher than the scientists in actual achievement and probably in intellectual caliber, for the scientists include all persons of that type regardless of age or distinction. On the left those of the *Who's Who* group who were born in New England and the Middle Atlantic States (*A*) and farther west in the North Central States (*B*) show the usual maximum in February (conceptions in May), and a minimum in May (conceptions in August at the

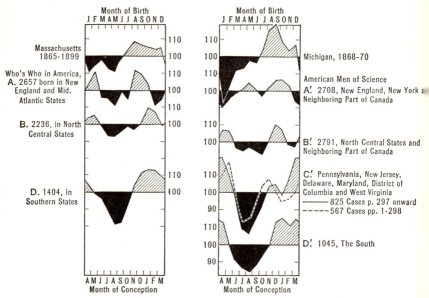

Fig. 73.—Season of Birth among Persons in *Who's Who in America* Compared with Those in *American Men of Science*.

end of the hot weather). They also show a second maximum —August in one case and October in the other (conceptions November and January). Here, as in other cases, the second maximum is more variable than the first, but in general it corresponds to what happens in the general population as illustrated by Massachusetts at the top of Figure 73.

Farther south the form of the curve of births changes just as it did in Figure 30 (page 116) where the season of birth among people as a whole in many states was illustrated. A deep summer minimum appears. In Figure 30, however, among people in general, this deep minimum did not occur until we were as far south as Florida. Among the people of *Who's Who,* on the contrary it occurs in Curve *D* among people born for the most part in the Virginias, Carolinas, Kentucky, and Tennessee. Moreover, in Curve *D* the maximum occurs very decidedly in September, October, and November, which means that the period when these leaders were conceived was concentrated more fully in the coldest weather from December to February than was the case among the ordinary Southerners on whom the curves of Figure 30 are based. Then, too, Curve *D* shows that the births of leaders in the southern states are at a minimum in May and June, corresponding to conceptions in August and September when the hot weather has had time to produce its maximum effect. Thus, taken as a whole, the leaders seem to be more sensitive to the weather than do other people.

Among men of science, on the right of Figure 73, those born in the relatively cool climate of New England, New York, and the neighboring parts of Canada show a curve of births (*A'*) a good deal like that of people in general, but with a tendency toward numerous births in May (conceptions in August) as well as in September and October (conceptions in December and January). The resemblance between this curve and the general curve may mean that the people who become scientists in New York and New England do not differ much from people as a whole. It is possible that the peak in May is accidental, but it may also represent the summer maximum of conceptions seen in Figure 30 in northern regions such as Maine and Canada. The rest of Figure 73 is clear. The curve for scientists in the North Central States (*B'*) is closely similar to that for persons in *Who's Who* in the same region (*B*). Only a little farther south, however, *C'* shows that in Pennsylvania, New Jersey, Maryland, West Virginia, and the District of Columbia, where many scienists are born, the tendency toward concentration of births in cold weather and toward few conceptions in hot weather is strong. When we divide the scientists of this region into two small groups we find that the two behave essentially alike, as appears from a comparison of the solid and the dotted lines in *C'*. Finally in the South, which means mainly the northern South, Curve *D'* shows essentially the same conditions as among the *Who's Who* group (*D*). The maximum of births occurs as the result of conceptions in the colder weather from December to April, and the minimum as the result of conceptions in July, August, and September. When Figure 73 is taken in conjunction with Fig-

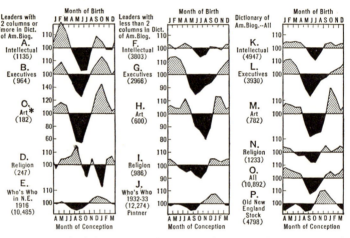

FIG. 74.—Season of Birth among Eminent Americans according to Occupation.

ure 30 (page 116) it seems quite clear not only that hot weather is unfavorable to conception, but that the conception of persons with unusual ability is much more hampered by heat and favored by cold than is that of ordinary persons.

It has been suggested (Kassel, 1929; Petersen 1936) that the season of birth may vary according to people's type of occupation or talents. In Figure 74 the persons in the *Dictionary of American Biography* have been divided not only according to the space allotted them, but also according to their occupation. Those called intellectuals include scientists, professors, authors, journalists, and others whose work consists mainly of pure intellectual effort; executives include business men, politicians, and soldiers; art includes music and the drama as well as painting, and so forth; the religious leaders have mainly been preachers, for abstract theologians are in many cases counted as professors. On the left, the intellectuals (*A*), executives (*B*), and artists (*C*) who are distinguished enough to get at least 2 columns of space all show essentially the same seasonal distribution of births. This is interesting because the artists number only 182, whereas the intellectuals number 1135. Yet the maxima and minima of the artists agree closely with those of the other groups. The amplitude of their curve, which is plotted on half the scale of the others, is 45 in comparison with 19 for the intellectuals and 15 for the executives. The curve for the religious leaders (*D*) differs from the others, but inasmuch as it is based on only 247 persons we cannot place much reliance on it.

The middle section of Figure 74 shows that among the people who receive less than 2 columns of space in the *Dictionary of American Biography* the curves of birth are not so well defined as among the more eminent leaders. The curve of the intellectuals is surprisingly flat, and its maximum is indeterminate. The minor executives, however, behave almost the same as the major ones; and the same is true of the artists except for a peak in April, which may be accidental since only 600 persons are concerned. The religious leaders behave much more nearly like the others than do their more distinguished men confréres. No group of eminent people, whether with much space or little, behaves in the same way as the less distinguished people who are represented at the bottom of Figure 74 by *Who's Who in New England* (*E*), *Who's Who in America* (*J*), and ordinary old New England stock (*P*).

Curves *K* to *O* on the right of Figure 74 include all the people in the *Dictionary of American Biography* and sum up the situation very clearly. Although based on varying numbers (782 to 10,892) they all agree in showing a decided winter maximum and summer minimum with no trace of the low level seen in January among less gifted people in Curves *E, J,* and *P* at the bottom of the three columns in Figure 74. The 5000 intellectuals and the 1200 religious leaders both show flat curves in spite of the difference in numbers. The artists show a sharp peak in October, but since less than 800 people are concerned, this may be pure accident. Perhaps it means that among artistic parents the husband is especially likely to be away from home and to return just at Christmas time, but such an idea may be farfetched. On the whole, the upper four curves of Figure 74 are so closely similar that in America, at least, there seems to be little to support the claim that one type of occupation differs from another in seasonal distribution of births.* In Europe, however, we shall find distinct evidence of such a difference. This is in harmony with the prevalence of strong class distinctions in Europe, and their absence in America.

The differences in the seasonal distribution of births according to degree of success or eminence appear to be highly significant. How great they are may be judged in Figure 74 from a comparison between Curve *O* for all the eminent Americans and Curve *P* for ordinary people. The distinguished people of Curve *O* show a pronounced maximum in January corresponding to conceptions in April, and an equally distinct minimum in June corresponding to conceptions in September. The ordinary people of Curve *P* show only a very inconspicuous winter maximum in March. This is one of four great differences between the two curves. A second is that, although the summer minima occur at approximately the same time, the minimum for the eminent people drops considerably lower than for the others. These two differences appear to be climatic. Two other differences, namely, the general low level of the curves for ordinary people in winter, and the high level in August, September, and October, may be partly cultural. During the eighteenth

---

* On pages 358 to 361 this conclusion is somewhat modified by data which came to hand at the moment when this manuscript was completed.

and nineteenth centuries, especially from about 1750 to 1875, seasonal migrations of husbands among the population as a whole may have restricted conceptions during the warm months from April to September, and increased them from October to February. Among the type of people whose children became leaders, on the contrary, the curves of birth, as well as our knowledge of social history, make it clear that there was relatively little of such migration. The majority of American leaders have come from the professional classes and from the more successful farm and business families, and these are the ones among whom there has been least seasonal separation of families. Thus, in spite of what was said in the last paragraph, a class distinction appears to have played a part in causing the season of birth among distinguished people to differ from that among people as a whole. But note that this applies only to the *degree* of distinction and not to the kind of occupation in which distinction is gained. The importance of this will appear when we see how the seasonal distribution of births among kings and prelates in Europe differs from that of certain other types of eminent people.

When we eliminate cultural influences, we are left with strong evidence leading to four conclusions: (1) in America the coming and going of the seasons has a greater effect upon the birth of very able people than of ordinary people; (2) the most able type shows a maximum number of conceptions and births at a lower temperature than do people as a whole; (3) the conditions of summer—presumably the heat—diminish the conception of able people more than of others; (4) the geographical distribution of births confirms the conclusions derived from the seasonal distribution.

These conclusions entail such far-reaching consequences that we must test them in every possible way. One such test lies in studying the births of women in comparison with those of men. This is done in Figure 75 where Curve *E* is reproduced from Figure 68, but the others are new. Curves *A, B,* and *C,* are based on women in *American Women: The*

Official Who's Who, 1935-6 They represent an occupational division in which Curve *A* corresponds approximately to the intellectuals of Figure 74; *B* to the artists, and religious leaders; and *C* to the executives. The persons included in *American Women* were selected with less care than the leading women of the nineteenth century (Curve *E*). Inasmuch

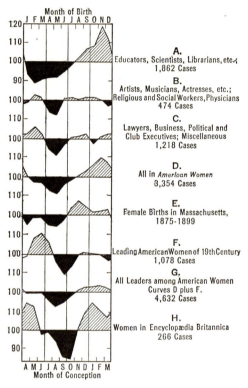

FIG. 75.—Seasonal Distribution of Births among American Women Compared with Women in the *Encyclopædia Britannica*.

as many of the most able women devote themselves to their homes and children, and hence have little chance to be included in reference books, it is doubtful whether the average caliber of the women of Curves *A* to *C* is as high as that of the men in *Who's Who*.

The first group of these women (*A*), including educators,

scientists, and librarians, shows a curve very much like that of early Michigan (F, Figure 25, page 102), as it would appear if plotted according to month of birth instead of conception. It bears some resemblance to the curve for all female births in Massachusetts from 1875 to 1899 (D). This seems to suggest that the women who become educators, scientists, and librarians do not differ much from ordinary women so far as their season of birth is concerned. Those who follow artistic or religious pursuits, or engage in social services (B), show a peak in February and a minimum in May, as does Group C which corresponds to the executives in Figure 74. In neither case, however, is the seasonal fluctuation as marked as among the men. Putting all these modern women together we get a curve (D) somewhat like Curve B in Figure 70 (page 308), but we have decided that that curve is not reliable. Going on to Curve F in Figure 75, we find that the leading women of the nineteenth century have a curve much like Curve D in Figure 70.

The great variation among these curves for American women leads us to think that none of them is reliable. They are based on too small a number of cases and perhaps include too many women who are not of outstanding mentality. When all the curves are combined, we get a very flat curve (G) which ought to be fairly reliable, as it is based on 4632 cases. This curve is much like Curve J in Figure 70 (page 308) based on 10,458 persons (practically all men) in Who's Who in New England. The chief difference is that in the women's curve the maximum comes in November and in the men's in September. Both curves are much like those for all births in early Massachusetts (E, Figure 69, page 305) and among old New England stock (E, Figure 68, page 300) except that these others show a greater amplitude than Curve G. From all this we are inclined to think that, if data for 10,000 leading women were available, they would show practically the same seasonal distribution of births as the men in Who's Who in New England. The differences between one group and another in Figure 75 appear to be accidental except in Curves *F* and *H.* In Curve *H,* representing the world's most distinguished women, we find a curve very much like that for men of corresponding caliber. Inasmuch as Curve *F* for leading women of the nineteenth century is intermediate between *G* and *H* and represents an intermediate type of woman, it seems that the data for women agree with those for men so far as they go.

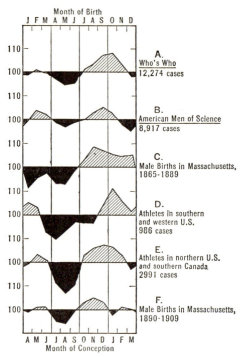

Fig. 76.—Seasonal Distribution of Births among American Men.

It is of interest to inquire whether people who are unusual in physical strength as well as in mental qualities display any special seasonal distribution of births. The data here used for this purpose are based on *Who's Who in Athletics.* Three-fourths of the persons whose birthdays are given there were born in the northern United States and Canada (*E* in Figure 76) and one-fourth in the South and West (*D*). The seasonal curve of the northerners shows approximately the same features as the curve for all males in Massachusetts (F) from 1890 to 1909 when most of the athletes were born. Among the southern and western athletes the winter maximum is pushed back to January, as in many other southern curves, and there is a sharp peak in October, but the number of persons is not large enough to give this feature much significance. A comparison of the athlete's curves with those of the other groups in Figure 76 suggests that so far as season of birth is concerned the athletes are like ordinary people. The resemblance of the curve of northern athletes to that of the general run of scientists (B) and to the people in Who's Who (A) is close. This merely means that the births of athletes are distributed through the seasons in much the same way as those of ordinary people. The fact that their February maximum is higher than that of the Who's Who group is probably due merely to the fact that they are much younger. We have seen that in Massachusetts, for example, there has been a strong tendency for the winter maximum of births to rise as time has gone on (Figure 24, page 100). The finest athletes, like the greatest intellectual leaders, may perhaps show a tendency to be born at some special season, but as to this we have no data.

The facts thus far before us suggest that persons of unusual mental ability show a stronger tendency than others to be born in winter. Pintner has assumed that, if this is true, the average intelligence quotient of people born in winter must be higher than that of those born at other seasons. This is not necessarily the case, as will appear from further analysis of Pintner's data. He obtained the I.Q.'s and birth months of thousands of children in and around New York and divided the children into three groups according to "social status." This first group (A in Figure 77) consisted of 7754 children of low social status with an average I.Q. of 92.5; his second of 4171 children of medium status with an average I.Q. of 100.9; and his third of 5586 children of high status, I.Q. 115.2. The solid lines in Figure 77 show the number of children born in each month and are plotted according to our usual method; the dotted lines show the average I.Q. The solid lines display the same kind of irregularity which we found in our five successive groups from *Who's Who in New England* (Figure 70, page 308). Their average, however (*D* in Figure 77), gives a consistent curve of standard form much like that of all the children born in New York City from 1915 to 1924 (*F* in Figure 77).

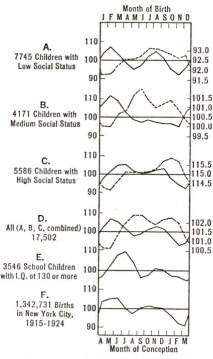

FIG. 77.—Intelligence Quotients of Children (dotted lines) Compared with their Season of Birth (solid lines)

The I.Q. curves of Figure 77 are as erratic as those showing the number of births. Nevertheless, when averaged, as in the dotted line of *D*, they probably represent the true state of affairs. The two curves of *D* fluctuate in almost opposite directions. Births are at a maximum in February, but the average I.Q. of children born in that month and in January is the lowest of the year. May and June have few

births, but the children then born have an average I.Q. about
1.8 points higher than that of the children born in January
and February. This difference is real, but very slight.
Among children born from May to November the I.Q. is
almost constant, although there is a drop of 0.5 in August
corresponding to a rise of about 5 per cent in the number
of births as compared with May.

The correlation between many births and low I.Q. is too
strong to be ignored, but its interpretation is difficult. Although Pintner does not exactly say so, his readers are likely
to interpret his data as disproving the idea that famous people tend to be born in the winter. This interpretation might
be correct if the number of births per day were the same each
month of the year, or if all types of people had the same
seasonal rhythm of reproduction. As things actually are,
however, the solid line of D in Figure 77 shows 9 per cent
more births in February, when the average I.Q. is lowest,
than in May, when it is highest.

A question at once arises as to the type of people among
whom the extra births occur. No exact data are available,
and we can merely make a few suggestions on the basis of
general probability. It seems probable that impulsive, unrestrained, and passionate parents are especially likely to
produce more than their usual percentage of children at this
season. They are especially prone to yield to the feelings
which arise because of the onset of the natural breeding season according to the basic animal rhythm. Unintelligent
parents are likely to behave similarly. They may practice
birth control more or less perfectly most of the year, but are
likely to become careless about it under the urge of the
increased sexual attraction which is characteristic of the
animal rhythm. Weak-willed parents form another group of
the same sort. Our study of conceptions year by year in
Massachusetts (Figures 27, 28, pages 106, 107) indicates that
birth control has greatly modified the animal rhythm of
reproduction, but has not destroyed it. It seems highly
probable that the three types here mentioned, namely, the

passionate, the unintelligent, and the weak-willed, contribute more than their proportional share to the excess of births which still occurs at the height of the animal rhythm. We should expect many of the children of such parents to have low intelligence, and they might well suffice to overbalance the unusually bright children who are born at the same season, thus giving a low average I.Q.

Still another type of parent must not be overlooked. This type consists of couples in which one or both is physically below par so that the production of children is impossible most of the year. At the height of the animal rhythm, however, their reproductive powers must rise like those of the community as a whole. Thus a considerable number of relatively weak parents may procreate children at the height of the basic animal rhythm, but not at other seasons. This does not exhaust the possibilities, but the four types already mentioned are enough to show the general situation. Among normal parents who produce most of the children of high intelligence, and who are in general the group that most carefully practices birth control, the number of extra children produced because of the annual surge of reproduction must be proportionally much less than among the passionate, the unintelligent, the weak-willed, and the physically weak types of parents. From this point of view we should expect a low average intelligence at the very time when the greatest number of children of unusually high intelligence are being born.

Although the preceding paragraph clears up some difficulties, it still leaves many points in doubt. One of the most puzzling things is seen when Curve E in Figure 77 is compared with the solid portions of A, B, and C. Curve E shows the seasonal distribution of births among 3546 school children with I.Q.'s of 130 or more. The data for these children were collected partly from school records in New Haven, but for the most part they are due to the kind cooperation of Dr. William Jansen and Dr. David J. Swartz of the public schools of New York, who gathered data from junior high and high schools in that city. The curve of birth of these children, when taken in conjunction with curves based on Pintner's data, shows us the season of birth among children with average I.Q.'s of 93 (Curve *A*), 101 (*B*), 115 (*C*), and approximately 135 (*E*). If all classes of the population showed the same seasonal variations of the birth rate, we should expect the month of maximum births to come earliest among children with high I.Q.'s, just as it does among eminent people of greatest distinction. Exactly the contrary is what actually occurs. Curve *A* for children of low social status and low average I.Q. has a sharp maximum in February, corresponding to conceptions in May. Curve *B*, based on children of a somewhat higher level, also has its maximum in February, but March is almost equally high. In Curve *C* we find the maximum almost equally shared by March and April; while in *D* the most intelligent children show a maximum in April.

There appear to be only two ways to harmonize this systematic change with the seemingly opposite type of change observed in Figure 69 (page 305) and elsewhere. One way is to assume that the apparently systematic relationships described above are in reality pure accident. The other, as explained above, is according to the hypothesis that in the spring the onset of the reproductive surge increases the number of conceptions more quickly among the types which have just been described as passionate, unintelligent, and weak-willed than among the finer types of parents whose children are likely to have a high intelligence quotient. This carries with it the corollary that mentally deficient children ought to show a maximum of births early in the season just as do the most intellectual types. We shall find some evidence for such a view in a later chapter. More puzzling problems still remain for future study. Nevertheless, it seems clear that Pintner's data as to intelligence quotients do not necessarily conflict with the abundant facts which indicate that persons who achieve unusual success show an exceptional tendency to be born in winter.

Chapter XIV

GENIUS AND SEASON

The relation between success and season of birth is the same in Europe as in America. This is shown not only by the birthdays of the most famous people, as given in the *Encyclopædia Britannica,* but by those of minor lights included in books which correspond to the *Dictionary of American Biography* or even to *Who's Who.* The *Encyclopædia Britannica* includes all the most famous people of the western world so far as we have knowledge of them. Thousands of others who may have had equal ability are omitted because lack of opportunity, physical weakness, or some other cause prevented their talents from coming to fruition or from being recognized. This is immaterial for our present purpose. The main thing is that, when once we have analyzed a list such as that in *Britannica,* it is impossible to obtain any other, similar list. Even if we could pick out the unknown geniuses, we should not be able to discover their birthdays. In fact, among the people in the *Britannica,* the birthdays are unknown for most of those who lived more than 300 years ago, or who were born outside Europe and the Europeanized parts of the other continents.

Inasmuch as few data are available elswhere, the following study of the *Encyclopædia Britannica* is restricted to persons born in Europe, the United States, and Canada. In those regions a few are omitted because their claim to fame lies in crime, physical strength, or purely accidental relationships involving no special ability. This leaves about 7000 persons, who have been divided by Mr. Ziegler into the following groups according to occupation:

> A. *Religious leaders,* including reformers and people in any
> walk of life whose main interest was altruistic.

B. *Intellectual leaders,* including persons engaged in literature, science, philosophy, education, engineering, etc.   Many ✓ jurists and theologians are included here if their work was primarily intellectual.   Lawyers whose main interest was politics, however, have been placed with the executives (D), whereas those who really contributed to the theory of the law are placed here.   In the same way, if the religious leaders were of the emotional type, or mainly interested in the betterment of mankind rather than in abstract reasoning, they have been placed in an earlier category (A).

C. *Artists,* including painters, sculptors, musicians, and actors.

D. *Executives,* including leaders in business, politics, and war.

E. *Hereditary rulers,* some of whom would doubtless have found places in the other four classifications, even if they had not chanced to be born to the purple.

These five divisions have been subdivided geographically:

1. *Western Europe,* including Great Britain, Scandinavia, Germany, the Low Countries, France, Switzerland, and Austria.

2. *Mediterranean countries* and allied regions, including Spain and Portugal, Italy, Greece, and all other countries bordering the Mediterranean Sea, both north and south. The great majority of this group come from Italy, with some from Spain, and only a few from elsewhere.

3. *Eastern Europe,* including Russia, Poland, the Baltic States, Finland, Hungary, Rumania, Bulgaria.

4. *The United States and Canada.*

Smoothed curves showing the seasonal distribution of births according to the combined occupational and geographical classification are shown in Figure 78.   Religious leaders and hereditary rulers are so scarce that those outside western Europe are omitted in this figure, although included in Figure 81.   Even with these omissions there are 14 curves. Under such conditions some of the curves are inevitably based on very few persons, the extremes being 71 artists in eastern Europe (Curve *M*) and 2517 intellectuals in western Europe (*B*).   It is therefore all the more remarkable that at least 10 of the curves show essentially the same standard form, with a maximum early in the year and a minimum in midsummer.   This lends weight to an idea which has already been suggested, namely, that the conception of highly intellectual and strong-willed types of people is peculiarly sensitive to the weather.

This same suggestion comes also from a study of the form and amplitude of the curves in Figure 78. On the left the artistic group of western Europe (C) displays an almost per-

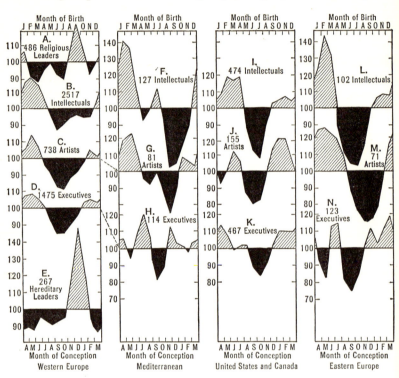

FIG. 78.—Seasonal Distribution of Births in the *Encyclopædia Britannica* according to Geographical Divisions and Occupation.

fectly typical curve based on 738 persons. From a sharp peak in February (conceptions in May) it declines to a pronounced minimum in June and July (conceptions in September and October). The only irregularity is a slight dip in December. The curve for intellectuals in western Europe (*B*) is almost the same except that in a mild form it shows the familiar peak in September, and does not show the December dip. It has the same amplitude as *C*, although based on three times as many persons, which would tend to flatten it. Does this indicate that purely intellectual achievement is more sensitive to weather than is artistic achievement, or are we dealing with a mere accident?

A comparison of the curve for executives in western Europe (D) with those for intellectuals (B) and artists (C) adds point to this inquiry. The curve for executives is almost a replica of that for artists except that its amplitude is less and its peaks not so sharp. This is what we should expect because it is based on twice as many cases. Is it, then, a mere accident that Curve *D* for executives is flatter than *B* for intellectuals? *B* is based on almost twice as many cases as *D*, and on more than three times as many as *C* for artists. One reason for raising this question is that in the other three portions of Figure 78 the curves for intellectuals display greater amplitude than do the others in their respective regions. They do this in spite of the fact that, with the exception of *L*, they are based on more persons than are the curves for executives as well as artists.

This does not end the matter. The curves for executives also have their own distinctive peculiarities. In each of the four sections of Figure 78, their amplitude is less than that of the curves for artists and intellectuals, regardless of whether they are based on many cases or few. Two possible explanations of this should be considered. One is that executives, unlike artists and intellectuals, frequently owe their position to the opportunities afforded by social position, even though they do not rank as hereditary rulers. Some of them also owe their position to traits of temperament which are emotional rather than purely intellectual. Thus as a whole the executives form a group in which genius burns less brightly than in the artists and intellectuals. The validity of such an explanation depends on our final conclusion as to the hypothesis that the weather at or before the time of conception has an especially close connection with intellectual capacities.

The other possible explanation is that executives tend to come in large proportion from the aristocracy. The seasonal distribution of births among the aristocracy, as we shall soon see, is not the same as among the rank and file. This second explanation finds support in the fact that two of the curves for executives (*H* and *N*) depart widely from the standard form. Both show maxima in April and again in August or September. Inasmuch as each curve is based on a very small number of persons (114 and 123) their departure from the standard form would have little significance were it not that it agrees with what we find in curves for the European aristocracy as a whole, as will appear later. It suggests that in the Mediterranean countries and eastern Europe, unlike western Europe and the United States, the executives who find a place in the encyclopedia come in large measure from a limited upper class which has a peculiar seasonal distribution of births. We believe that both of these explanations play some part in causing the curves for executives to differ from those of artists and intellectuals.

Another noteworthy feature of Figure 78 is the astonishingly regular form of the curves for artists (*M*) and intellectuals (*L*) in eastern Europe. The curve for artists is based on only 71 persons, and the other on 102. These curves do not stand in a class by themselves, however, for we have already found a parallel case in the curve for 95 starred American scientists who are also included in the *Encyclopædia Britannica* (Figure 72, page 312). The curve of the scientists, to be sure, is less regular than that of the artists and intellectuals, presumably because the scientists are of lesser intellectual stature. A closer parallel is seen in the upper solid line of Figure 79. This is the smoothed seasonal curve of births for 67 persons in the American Hall of Fame at New York University—all for whom the date of birth is available. These persons have been selected by highly competent judges as the most outstanding Americans. The form of the curve is almost perfect although it is based on only 67 persons. The range is so great that there is only one chance in 740 that February, March, and April would show so high a maximum by accident, only 1 in 80 that June, July, and August would be so low, and of course only one in many thousands that the general form would agree so closely with that of other curves of eminent people.

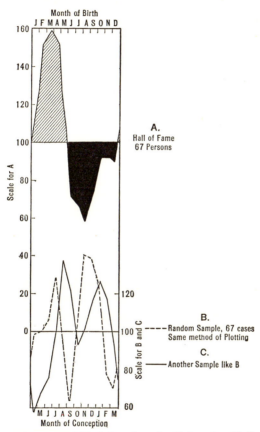

Fig. 79.—Seasonal Curves of Birth based on Small Samples: Hall of Fame and Ordinary People.

The systematic quality of the curve for the Hall of Fame becomes still more evident when we compare it with the lower lines of Figure 79. Each of these is based on 67 birthdays selected haphazard at the top of 67 pages of an American genealogical memoir, and is computed and smoothed exactly like the curve for the Hall of Fame. These curves for ordinary people do indeed show the two main features of the curve of births in the eastern United States during the last century (Figure 24, page 100, lower curves; and Figures 68, 70, 74, pages 300, 308, 316, lowest curves), but they lack the clear-cut quality of the curve for the Hall of Fame. Nor do they display the basic animal rhythm as does that curve, and they differ from one another much more than do pairs of curves like F and G, or L and M in Figure 78.

Returning to Curves L and M, we know that the backward condition of old Russia and of eastern Europe in general has imposed such handicaps that only persons endowed with extreme ability have been able to overcome them, and win a place in the *Britannica*. Hence the curves for the artists and intellectuals of eastern Europe represent a peculiarly high intellectual selection. The curve for executives (N) does not represent so high a selection, for even in backward countries generals and politicians find it easy to come to the front. All this seems to lend weight to the idea that, the higher we go in the scale of intellectual ability, the greater and more persistent the tendency toward birth in accord with the basic animal rhythm, or with a slight modification of it which will soon be discussed.

This does not mean a direct effect of the weather upon the mind. It means that high achievement, if our hypothesis is correct, depends primarily upon innate capacities, but that these capacities can come to full fruition only if the physical as well as the social environment gives them opportunity to develop. Among the environmental factors the first in point of time is the condition of the parents before a child's conception. If the weather, as well as other factors, is favorable, the embryo begins life under conditions which are especially favorable to the smooth functioning of the glands, nerves, and other organs. This does not create genius, but it is an important factor in permitting genius to express itself.

Returning once more to Figure 78 let us inquire into the

peculiar form of Curves *A* and *E*, which illustrate the season of birth among the most distinguished religious leaders and hereditary rulers of western Europe. Both curves show a strong maximum in September, which is especially remarkable in the curve for rulers. Religious leaders include three distinct types: first, supreme intellectual and moral leaders such as Jesus, Mohammed, St. Augustine, and Luther; second, mystics, and emotional preachers such as Peter the Hermit; and third, many ambitious and able, but not especially religious, sons of noble families. These last are men for whom there was no place in the hereditary scheme of Europe, but who were appointed to benefices as bishops, archbishops, and lords spiritual. They might almost be included among hereditary rulers. They are fairly numerous in the *Britannica,* and almost certainly account for the way in which the September peak of Curve *A* repeats on a smaller scale the peak of Curve *E*. Hence if we can explain the peak in the hereditary curve (*E*) we shall understand the similar peak in the religious curve (*A*).

Let us inquire into the reasons for such an excess of births in September. Such births indicate conceptions in December. Among royal families they include a high percentage of first births, but among religious leaders they include a correspondingly low percentage of first-born. Therefore, it does not appear probable that the September maximum is due wholly to season of marriage. This leaves two other possibilities. One is that the September births are due to a relaxation of marital restraint at Christmas time. The other is that at that season many married couples who have been separated are reunited. On the continent of Europe such separations may be social as well as physical. Where marriages are contracted on the basis of public policy rather than personal choice, and where the accepted standards permit leading men to keep mistresses without losing caste, legitimate husbands and wives often remain apart even though living in the same palace or castle. The Christmas season is a time when they are especially likely to be reunited.

In England, where family life is more highly regarded than on the continent, a somewhat different situation prevails. Husbands and wives are much more likely to live together at all times of the year. This is perhaps the reason why Curve *E* in Figure 84 (page 353) disagrees with Curve *E* in Figure 78. Figure 84 deals with the births of hereditary rulers in Britain instead of in western Europe as a whole. The British rulers show a maximum of births in April and May, corresponding to conceptions in July and August. In this respect the British rulers agree with the people of Scotland as a whole (Curves *J* and *K*, Figure 83), and probably with those of Great Britain as a whole, although data by months are not available for England. Nevertheless, the abrupt spring maximum of the curve for hereditary British rulers (*E*, Figure 84) may be due in part to social customs. "The season" in London lasts from April to about the middle of June. It is possible that this prevents husbands and wives of the highest station from being together as much as usual. The relaxation which comes when it is over may result in many conceptions. British executives, who are mainly political and military figures, come in large measure from the upper classes. Curve *D*, Figure 84, shows that they, too, are conceived in maximum numbers in July and August and born in April and May, but have a second maximum of births in September.

An interesting light is thrown on this whole matter by Steiger (1929), who compiled data as to 1145 births in the princely and royal families of Europe during the nineteenth century. Because of the multitude of little German states at that time the majority of these births were German. Curve *B* in Figure 80 shows that as a whole the princely births rise to a strong summer maximum which lasts from June to September, thus indicating conceptions from September to December. A closely similar situation exists among the landed gentry of England, as in Curve *I* of Figure 83 (page 349). There the minimum of births occurs in January (conceptions in April), and there is a steady rise to a prolonged maximum from July to October (conceptions from October to January).

These prolonged maxima of births cannot be due to the season of marriage.   Conclusive proof of this is available because Steiger has divided the princely births into first-born and later-born.   The first-born, Curve *A* in Figure 80, show an irregular curve with maxima of births in March and November, corresponding perhaps to marriages in June and February. The later-born (Curve *C*), on the contrary, show a much more regular curve with a minimum in March (conceptions in June) and a maximum in August (conceptions in November). This is like the curve for the British landed gentry except in minor details. The two curves together make it quite clear that among the titled aristocracy of western Europe the seasonal distribution of births has been quite different from the distribution among the population as a whole.

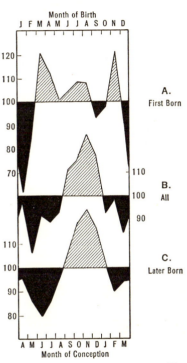

Fig. 80.—Births in Princely Families of Europe during the Nineteenth Century.

Von Alter (1930) makes an interesting suggestion as to the cause of the August maximum.   He says that when he was a child he heard the high-born August children referred to as "Jagd kinder" or "hunt children."   Therefore for a long time he supposed that the hunting season came in August, not knowing that the children's designation referred to conception rather than birth.   On this basis he suggests that the hunting season, which was universally observed among the princely families, as well as among the British landed gentry, encouraged conception. It might do this by increasing the vigor of both sexes, or by creating social conditions which bring husbands and wives together under especially favorable conditions.

But why should the minimum of births among the British landed gentry occur from February to May (conceptions from May to August) at the very season which is best according to the basic animal rhythm? One possibility is that the London "season" formerly separated many families of the gentry. In former days, when agriculture was important in England, many country squires and knights sent their wives and daughters to "town" during the spring, but remained at home themselves to look after their estates. This might account for few births from February to April (conceptions from May to July) but not in May. Unfortunately, we have no means of testing this suggestion statistically, and it may be without value.

It seems clear from all this that, when a seasonal curve of births departs systematically from the basic animal rhythm, a study of social conditions is in order. In Figure 78, for example, we have found a reasonable, although as yet unproved, social cause for the September maximum among religious leaders and hereditary rulers, even though there may be no physical separation of married couples like that which influences the curves of birth in Russia. Again, among the aristocratic families of western Europe, the season of birth may be influenced by the almost universal custom of gathering in the country estates for the hunting season. Other social customs which are not here investigated must also play some part. Even if we cannot place our finger on the exact social custom involved, it seems clear that the seasonal curves of birth among diverse social classes show a real and pronounced difference. The politicians, soldiers, and kings of Europe have come predominantly from a small section of the upper classes. The scientists, authors, and other intellectuals have come more largely from the professional and middle classes where there are no such pronounced seasonal variations in mode of life as are found among the aristocracy. In Great Britain, at least, the artists and actors, according to Ellis (1927), have tended to come from still lower in the social scale.

In the present incomplete state of knowledge it is very necessary to hold an even hand between social customs and the weather in attempting to explain seasonal variations in the distribution of births. Therefore it seems wise to recall the fact that in studying Figure 30 (page 116) we noted that a persistent maximum of births culminating in August seems to occur only as the result of conceptions which take place after a summer which is fairly warm, but not hot enough to be depressing. We also saw (Figure 26, page 104) that in Massachusetts the conceptions which give rise to the August maximum occur at the season when the ability to work also reaches a maximum. We saw, too, that among rats which have an abundance of nutritious food at all seasons for generation after generation, the normal seasonal cycle of reproduction not only becomes less pronounced as time goes on, but changes its form somewhat. A comparison of Curves C and E in Figure 3 (page 36) shows that when Dr. King kept gray rats in captivity and fed them abundantly and wholesomely at all seasons the relative importance of their April maximum of births declined, while that of their August maximum increased. The well-fed tame rats may be analogous to the well-fed upper classes of man.

It would be dangerous to insist on this analogy, but it is interesting to note that the human groups in which the August maximum is strongly developed are extremely well fed, well housed, and well cared for in other ways. Among a large part of them these favorable conditions have prevailed for several generations. So far as survival is concerned, the biological advantages of birth according to the basic animal rhythm have practically disappeared. Therefore these people may have reached a stage where the chief determinant of the seasonal course of conceptions is not the stimulation to reproduction which accompanies the improvement in health on the advent of the optimum temperature in the spring, but the still greater physical and mental stimulus which comes with the approach of cool weather in the autumn after a mild summer.

The autumn stimulus makes people work faster than at any other time. In studying factory workers in New England (Figure 26, page 104), we found that if the summer is cool the amount of work per hour increases steadily from a minimum in February to a maximum in late October or November. There is a marked contrast between the pronounced drop in vigor which occurs among factory workers in hot summers, such as 1911, and the steady gain in efficiency during cool summers, such as 1913 (Huntington, 1915, 1924).

Cool New England summers are comparable to ordinary summers in western Europe. It may be that such summers, together with the best available food and care at all seasons, change the basic animal rhythm in such fashion that the maximum of conceptions occurs in the fall. In other words, we are confronted by the hypothesis that the attainment of a certain economic and social level among a given group may change the effect of the seasons so that a new seasonal distribution of births occurs. We know very well that such a change has taken place in infant mortality. We saw this in Massachusetts (Figure 27, page 106). We saw at the same time that with this change went the beginning of a similar change in the seasonal distribution of conceptions. Among the aristocracy of Europe such a change may have gone still further. We suspect that the importance of the hunting season among the titled aristocracy of Europe is largely a response to a feeling of physical vigor which would increase the number of conceptions even if there were no especially favorable social conditions.

In this connection it seems worth while to add certain data which were sent to me by Dr. Neil A. Dayton the day before the manuscript of this book was scheduled to go to the printer. The data were procured through Dr. Joseph De

Porte of the New York State Bureau of Vital Statistics. They include all births during 1935 in New York State outside of New York City, and are divided into first-born, second-born, and so forth, according to birth-rank. They illustrate two main facts. One is that each new set of data thus far obtained is in harmony with our general hypothesis. The other is that in order to get dependable results, large numbers of cases, and statistics for several years, are necessary. Curves derived in the usual way from the New York data are plotted in Figure 81. Those on the right have been smoothed because some birth ranks include less than 10,000 births, and all represent only a single year.

The general aspect of all except the first two upper curves in Figure 81 appears to depend upon the particular kind of weather experienced in New York in 1934 and 1935. The weather doubtless influenced the number not only of conceptions, but also of abortions and stillbirths. Births in January, 1935, represent conceptions in April, 1934, immediately following the coldest February on record, but whether this influenced conceptions as late as April we do not know. April and May, 1934, were warmer than usual, which would tend to hasten the coming of the spring maximum of conceptions. June was very warm, the warmest since 1919. This presumably checked conception, throwing the maximum of births into February or March. At least a minor maximum occurs then in 4 of the 6 smoothed curves of Figure 81. If we could correctly estimate the effect of the weather on abortions and stillbirths it would help still more in explaining the curves of birth. The effect presumably becomes greater as the mothers become older.

Aside from Curves A and G for first births, all the others in Figure 81 are composed of two main elements. One is the basic animal rhythm with a maximum in the late winter; the other is the rhythm which culminates in the August maximum discussed in previous paragraphs. The dotted lines show that the basic rhythm is almost the same for all birth ranks except the first. It is like that of Belgium and many other countries, as is especially clear in Curve *I* for the third child and Curve *L* for the sixth and later children. Curve *K*, which departs farthest from the standard form, is the one based on the smallest number of cases, less than 5000.

The second element in the smoothed curves of Figure 81 is the one in which we are most interested just now. It ap-

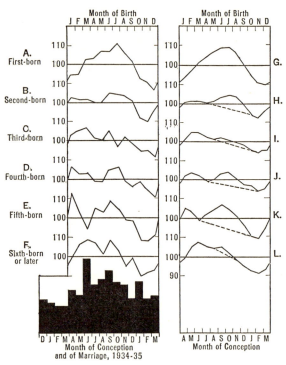

FIG. 81.—Births by Birth Rank During 1935 in New York State Excluding New York City.

pears in almost pure form in Curve *A* for first births. It is like what we have observed again and again in middle latitudes among well-nourished and carefully protected people, as well as among Dr. King's well-nourished and carefully protected rats. It is even more perfectly developed in the curve for first births in New York State than in those for the German "hunt children," the English landed gentry, and the well-fed Americans in the most-favored parts of the United States. Among such people conception appears to be stimulated even more by a return to cool weather after a fairly warm summer than by a rise to the optimum temperature in the spring. Nevertheless, the children born in past generations as the result of the autumn stimulus have not shown so great a tendency toward a low sex ratio, long life, and eminence as have those born in February and March at the height of the basic animal rhythm.

In order to remove all doubt let us inquire whether the peculiar shape of the curve for first births in Figure 81 can be due to the seasonal distribution of marriages. We have already seen (Figure 7, page 47) that births do not follow marriage so closely as would be expected, and that the seasonal distribution of births (Figures 6, 16, 17, pages 46, 70, 72) shows surprisingly little relation to the season of marriage. In the present case this is as true as anywhere else, as appears in the bars at the bottom of Figure 81. During 1934 and 1935 the seasonal distribution of marriage was wholly unlike that of conceptions leading to first births. Curiously enough, it was much the same as that of conceptions leading to births from the sixth child onwards.

Here, as in other cases, a social condition may enter into the seasonal distribution of births. In these days of birth control and of uncertainty as to the future, the conception of first children may depend very largely upon the psychological attitude of young married people. October and November are the period not only when people feel most inclined to work, but when industry as a whole is most active, jobs are most plentiful, the farmers have the most money, and people feel willing and able to undertake new responsibilities. The physical optimum in September is followed by a mental optimum in October or November, as will be explained more fully later. As the autumn goes on, the two together cause the young people who have been married during the preceding months to feel a psychological impulse in addition to the physical urge which accompanies the good health that prevails at the time when the temperature returns to the optimum. Hence they are optimistic and confident. Accordingly, they decide in increasing numbers that the time has come to have a child. Another psychological factor may account for the absence of any maximum of first conceptions in May and June. The present widespread knowledge of birth control permits a great many newly married young people to postpone pregnancy because they want to enjoy a summer vacation together unhampered by the limitations of pregnancy.

It seems clear that the statistics for New York by birth rank re-enforce our conclusion as to the intimate interrelation of psychological, social, and climatic factors. The maximum of births in July and August depends primarily upon the return of the temperature first to the physical optimum and then to the mental optimum. This brings both physical health and a mental attitude which creates not only a spirit of confidence in the future, but also a feeling of harmony between husband and wife. An important increase in the birth rate, however, springs from this only in regions where the summer is warm but not enervating and among people who are so well fed and well sheltered that the approach of winter does not entail any immediate deterioration of diet. Many cultural and psychological effects are brought into play by the march of the seasons at this same time. Such effects include the migration of farm laborers in Russia, the hunting season in Germany and England, and the industrial activity of America in order to fill orders for goods to be sold before Christmas. The birth rate is so sensitive that it is almost impossible to sort out the exact effect of each of these and other factors.

Let us now resume our inquiry as to the seasonal distribution of births among highly distinguished people compared with ordinary people. For this purpose let us combine all the *Encyclopædia Britannica* data for each of the four regions shown in Figure 78. The results appear in the shaded curves of Figure 82. In order that we may see how these curves vary from one geographical region to another, they are arranged according to the severity of the respective climates, the mildest being at the top on the left. Below each solid curve the dotted lines indicate the seasonal distribution of births which seems to be most nearly typical among the general population in the regions where the leaders were born. At best, however, these general curves are only approximate because they do not cover exactly the same region or period as the encyclopedia curves. Their weight is therefore not so great as that of curves of individual countries, which we shall consider later.

The encyclopedia curve for the Mediterranean region (*A*) in Figure 82 agrees with that for Italy as a whole from 1864 to 1867 (*B*), except that its maximum comes a month earlier

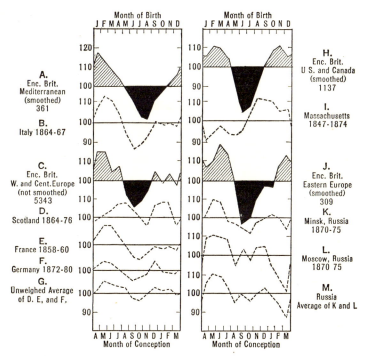

Fig. 82.—Seasonal Distribution of Births of Persons in the *Encyclopædia Britannica* Compared with That of People in General in Four Geographical Regions.

(in January), and its minimum a month or two later (July and August). The population of western and central Europe as a whole is represented by curves for Scotland (*D*), France (*E*), and Germany (*F*), taken from Figures 22 and 23 (pages 97 and 99). The average of these three curves (*G*) is much like the encyclopedia curve (*C*) for that same part of the world, except that it is much flatter. Moreover, here, just as in the preceding case, the maximum comes a little earlier in the encyclopedia curve than in the other. The minimum also comes a little earlier, thus introducing a point of divergence from the curves for Mediterranean countries.

On the right-hand side of Figure 82 the curve for Americans (*H*) is almost the same as for western Europeans except that it rises higher in the autumn. The corresponding curve for the population of Massachusetts as a whole (*I*) is quite different, as are all other available curves representing ordinary people in the United States half a century or more ago. We have already discussed the probable reasons why the curves for Americans in general depart so far from the standard form (Chapter VI). The important point is that, although the Americans of the encyclopedia depart from their fellow countrymen, they show a curve closely similar to those for corresponding people in Europe. The similarity goes so far that the maximum again comes earlier than the corresponding (minor) maximum for people as a whole.

Coming back now to the Old World, the encyclopedia people in eastern Europe show a curve (*J*) almost like that of the Americans, but with a more pronounced dip in January, perhaps because of colder winters. The curves of Minsk (*K*) and Moscow (*L*), which have been taken to represent the general population, may not be very reliable for this purpose, but nothing better seems to be available. The combined curve of these two (*M*), with its minimum in December, differs a good deal from the encyclopedia curve. The maxima, however, occur at nearly the same time as in the encyclopedia curve, and the agreement would be still better if the points for each month in Curves *K* to *M* had been placed half a month later to allow for the fact that they are based on the old Julian calendar. Even so, however, the maximum would come earlier in the general curve than in the one for the encyclopedia, thus being out of harmony with the other curves.

In spite of this discrepancy, the seasonal distribution of births among the most eminent people seems to respond to the weather in diverse regions much more closely than among people in general. Taken as a whole, the four encyclopedia curves of Figure 82 are much alike. Nevertheless, their form changes in harmony with the climate. The date of the maximum, for example, varies just as we have seen in other cases. The Mediterranean curve has its maximum in January (conceptions in April). In western and central Europe, where the climate is somewhat cooler than in Mediterranean lands, the maximum is divided between January and February. In America, with still colder winters, it comes in February; and in eastern Europe, where the winters are coldest, in March.

Another point which may be significant is that the maximum for the eminent encyclopedia people comes about a month earlier than the maximum for ordinary people in the first three sections of Figure 82, that is, in the sections where reasonably good curves for ordinary people are available for comparison. This means that the maximum of conceptions occurs at a slightly lower temperature among eminent people than among others. The extent to which the temperature is lower may be roughly estimated by obtaining the average temperature during the month of maximum conceptions in cities which represent each of the four geographical divisions of Figure 82. Table 22 shows that the mean temperature of the month in which men of genius are conceived in maximum numbers ranges from 13° C. (53° F.) in western Europe to approximately 18° C. (64° F.) in eastern Europe, and averages 14.7° C. (58.4° F.). This average may be compared with the median temperature 16.7° C. (62° F.), obtained from a study of over 80 curves for people in general in many countries (Figure 59, page 262). The fact that the temperature for eminent people is 2° C. (3.6° F.) lower than for people as a whole suggests that intellectuality may be fostered by temperatures below those best for bodily vigor alone. It should be remembered, however, that each encyclopedia curve covers many countries, so that our estimates of temperature may be considerably in error. Therefore, we must defer judgment until the data for individual countries can be examined.

TABLE 22

Estimated Mean Temperature of Months during Which Persons in the *Encyclopædia Britannica* were Conceived in Maximum Numbers

Mediterranean Europe	Western Europe	North America	Eastern Europe
Milan...... 13.0	London... 11.9	Montreal.. 12.1	Warsaw.. 17.2
Venice..... 12.7	Paris...... 13.2	Boston.... 13.5	Kiev..... 17.6
Florence.... 13.4	Berlin..... 13.7	Cleveland. 14.4	Moscow.. 16.4
Rome...... 13.6	Copenhagen 11.0	New York. 15.5	Leningrad 14.8
Naples..... 13.8	Vienna.... 14.0	Washington 17.5	Riga..... 15.7
Madrid.... 12.3	Lyon..... 14.4		
Barcelona.. 13.6			
Average 13.2° C. =	13.0° C. =	14.6° C. =	17.9° C. =
55.8° F.	55.4° F.	58.2° F.	64.2° F.

Average of all, 14.7° C. (58.4° F.)

Chapter XV

A TEST BY COUNTRIES

The births of eminent people in the individual countries of Europe show a seasonal distribution like that of the corresponding but more highly selected people in the *Encyclopædia Britannica*. Figure 83 illustrates the seasonal distri-

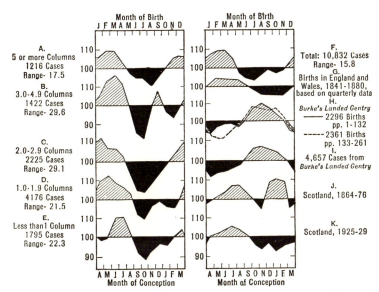

Fig. 83.—*Dictionary of National* (British) *Biography*. Births arranged according to length of biography.

bution of births among nearly 11,000 eminent British who are included in the *Dictionary of National Biography*. Here, just as in the corresponding *Dictionary of American Biography*, a division has been made according to the length of the biographical sketches. It is by no means certain, however, that Group A, with 5 columns or more of space, consists of such gifted people as Group B with 3 or 4 columns. Our British friends, especially a generation ago when the first part of the *Dictionary of National Biography* was compiled, still cling rather strongly to the aristocratic ideal. To them a king is a king and a duke a duke, and as such they deserve longer biographies than would be allotted to untitled people of similar achievements.   Nevertheless, as a whole the people with 5 or more columns are much more distinguished than those with only 1 to 3.

The left-hand side of Figure 83 makes it evident that all 5 groups into which we have divided the British leaders show essentially the same type of seasonal curve of births.   The maximum in every case falls in some month from January to April, and the minimum in July or August.   In three cases, a hint, at least, of a minor maximum is seen in September.   In Group E, comprising persons with less than 1 column of space, another minor maximum in December is followed by a minor minimum in January.   Aside from this last feature, the agreement with America, as illustrated in Figure 69 (page 305), is close.

If we disregard Group A because it includes so many hereditary rulers, the other four curves also agree with the corresponding American curves in showing a diminution of amplitude as the degree of eminence declines.   Curve E, to be sure, representing persons with less than 1 column of space, has a slightly greater amplitude than Curve D, with 1 to 2 columns.   It is based, however, on only 1793 persons, and its amplitude would presumably be lessened if it were based on as large a number as Curve D (4176).   When we turn to the month of maximum birth the change in date from the more to the less eminent is not so systematic as in America.   Among the persons receiving less than 3 columns of space, to be sure, the date of the maximum is later as the degree of eminence declines, just as in America.   Curve C has its maximum in January, D in February, and E in March or April.   In Curve A, the maximum comes in February or March, thus putting it between D and E.   Such a position may be in accord with the real abilities of the persons in Group A when allowance is made for hereditary rulers. The March maximum of Curve B, however, for persons with 3 or 4 columns, is out of line with the rest. This may be accidental, for Curve B is based on only 1422 cases, but we do not feel at all sure. Nevertheless, when we consider the large number of cases needed to give fully reliable curves, the 5 curves of eminent British births not only agree with one another and with the corresponding American curves in their general aspect, but are somewhat like the American curves in showing that the births of the more eminent people occur earlier in the season than those of the less eminent.

The right-hand side of Figure 83 illustrates an attempt to determine how far the season of birth among eminent persons in the British Isles agrees with that of ordinary people. Curve F includes all of the 10,832 persons for whom data are available in the *Dictionary of National Biography* (Curves A to E). Curve G shows the seasonal distribution of births in England from 1841 to 1880. Unfortunately, the English publish their births according to quarters, and data by months are not available. In an attempt to remedy this defect, we have compiled seasonal curves from *Burke's Landed Gentry*, which appears to be the best available source of data as to birthdays in the last century among people who are not distinguished.

Two groups of people culled from successive portions of that book give curves which resemble one another but are different in February and March (H). In *Who's Who in New England* we found that the first two groups of similar data (2000 persons per group, Figure 70, page 308) failed to show an important winter maximum. Therefore, we surmise that further data might increase the importance of the winter maximum which is suggested in the solid curve of H (Figure 83), but is not evident in the dotted line, nor in Curve I where the two parts of H are combined. The important fact about the data as to the *Landed Gentry* is that they show a strong maximum in August, as has already been explained, whereas a similar feature in the curve for eminent people on the left of Figure 83 is absent or inconspicuous.

Another way of compensating for the English failure to publish monthly statistics is to use data for Scotland, where many persons in the *Dictionary of National Biography* were born. The climate of Scotland is so similar to that of England that it can have only a slight effect in producing a different seasonal distribution of births. Scotch data for 1864 to 1876 (*J*) show two well-developed maxima. The first is the usual maximum according to the basic animal rhythm. The second appears to be due to the migration of workers back to their homes from December to February. In modern times (*K*) it has almost disappeared.

Judging from all the curves on the right of Figure 83 we conclude that, if monthly data for England, Scotland, and Ireland were available for the period covered by the births recorded in the biographical dictionary, we should have a curve about midway between the two Scotch curves, *J* and *K*. Such a curve would be a good deal like Curve *F* for all the people in the *Dictionary of National Biography*. There may be some difference between the seasonal distribution of births among eminent people and the British in general, but the data presented thus far do not establish such a conclusion. This agrees with what we found as to length of life. Among eminent Britons, unlike Americans, the season of birth shows little relation to longevity. We interpreted this as meaning that the climate of Britain is so excellent that nearly the same degree of vigor prevails among people born at all seasons. A similar explanation seems to fit Figure 83.

In spite of what has just been said, certain facts suggest that the more intellectual types of British tend to be born earlier in the season than do others, just as in America. This is illustrated in Figure 84 where the persons in the *Dictionary of National Biography* have been divided according to the occupational classification employed for those in the *Encyclopædia Britannica*. The occupations are arranged according to the date of the winter or spring maximum of births. Curve *A*, representing religious leaders, has a sharp maximum in February. The intellectual group (*B*), composed of scientists, educators, and students of the humanities, comes next with a maximum in March, but with February at practically the same level. Then come the artists, including actors, and musicians (*C*), with a sharp maximum in March. These are followed by executives (*D*)—the leaders in politics, war, and business—with a maximum in April, but with May only a little lower. Finally, among hereditary rulers (*E*), April and May share the maximum.

In a general way the order just given represents the rank to which a rating based on intelligence and strength of character would entitle the various groups. Let us begin at the bottom of Figure 84 with the hereditary rulers. On the basis of both intellect and character there is little doubt that the rulers as a whole rank lower than the other groups. Many of them, to be sure, were really eminent, but

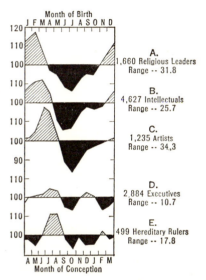

FIG. 84.—*Month of Birth. Dictionary of National* (British) *Biography.* According to occupation.

many others are included in reference books merely because of their position. Successful soldiers, political leaders, and others, who compose the major part of our next, or executive, group, excel in power of organization and in the personal qualities which attract followers rather than in sheer intellect or moral stamina. Artists (*C*) form a professional group of high talent, but their talent is of a special type. They are often emotional rather than intellectual. The power of intense concentration and prolonged exact thought is not demanded among them to so great a degree as in the so-called intellectual pursuits. Of course the greatest artists have these qualities, but Leonardo d'Vinci and Michelangelo are shining exceptions, not the rule. Moreover, in the artistic group strength of character in the sense of standing up against opposition is rarely required. The literary leaders, scientists, educators, historians, classical scholars, and other eminent persons of the next group (the intellectuals) all possess high intellectual qualities. On the whole, such people generally stand high in moral qualities, and only in rare cases can they succeed without the power of intense application to their work. Nevertheless, there is no special moral selection, and great success is sometimes achieved by men whose characters show comparatively little strength.

The religious leaders, at the top in Figure 84, include only a handful who were of the continental type that received high clerical positions because of their birth. The majority are especially representative of the Reformation and of the stormy seventeenth century. The leaders of the Protestant movement, the Puritans, and the founders of such sects as the Wesleyan Methodists and Quakers are prominent among them. Some were distinguished for the profound character of their theological writings. In intellectual caliber these religious leaders ranked high, but their most distinctive qualities were moral courage and persistence in the face of difficulty. This does not mean that the highest type of religious leader is more courageous or determined than the highest type of historian, musician, soldier, or king. What it does mean is that in the very nature of the case people who lack moral courage and high character are almost excluded from religious leadership.

We do not wish to press this point, but in general the curves of Figure 84 arrange themselves in the order which thoughtful students would choose if they were classifying the five groups there given according to their combined standing in intelligence and character. As a rule the season of maximum births comes earliest among the people in whom these two qualities are most fully combined.

The peculiar conditions that have just been described are a more or less faithful repetition of certain features which we have already seen among the persons in the *Britannica,* but have not sufficiently studied. In Figure 78 the five groups of occupations stand in the same order as in Figure 84. Turn back to page 330 and note that in western Europe the religious leaders (Curve *A*) show a minor maximum in January; the intellectuals (*B*), artists (*C*), and executives (*D*) have their maxima in February; and the hereditary leaders (*E*) have a very minor maximum in March. In the next column, the Mediterranean intellectuals (*F*) have a maximum in January; the artists (*G*) in February; and the executives (*H*) in April. In the United States and Canada the corresponding order is: intellectuals, February (and April); and artists, March; but the executives fall out of line, with a decided maximum in January. Finally, in eastern Europe the order is, intellectuals, February; artists, February, with January almost equally high; and executives, March and April. Among the less eminent leaders mentioned in the *Dictionary of American Biography* (the right-hand section of Figure 74, page 316) the order is almost the same: religious leaders, December; intellectuals, March, but with January and February almost as high; artists, January; and executives, February. Thus six regional groups agree more or less closely. Their agreement is by no means perfect, but it is close enough to warrant investigation. The whole thing is summed up in Table 23 where *1* means the earliest maximum, *2* the second, and so on. Inasmuch as religious leaders and hereditary rulers do not appear in all groups, it has been assumed that where they are missing they hold the first and fifth places respectively.

It is not easy to determine whether differences such as appear in the averages on the right of Table 23 are significant. Nor are we sure that our estimate of the intellectuality and character of the various groups is correct. Nevertheless, it is almost certain that the most intellectual types tend to be born earlier in the year than do those of lesser intellect.

TABLE 23

	British Biographical Dictionary	Western Europeans in the Britannica	American Biographical Dictionary	Americans in the Britannica	Mediterraneans in the Britannica	Eastern Europeans in the Britannica	Average
Religious leaders..	1	1	1	....	....	....	1.0
Intellectuals.....	2	3	4	2	3	3	2.8
Artists..........	3	4	2	3	4	2	3.0
Executives......	4	2	3	4	2	4	3.2
Hereditary rulers.	5	5	....	....	....	....	5.0

This last statement is confirmed by the work of Havelock Ellis in *A Study of British Genius* (1927). Estimates of intellectual ability by means of the space in reference books suffer from a serious disadvantage. The picturesqueness of a man's life, its connection with great historical events, and the popularity of the subjects with which he deals all have a great effect upon the amount of space allotted by editors. A profound mathematician may receive half a column, while a popular author of far less intrinsic ability may receive several pages. In order to overcome this difficulty Ellis went through the *Dictionary of National Biography* and other reference books, and on the basis of the best estimates that he could make selected approximately 1000 persons who appear to have been genuinely the greatest products of Great Britain. Royalty and persons who appeared to owe their position in any large degree to birth or special opportunity were omitted. The resultant list may not be perfect, it is decidedly better than a classification according to amount of space in reference books.

Using the occupational classification given by Ellis, I have divided his eminent people into two groups, one primarily intellectual, and the other distinguished for qualities other than pure reason. The 265 men of letters, scientists, scholars, philosophers, lawyers, and doctors for whom data are available are to be compared with 327 actors, artists, divines, musicians, poets, politicians, sailors, soldiers, and travelers. The divines ought to have been placed in the first group, but if this were done, it would merely accentuate the contrast which appears in Figure 85. There the smoothed curve of birth of the intellectual group shows a main maximum in November, a minor maximum in February, and a well-developed minimum in June. If more abundant data as to men of similar caliber were available, we should probably find a single major maximum in December or January. The other group (*B*, Figure 85) shows a decidedly different curve,

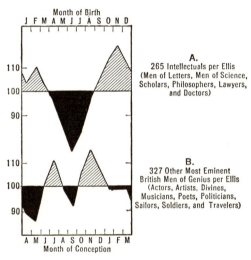

FIG. 85.—Births of Ellis' List, *Men of Genius.*

with maxima in April and August. In other words, even when we follow the exact method of Ellis, we still find a marked contrast between the seasonal distribution of births among the most intellectual group and among other eminent people who are less purely intellectual. Moreover, this more exact method confirms our observation as to the tendency for the births of the most highly intellectual type to reach a maximum in cold weather and to show a very decided dip in warm weather.

The effect of the weather is especially clear in the curve

for the intellectuals selected by Ellis. Social factors seem to play no appreciable part in determining the form of the curve. If we assume that the true maximum of Curve *A* in Figure 85 is equally divided between December and January, the maximum of conceptions takes place when the temperature averages about 45° F. If the true maximum is in November, the temperature at the time of maximum conceptions averages about 40°. The important point is that in either case it is lower than would appear from less accurate methods. On the other hand, quite a different set of conditions appears to determine the form of Curve *B* for the births of the less intellectual types of genius. The August maximum is doubtless the same as the one which we found in the curve for the landed gentry (*I*, Figure 83), and the April maximum is presumably the same as the spring maximum for Scotland as a whole (*J* and *K*, Figure 83). Thus the work of Ellis supplies additional evidence that the seasonal distribution of births among people of supreme intellectual ability is different not only from that of people as a whole, but even from that of highly eminent people in whom the intellectual quality is less pronounced.

Let us return once more to the United States. A few days before the manuscript of this book was ready for the printer, Mr. C. P. Tobey of the American Astrological Society sent me an extensive tabulation of birthdays. These proved so interesting that their smoothed curves, calculated according to our regular method, are presented in Figure 86. If this figure had been available when Chapter XIII was written, pages 316 to 318 might have been a little different. It has seemed of interest, however, to leave the entire text up to this point exactly as it was written. The 8 solid lines of Figure 86 (*B* to *I*) represent *Who's Who in America* (1929) and 7 distinct occupations. A large proportion of the persons in the occupational groups are successful people with a local reputation, but are not in *Who's Who*. Although some foreigners, as well as Southerners and Westerners, are included, the great majority were born in the northeastern United States from Missouri northward and eastward. The date of birth is usually from 1850 to 1890.

Curves *B* to *I* all show a winter maximum in January or February; a spring minimum in May, or possibly June; a more irregular autumn maximum, coming anywhere from August to October; and a winter minimum, usually in November or December. Most of the curves dip deeper in April and May than do the corresponding curves for people in general, thus suggesting that the hot weather of July and August is more unfavorable to the conception of successful people than to that of ordinary people.

Curves *B* to *I* are arranged according to the amount by which the winter maximum exceeds or falls below the autumn maximum. In curve *B* for clergymen the winter maximum shows the greatest excess, whereas in *I* for industrialists it almost disappears. This brings out the most significant feature of Curves *B* to *I*, namely, the change from a curve of the eminent type at the top to one of the ordinary type at the bottom. To begin at the bottom, Curves *I* and *H* for industrialists and engineers closely resemble those for old New England stock in general (*E*, Figure 68, page 300), and are practically identical with the curve for 10,000 persons in *Who's Who in New England* (*J*, Figure 70, page

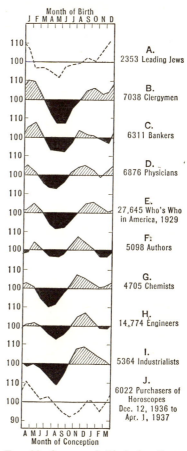

FIG. 86.—Season of Birth by Occupation in the United States.

308). On the other hand, the curve for bankers (*C*) is almost the same as that for leading American women of the nineteenth century (*D*, Figure 68); and the curve for clergymen (*B*) resembles that for Americans in the *Encyclopædia Britannica* (*B*, Figure 68). Does this change in form indicate a corresponding variation in mentality? We cannot answer positively, but it is interesting to find that the industrialists, like the corresponding executives of our previous tabulations, depart farthest from the type of curve associated with the highest mentality. Moreover, here, just as in Great Britain (*A*, Figure 84, page 353), the clergy show the greatest tendency toward the type associated with real eminence.

Must we therefore infer that from the lower to the upper of the solid lines of Figure 86 there is a gradual increase in mentality? In order to judge of this fairly we ought to take account not only of pure intellectuality, but also of strength of character—will power—and of the degree to which the people in our various lines of effort are selected. In order to obtain 5000 leaders in commerce and industry (Curve *I*), one must include the owners or managers not only of all the largest concerns, but also of a good many moderate-sized ones. Although engineers and chemists are often considered rather intellectual, to get nearly 15,000 engineers and 5000 chemists one must scoop quite far down into the common herd. To get 5000 authors, one must take not only the cream, but a great deal of thin milk. Among physicians, on the contrary, 7000 represent only the cream, and among them, more than among the other occupations thus far mentioned, a moral factor is involved. Society is much more exacting in its demands for high character among leading physicians than among engineers, for example. Therefore the physicians presumably represent both intellect and will power more fully than do the groups in the curve below theirs in Figure 86.

As to the bankers, the case is not clear. Their list dates from 1911 and is therefore a quarter of a century older than the others used in Figure 86. They are undoubtedly an able group. A selective process may perhaps eliminate moral weaklings more effectively than among chemists and authors, who are not exposed to great financial temptations. It is the custom nowadays to depreciate bankers, but taken as a whole, they are very trustworthy. Among clergymen, the case is clearer. They may not stand at the top intellectually, but they certainly stand there morally. It requires much strength of will to make the sacrifices that they do, and live up to the very stringent moral code which society imposes upon them. Moreover, the 7000 here used represent the cream as fully as do the physicians. Thus a tabulation of American occupations seems to agree with our study of the encyclopedia and of British leaders.

The dotted lines at the top and bottom of Figure 86 seem to confirm our conclusions as to the sensitive quality of seasonal curves of birth. The 2353 Jews of Curve *A* are taken from the *Biographical Encyclopædia of American Jews, 1935.* Including, as they do, all occupations and all periods among a social group in which high achievement is common, they represent a more rigid selection than do the other curves of Figure 86. Therefore it is not surprising that their curve approaches that of the most eminent people (*A*, Figure 68). The occurrence of the maximum in December rather than January may be accidental, for the difference between the two months is not great.

Curve *J*, representing people who purchased "horoscopes" from an astrological publisher, is interesting in quite a different way. Here for the first time we meet a curve based on individuals whose selection as subjects of study may have been influenced by the month of birth. When we choose chemists, or Frenchmen, we take them as they come, regardless of their date of birth. The Americans who purchased astrological "horoscopes," however, are very much concerned with their birthdays. I do not know how important January may be astrologically, but during the winter of 1936-1937, when these purchases were made, the newspapers had a good deal to say about the advantages of birth in winter in contrast to the disadvantages of birth in summer. Therefore people whose birthdays were in winter were encouraged to inquire into the mysteries of the stars, whereas many of those born in summer said, "What's the use?" For this reason Curve *J*, with its January maximum and July minimum, is distinctly different from the rest of Figure 86. The readiness with which seasonal curves of birth respond to social conditions, and therefore may be misinterpreted, is very evident.

From this excursion into astrology, let us return to our

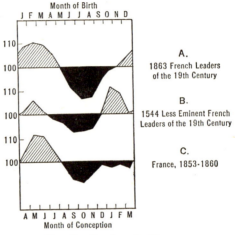

A.
1863 French Leaders
of the 19th Century

B.
1544 Less Eminent French
Leaders of the 19th Century

C.
France, 1853-1860

FIG. 87.—Leaders in France.

main problem. Let us test our conclusions as to eminence and season of birth by means of other countries as well as Great Britain and the United States. France is the first country to be examined in this way. For this purpose we have employed the *Dictionnaire national des contemporains* (1899), which is practically a rather select *Who's Who*. The 3000 leaders of France during the nineteenth century whom it includes have been divided into two groups according to the length of their biographical sketches, as appears in the upper two curves of Figure 87. The lower curve shows the seasonal distribution of French births as a whole during the nineteenth century. In general the three curves are alike, but two differences may be noted. First, the curve for people in general (*C*) is much lower during the second half of the year than are those for the leaders. Second, the time of maximum births varies very slightly according to the degree of eminence. Among the most famous it is February, but January and March stand at practically the same level. Among the less eminent the maximum occurs conspicuously in February; among people in general, February and March share the honors. Thus the most eminent Frenchmen of the nineteenth century agree with other leaders in having their maximum of births earlier than people in general.

In Germany a similar situation is seen. Using curves based on Kruger's *Deutsches Literatur Lexikon* (1914), we find that the most distinguished people (*A* in Figure 88) show a maximum of births in January. Since this curve includes only 310 persons it would not be important, were it not that its data agree with those of many other regions. The 2000 less eminent Germans of Curve *B* show a maximum in February. This agrees with that of Germans as a whole from 1872 to 1880, and again in 1903, as shown in Curves *C* and *D*. Since the World War the maximum for people as a whole has shifted to March (*E*).

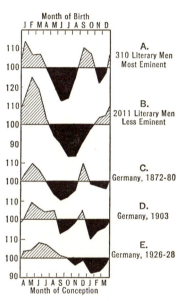

Fig. 88.—Leaders in Germany.

Sweden is another country for which data are available. The number of leaders is small, but again there is remarkable agreement with other countries. The 154 most eminent people listed in the *Sveniskt Biografiskt Lexikon* (1918) show a very sharp maximum in February, as appears in the heavy solid line of *A* in Figure 89, and in the finer solid line which is plotted on half as great a scale. Less eminent leaders (625 in number) show a similar maximum, but with March almost as high as February (*B*). The 779 least eminent leaders defer their maximum until April. Amongst Swedes as a whole the maximum comes in March as appears in the dotted line of Section *A*. Thus here, as in so many

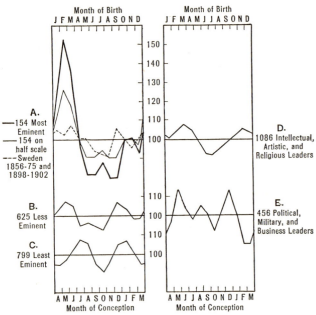

Fig. 89.—Seasonal Distribution of Births among Eminent Swedes, 1856–1875.

other cases, the most eminent people tend to be born earlier in the season than the others.

Another interesting feature of Figure 89 is that the September maximum, due to conceptions in December, is strong in the curves for the two groups of minor leaders (*B* and *C*). and among people as a whole (the dotted line), but almost disappears in the curve for the most eminent people, as is the case in several other countries. It also disappears in Curve *D* where intellectuals, artists, and religious leaders have been grouped together. On the other hand it is strongly developed in Curve E for the executive and hereditary group. It is very strange that people of these types so often show a much more irregular seasonal curve of births than do the leaders whose position depends more intimately upon intellectual achievement. But note that in this case, unlike some others, the maximum for the executive type comes earlier than for the intellectuals.

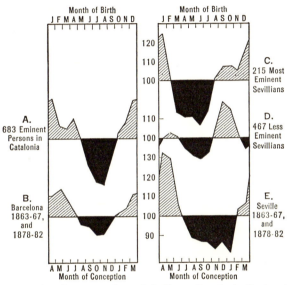

Fig. 90.—Births of Eminent People and Ordinary People in Spain, 1863–1867, and 1878–1882.

Spain, again, repeats the conditions which we have seen repeatedly. Taking our data from two Spanish dictionaries of biography * for the provinces of Seville and Catalonia respectively, we get the results shown in Figure 90. In Catalonia the curve for 683 eminent persons (A) has a maximum in January, but December is almost equally high. This means that in a region so warm as Spain the concep-

---

* *Diccionario de escritores, maestros, y orodores naturales de Sevilla y su actual provincia,* Sevilla, 1922, 3 vols. *Diccionario biográphica de escritores y artistes catalones de siglo XIX,* Barcelona, 1889, 2 vols.

tions of eminent people show a decided tendency to be much more numerous in March and April than at any other time of the year. Among the people of this region in general, as is illustrated by the curve for the province of Barcelona (*B*), births are at a maximum in February. Among both the eminent and the others the minimum of births occurs in July and August, which corresponds to conceptions in October and November. This agrees with the basic animal rhythm. In Seville, on the right of Figure 90, a similar situation is found. The maximum of births among the most eminent leaders is strong in January. Among the 467 who are less eminent it shifts to February. Among the people of the province of Seville as a whole the maximum comes in January, but February is almost equally important. In Seville, unlike most places, the eminent people, especially the less eminent, show a strong maximum in September due to conceptions at the holiday season in December, but ordinary people show it very faintly. We do not understand this, but it may be the same sort of thing as the bulge for the German "hunt children" in Figure 80 (page 337) but shoved a month later because of the warm climate. The important fact for our present purpose, however. is that, even though the number of people is small, those who are most eminent show practically the same kind of curve as the corresponding people in other countries.

The last country which we shall use to illustrate the season of birth among eminent people is India. By consulting many books we have been able to ascertain the birthdays of 1106 eminent Indians, of whom 333 may be classified as intellectual leaders, and the remainder as political or commercial leaders, or hereditary rulers. In Figure 91, Curve *A* shows the seasonal distribution of births among intellectual leaders. In *B*, the solid line is the same as *A* except that it has been smoothed. There we see that in March the births fall to a minimum and in August rise to a maximum. A minor minimum in October is followed by a minor maximum in November. At first sight it seems as if this curve were directly the opposite of the other curves which we have studied, aside from those for the European aristocracy. Its minimum occurs when the European and American curves for eminent leaders are near the maximum. As a matter of fact, however, it agrees with them perfectly. This is evident when we recall that in India the temperature is so high that only in the coolest months and in the northern half of the country does the average for even a single month drop to the optimum.

The majority of the Indian leaders, especially those of the intellectual type, come from the northern part of the country. Therefore, it has seemed legitimate to use the temperature of Delhi, the capital, for purposes of comparison. The line of crosses in Section *B* of Figure 91 indicates the amount by which the temperature of Delhi *departs* from 62° F. *during the month of conception*. We use a temperature of 62° because this appears to be the optimum temperature for conceptions. It is the median temperature of the month of maximum conceptions in 84

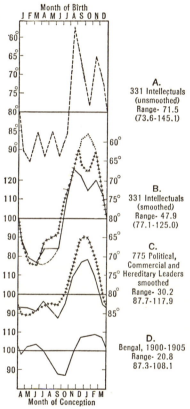

FIG. 91.—Season of Birth in India.

regions, as we saw in Figure 59 (page 262). The *highest* point in the line of crosses represents a monthly average temperature of 62°. Using the scale of months at the bottom of Figure 91 we see that during June, as indicated by the *low* point of the line of crosses, the mean monthly temperature at Delhi rises to 92° F. During that month, according to our usual scheme of index numbers, the conceptions of Indian leaders who were born the following March numbered only 77. In November, however, the temperature at Delhi drops to 62°, and conceptions of eminent people reach a maximum of nearly 126 according to the smoothed averages. Thereafter, as indicated by the fine dotted line and the inverted scale on the right, the temperature falls a little further. At the same time the line of crosses drops once more because the temperature again departs from 62° F., this time, of course, in an opposite direction from before. The significant fact is that with a drop to a temperature below the optimum the number of conceptions at once declines. It reaches a minimum in January, thus producing a corresponding minimum of births in October. In February, the temperature at Delhi once more rises to 62°, and with this rise comes an increase in the number of births. Then, when the temperature passes the optimum and goes on rising, the number of births falls rapidly.

Another minor feature of Section *B* in Figure 91 emphasizes the close agreement between the conception of men of eminence and the departure of the temperature from the optimum. The hottest time in northern India, it will be remembered, is May and June. July and August are cooler than June because the southwest monsoon brings abundant clouds and rain. Perhaps the most remarkable feature of Figure 91, and one of the most remarkable features of this whole book, is the fact that in July and August, according to the scale at the bottom, the smoothed curve of conceptions (the solid line in Section *B*) shows a little step closely resembling a similar step in the line of crosses which here represents the temperature inverted. Under ordinary conditions one would expect that the temperature in July and August would rise higher than in June and that this would be accompanied by a further decline in conceptions, as suggested by the dotted line. Nothing of the kind occurs. The coming of the monsoon with its clouds, rains and breezes is accompanied by a slight drop of temperature in July and by only a slight change in August, thus forming a sort of step in Figure 91. In harmony with this there occurs an increase in conceptions that give rise to intellectual leaders. Thus the solid line in Section *B* does not follow the course indicated by the dotted line, as one might expect, but forms a sort of step almost parallel to the inverted course of temperature. Taken as a whole the seasonal fluctuations in the conceptions of eminent intellectual leaders in India agree almost perfectly with the departures of the temperature from the optimum for physical vigor, as determined in many other countries. This agreement with distant countries having very different climates is most extraordinary.

We have not yet finished with India. The solid line of Section *C* (Figure 91) shows the curve of births among the less intellectual type of Indian leaders. For comparison with this the inverted curve of temperature for Calcutta during the month of conception is inserted as a line of crosses. Calcutta has been chosen rather than Delhi because leaders of the political, commercial, and hereditary types are represented more fully in south India than those of the more intellectual types. Here again we find an extraordinarily close resemblance between the curve of births and the inverted curve of temperature at the time of conception. In the cooler weather there is no decline in conceptions, such as we have seen among the intellectual leaders. This is presumably because the coolest month averages 65° F., and is therefore above the optimum.

In Bengal, as a whole (Curve *D*) the births follow approximately the same course as among the less intellectual types of leaders (Curve *C*). There is one important difference, however, for among ordinary people there is a strong minimum of births in June and July. This is faintly seen among the less intellectual leaders, but can scarcely be detected among the intellectuals. The gist of the whole thing is that in India, just as in other countries, the births of leaders, especially those of the intellectual type, show a much stronger tendency than those of people in general to occur in harmony with the basic animal rhythm. The most highly gifted persons seem in a certain way to be a response to ideal conditions of weather. They seem also to be a response to temperatures slightly lower than those associated with the greatest number of births among people in general. This last point is so important that it will form the subject of the next chapter.

Chapter XVI

TEMPERATURE, HEALTH AND GENIUS

Throughout this volume the importance of temperature is repeatedly emphasized. This is in harmony not only with universal experience, but also with the conclusions of specialists. No phase of human physiology is more vital than the mechanism whereby the body maintains a uniform temperature. Hill, Winslow, and Mills, although differing considerably otherwise, represent types of investigators who stress this point. The importance of temperature is obvious from the fact that within the body a departure of a single degree from the normal is accompanied by discomfort. Outside the body a change of a single degree in the temperature of the air can easily be detected. Movements of the air and changes in its humidity are detected by the body mainly through their effect on temperature. The optimum temperature is evidently that at which the body maintains the normal level of internal temperature with the least effort. The heart, lungs, and other organs then function with a minimum of strain, thus giving a feeling of well-being, and leaving the maximum amount of energy available for other purposes.

Such being the case, it is not surprising that reproduction takes place most effectively when the optimum temperature prevails. Mills has made a special study of this matter. His statistical studies, many of which are not yet published, agree essentially with those set forth in this book. His experiments show that, when white mice are kept at high temperatures, their powers of reproduction decline rapidly, and the stock tends to die out. On the other hand, mice kept at relatively low temperatures retain their full vigor generation after generation. Among other evidences of the injurious effect of heat upon reproduction Mills cites the case of a valuable stallion which was shipped in a closed box-car in very hot weather. The stallion was mated repeatedly thereafter, but never produced foals. His germ cells had apparently been destroyed. I have observed that in certain parts of Central Africa the natives swathe the scrotum of the he-goat in a woollen bag at certain seasons. They have learned that when the testicles are kept at the same temperature as the rest of the body, the germ cells are impotent, even though mating may take place. There is abundant medical evidence to this same effect. Mills thinks that hot baths may impair men's powers of reproduction and be one cause of the high percentage of sterility in modern families. Whether this be true or not, there is abundant evidence that heat is especially injurious to the germ cells of the male. Hence it is not surprising that in so many of our diagrams conceptions decline greatly during and especially after hot seasons. Nor is it surprising that under such conditions a diminution of vigor is especially noticeable in the most delicate and most important of distinctively human functions, namely, the power of creative thought.

The explanation of how both physical and mental activity are influenced by the temperature and other conditions to which parents are subjected before the birth of a child presents a very pretty problem for the physiologist. One important line of research is foreshadowed in the statement of W. A. Price that among a certain tribe in Africa a woman who is expected to conceive a child is subjected to certain rigid rules of diet for two months before cohabiting with her husband. From another angle we may expect much light from careful daily measurements such as those made by Petersen. His graphs show that in Chicago, Detroit, and Milwaukee the response of the death rate to daily changes in the weather is of precisely the same clear-cut kind which I found for a much earlier period in New York. Each cyclonic storm, or in the newer parlance, each alternate advance of a polar front and a tropical front, is accompanied by a pronounced wave-like change in the death rate. The way in which health and storms go together year after year at all seasons is astonishing. Petersen has gone far beyond the mere measurement of the number of deaths. By means of careful daily measurements of his patients he has found that practically every measurable function of the body is subject to constant fluctuations which evidently bear a close relation to the weather. Respiration, pulse, blood pressure, the chemical composition of the blood and urine, the concentration of ions, and the general rate of metabolism all pass through rapid changes from day to day in the same wave-like fashion as the general death rate.

The physiological cause of these fluctuations in bodily functions and in health is not yet clear. Some light may be derived from an investigation made by the Metropolitan Life Insurance Company under the direction of the National Research Council's Committee on Atmosphere and Man, and published under the title *Weather and Health* (Huntington, 1930). Using the daily deaths in New York City for a period of six years, we found that when the temperature falls, the death rate also tends to fall on that same day and on the next. When the temperature rises, the death rate rises in similar fashion. The effect in both cases, however, is only temporary. If the temperature stays near a certain level, the deaths soon adjust themselves to the rate appropriate to that particular temperature.

Such a state of affairs is easy to understand when the temperature is above the optimum. No matter whether people are well or ill, a fall in temperature brings conditions more closely approaching the optimum. It therefore makes it easier to maintain the proper balance between the production and outgo of heat. For people who are in good health this means more energy for work. For those who are ill it means less strain in order to keep the body at the right temperature, and therefore more strength to use in resisting disease. The difficulty comes when we try to explain the conditions at temperatures below the optimum. When the average temperature for day and night together drops, let us say, from 50° F. to 45° F., why should this mean a drop in the death rate on that day and the next? The lower temperature is less favorable than the other, as soon becomes evident after it has prevailed for a few days. And why should a rise of temperature raise the death rate when it brings the temperature to a level nearer to the optimum?

We cannot answer these questions yet, but an analogy will make the matter clearer. On entering a cold bath a person in good health feels a stimulating shock which brings the blood to the skin, produces a sensation of warmth and exhilaration, and promotes activity. If the same person remains long in a cold bath, however, he becomes chilled and may suffer seriously. On the other hand, a hot bath immediately produces a feeling of relaxation and drowsiness. It depresses one's activity as markedly as the cold bath stimulates it. Changes in the temperature of the air, as we know from common experience, produce a similar effect. A mild breath of cool air from a window will often arouse a sleepy audience to alert attention. On the other hand, if the air grows gradually warmer, many of the audience may fall asleep before the end of the lecture.

Among people who are ill the situation is somewhat different because they are more or less completely protected from changes of temperature, especially in winter. Nevertheless, they respond with remarkable readiness to changes in the weather. This suggests that some other element of the weather, such as atmospheric pressure, relative humidity, or atmospheric electricity, may produce the observed effect. Both Mills and Petersen ascribe great importance to atmospheric pressure, but neither of them appears to have made a detailed statistical analysis of the matter. It is obvious that changes in pressure are very closely associated with those in temperature and other elements of the weather. So far as I know, however, no one has yet found any important direct relation between atmospheric pressure and health through an analysis of daily changes. My own attempts to find such a relationship proved so unconvincing that I have never published them. Nevertheless, the question still remains open.

The case as to atmospheric electricity remains equally unconvincing. Yaghlou and others have shown that there are great fluctuations in the number of atmospheric ions of different sorts from day to day, as well as from hour to hour. Winslow and his colleagues, however, have been unable to detect any effect of these upon physiological reactions. Again, there is plenty of evidence that atmospheric humidity and the movement of the air have a close relation to health and comfort. This relationship, however, is largely, although probably not entirely, a matter of temperature. So long as there is no condensation of droplets, air of high humidity feels warmer than dry air. Moving air creates a sensation of coolness by means of evaporation. The net result, then, seems to be that an enormous body of evidence indicates the extreme importance of temperature. We are not yet certain, however, that other climatic factors exert much direct effect upon health except as they influence the rate at which heat is lost from the body. The effect of changes of temperature upon sick people in cold weather may be produced through changes so slight that they have hitherto passed unnoticed or through variations in the cooling effect of the air by reason of changes in its movement and humidity after it enters the house. Careful experiments are needed before there can be any certainty either on this point, or as to the effect of atmospheric pressure.

Meanwhile the one great certainty is that the maintenance of the temperature of the body at a very definite level is of supreme importance, and that any change in the temperature, humidity, or movement of the air alters the physiological reactions which control the temperature of the body. Moreover, any change in barometric pressure at once leads to alterations in the movement and hence in the temperature and humidity of the air. Thus a great chain of connected events is set in motion by variations in barometric pressure, and each storm—each advent of a polar or tropical front—involves a vast network of physiological changes.

With this point of view before us, let us turn to the problem of the relation between mental activity and temperature. We shall not attempt any physiological explanation, but shall merely aim at a clear picture of the facts.

If we were to construct a diagram showing the distribution of the births of distinguished people in relation to temperature it would resemble Figure 59 (page 262), but would show a much greater concentration of the maxima of both conceptions and births around the median. Moreover, the median in both cases would be at a lower temperature than in Figure 59. A better way, however, is to compare the seasonal curves of birth of the most eminent people with corresponding curves for the population as a whole. For this purpose we can use the American and Mediterranean groups from the *Encyclopædia Britannica,* and the distinguished people of Britain, France, Germany, Sweden, and Spain, as appear in Table 23. We exclude the eastern Europeans of the *Encyclopædia* because no curves for the population as a whole provide a correct standard of comparison. India is likewise excluded, not only because its curves for the population as a whole are not comparable geographically with the curve of the leaders, but also because they are dominated by malaria.

Spain gets too much weight in Table 23 because data from two biographical dictionaries are given separately. The French and Spanish used there do not represent so great a degree of eminence as do the others, but they are probably of a higher caliber than the average in a modern *Who's Who.* In order to balance this, and also because of their intrinsic value, the data of Ellis (1927) for the most intellectual group of British geniuses have also been included. Averages have been calculated omitting these and also including them. The comparison of the 9 curves mentioned in Table 24 with the corresponding curves for people in general appears to

TABLE 24

TEMPERATURE RELATIONSHIPS OF EMINENT PERSONS COMPARED
WITH PEOPLE IN GENERAL

Fig-ure	Curve	Type of Eminent Persons	Temperature at Time of Maximum				Excess of Temperature for Ordinary Compared with Eminent Persons	
			Births		Conceptions		Births	Concep-tions
			Emi-nent	Other	Emi-nent	Other		
			A	B	C	D	E	F
84	A	361 Mediterrane-ans in *Encyclo-pædia Britannica*	4.3	7.2	14.2	18.2	2.9	4.0
84	H	1137 Americans in *Encyclopædia Britannica*......	0.0	2.3	16.1	19.4	2.3	3.3
85	A	1216 most emi-nent British.....	4.5	9.5	12.5	16.0	5.0	3.5
87	A	265 most eminent British (Ellis)...	4.0	9.5	5.1	16.0	5.5	10.9
88	A	1863 French lead-ers of nineteenth century........	4.1	4.5	14.2	14.4	0.4	0.2
89	A	310 most eminent Germans.......	−0.3	1.5	8.3	14.5	2.8	6.2
90	A	154 most eminent Swedes.........	−2.8	−1.3	9.7	14.1	1.5	4.4
91	A	683 eminent Cata-lonians.........	8.5	9.0	12.2	15.7	0.5	3.5
91	C	215 eminent Sevil-lians..........	11.2	12.1	18.2	19.3	0.9	1.1
Average in degrees C. omit-ting Ellis.................			3.7	5.7	13.2	16.5	2.0	3.3
Average in degrees F. omit-ting Ellis.................			38.7	42.3	55.8	61.7	3.6	5.9
Average in degrees C. includ-ing Ellis.................			3.7	6.1	12.3	16.4	2.4	4.1
Average in degrees F. includ-ing Ellis.................			38.7	43.0	54.1	61.5	4.3	7.4

give an approximately accurate picture of the differences between the seasonal distribution of births among people of high intellectual caliber and people in general.

The first point to note in Table 24 is that the average temperature at which ordinary people are conceived in these 8 regions (Column *D*) is approximately 62° F., which is practically identical with the corresponding median temperature in the 84 regions of Figure 59. This shows that we are dealing with average communities in which conceptions are most numerous at the temperature which many lines of research have indicated as the optimum for physical health and efficiency. The next point is that in every case the births (Column A) and especially the conceptions (Column C) of the leaders reach a maximum at a lower-temperature than do those of the rank and file (Columns B and D). In the case of births, the average temperature for the leaders is 38.7° F. (Column A) and for the others 43° (Column B), a difference of about 4° (Column E). The average temperature of maximum conceptions is 54.1° F. for the leaders, and 61.5° for the others if we include the data of Ellis, thus making a difference of 7.4° F. (Column F).

Even if this difference is only 5.9° F., as it becomes if we omit Ellis, it is too large and too consistently present to be an accident. Column F shows that it occurs in each of the regional groups. It falls below 6° F. (3.3° C.) only in the case of the French and the Sevillians. These are the two groups which are limited to contemporaries. They therefore comprise a smaller proportion of great minds than does any other group. If they are omitted, the difference between the temperatures at the time when the great leaders and the rank and file are conceived rises to 10.2° F. (5.7° C.) and the optimum temperature for the conception of leaders becomes 50.7° F. (10.4° C.).

The question at once arises whether this difference between eminent people and others has any connection with the fact that people display the greatest mental activity at a temperature considerably below the optimum for physical activity and comfort. The existence of a mental optimum of temperature was first demonstrated by Lehman and Pedersen in *Das Wetter und unsere Arbeit* (1907). From daily tests of school children they concluded that mental activity varies with the outdoor temperature in the same way as physical work, but reaches its highest efficiency at a lower temperature. *Civilization and Climate* (Huntington 1915, 1924) contains fuller and more definite evidence to this effect based on the marks of hundreds of students at West Point and Annapolis. Rossman (1929) carried the matter further by showing that applications for patents, and especially for amendments of patents, follow the same rule. Later data (Huntington, 1933) show that success in passing civil-service examinations does likewise.

Part of the evidence as to the optimum temperature for mental activity is illustrated in Figure 92. Curve *A* shows that in April about 75 per cent of the young people who take the educational tests for civil-service positions in Massachusetts pass the examinations; in August the percentage drops to about 58; in November it rises to another maximum of 73. In New York State (*B*, Figure 92) the same thing occurs except that the autumn maximum comes in October instead of November. New York City (*C*) repeats the Massachusetts curve with a shift of the minimum to July.

Amendments to patents (*D*) behave very closely in the same way as civil-service examinations. They are particularly interesting because they represent a widespread cross section of the people in the manufacturing regions of the northeastern United States and the Great Lakes. Moreover, as Rossman points out, they represent an immediate expression of mental activity. The original application for a patent is usually the result of prolonged thinking. After the application has been filed many months elapse before the patent is granted. During that time the inventors mull over their work, and in many cases get new ideas which they wish to incorporate in their patents. Immediately there is a furor of activity. Unless the new idea is forwarded at once to the Patent Office, the patent may be granted without it. Therefore amendments to patents represent a very prompt response to the highest kind of mental activity, the creative faculty which is the root of all progress. Curves *E* and *F* at the bottom of Figure 92 show that when such activity is at its height and when people have the greatest success in pass-

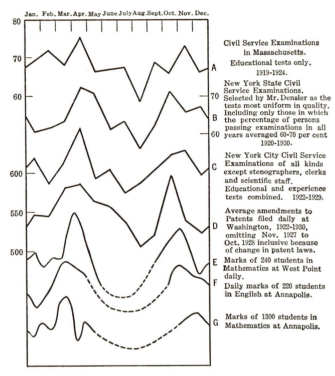

Civil Service Examinations in Massachusetts. Educational tests only. 1919-1924.

New York State Civil Service Examinations. Selected by Mr. Densler as the tests most uniform in quality. Including only those in which the percentage of persons passing examinations in all years averaged 60-70 per cent 1920-1930.

New York City Civil Service Examinations of all kinds except stenographers, clerks and scientific staff. Educational and experience tests combined.   1922-1929.

Average amendments to Patents filed daily at Washington, 1922-1930, omitting Nov. 1927 to Oct. 1928 inclusive because of change in patent laws.

Marks of 240 students in Mathematics at West Point daily.

Daily marks of 220 students in English at Annapolis.

Marks of 1300 students in Mathematics at Annapolis.

Fig. 92.—Mental Activity and Temperature.

ing civil-service examinations, the students at West Point and Annapolis do their best work.   The agreement among these diverse types of intellectual activity is remarkable.   The only reasonable explanation seems to be that the weather at a certain time in the spring and again in the autumn stimulates the nervous system to an unusual degree.

Let us examine Figure 92 in order to discover what conditions of weather prevail when the greatest mental activity occurs. The effect of light may be dismissed at once. In April the noonday sun is comparatively high; in October and November it is about three-fourths of the way from its highest to its lowest position. The height of the sun in mid-April is about the same as at the beginning of September, fully two months before the autumn maximum of mental activity. Humidity may also be dismissed. The variations in the relative humidity for the year as a whole in the eastern United States are of relatively small importance and their course is quite different from that of mental activity. The same may be said of barometric pressure. When we come to temperature the degree of variability from day to day may be important, but the available data do not permit us to test this.

Quite a different situation prevails as to mean temperature, as appears in Table 25. There we have chosen certain

TABLE 25

TEMPERATURE RELATIONSHIPS OF MAXIMA OF MENTAL ACTIVITY

Type of Activity	Temperature of Month of Maximum Activity			
	Representative Cities	Spring Maximum A	Autumn Maximum B	Average C
A. Civil Service examinations, Mass..........	Boston	8.7° C	7.0° C	7.9° C
B. Civil Service examinations, N. Y. State....	Albany	10.2	10.9	10.6
C. Civil Service examinations, N. Y. City....	New York	9.2	9.2	9.2
D. Amendments to patents........	Boston, N. Y., Philadelphia	8.1	13.2	10.7
E. Marks in mathematics........	West Point	5.6	8.4	7.0
F. Marks in English	Annapolis, Md.	4.7	11.9	8.3
G. Marks in mathematics........	Annapolis, Md.	6.2	5.5	5.9
Average.........		7.5° C. (45.5° F.)	9.6° C. (49.3° F.)	8.6° C. (47.4° F.)

cities to represent the respective curves of Figure 92. Columns A and B show the temperature of these cities during the months of maximum mental activity.

In view of the many sources of error which must influence any set of figures such as those on which Figure 92 is based, the temperatures in each column of Table 25 show a rather close agreement. The spring maximum of mental activity occurs at temperatures ranging from 4.7° C. to 10.2° C., and the autumn maximum at 5.5 to 11.9°. Thus the greatest difference between any two maxima is only 7.2° C. or 13° F. Inasmuch as the possible range is about 28° C. or 50° F., it is evident that the maximum mental activity has a strong tendency to occur within a definite and limited range of temperature. On the basis of the data now before us the physical optimum occurs at a temperature of approximately 17° C. or 62° F., while the mental optimum occurs at approximately 8° C. or 47° F. Thus the difference between the two is roughly 8° C. or 15° F.

The mental optimum which we have now determined appears to be about the same as the temperature at the time of maximum births according to the basic animal rhythm. In Figure 59, Section *H* shows that the median temperature of the month of maximum births is 38° F. The average is higher, being 48° F. In Table 24, where the data are less abundant than in Figure 59 but more reliable, the average temperature of the month of maximum births among people in general is 44° F. None of these figures is far from 47°, which is the mental optimum according to Column C in Table 25. If we restrict ourselves to the marks of students, which represent the most accurate of the methods employed in Figure 92, the optimum temperature for mental activity appears to be 45° (7° C.). Much more work is needed before we can be sure of the exact optimum temperature for mental activity. Undoubtedly the optimum must vary somewhat according to a great variety of circumstances. It seems clear, however, that it lies somewhere in the neighborhood of 47° F. It is approximately 15° F. below the physical optimum, and not far from the temperature at which the maximum number of births takes place according to the basic animal rhythm.

This leads to the interesting possibility that the mental optimum of temperature became established in much the same way as the physical optimum. We have already seen that the physical optimum appears to owe its origin to an adaptation whereby health in general and reproductive vigor in particular reach their highest level at a particular time of the year. That time is 9 months before the season at which it is most desirable for children to be born. The most desirable season for birth is, of course, the one which gives the child the best chance of survival. Accordingly, the primitive parents who responded most fully to the stimulus of a particular kind of weather were presumably the ones whose children were most likely to grow up. In this way a rise of temperature to a mean of about 62° F. apparently became established as the physical optimum. Parents who were stimulated to special vigor by such temperatures produced not only more children, but also more vigorous children, than others. This vigor, we suppose, as well as the favorable season of birth, enabled an unusually large proportion of the children to survive and hence to pass on to their offspring an inherited reaction to the weather like that which had been a factor in their own survival.

In this way primitive man, like other animals, appears to have become endowed with an hereditary response to a climatic optimum which gives him unusual vigor at the season when conception is most desirable. The exact level of the optimum appears to be the result of the particular climate in which *Homo sapiens* originated as a species. A response to it still remains with us as a very deep-seated primitive inheritance. Therefore when the temperature either rises or falls to approximately the level at which it was most desirable for conception to take place in primitive times, people of all races, so far as is yet known, enjoy increased vigor which is reflected in good health, comfort, physical activity, and numerous conceptions. Among civilized people who live in houses and wear clothes, the physical optimum of temperature is found when the noonday temperature is about 70° F., that is, when the average for day and night is about 62° or 63°. Even among tropical people we have no evidence that the optimum temperature is ever higher than a daily average of 70°.

The mental optimum of temperature appears to be connected with the most favorable season for birth in the same way that the physical optimum is connected with conception. At the time of a child's conception the most important factor in promoting its survival is the physical vigor of both parents. When a child is born, physical vigor is still highly desirable, but another element now enters into the picture. In our species evolution has become mainly mental rather than physical. Survival depends upon intelligence and alertness more than upon physical strength. If the primitive parents of a helpless infant are alert and wise, the child is far more likely to survive than if they are inert and stupid. An alert, intelligent father protects the mother and child and supplies them with food. An alert, sensible mother does all manner of things which make her baby's chances of survival better than those of the child of an inert, stupid neighbor. Hence if the mental activity of parents is stimulated when the child is born, the child's chances of survival are increased. This leads to the hypothesis that such a stimulus is supplied by the temperature. The mental optimum is apparently the result of a climatic adaptation. When our species originated, the mental activity of people of a certain mutant type was presumably stimulated to useful activity by mean temperatures of 45° to 50° F. This type succeeded better than others in preserving the lives of its newborn babes. The others perhaps lost their babies because of inability to protect them from the wet, cold weather which the last glacial epoch then imposed upon regions that had previously been warm and dry. Modern inventions have now caused this adaptation to lose much of its value as a factor in survival. It still remains, however, as part of our biological inheritance. It may have great, though unrecognized, importance in other respects.

Having reached this conclusion concerning people in general, we may now turn once more to the tendency of highly gifted persons to be born at relatively low temperatures. We saw in Table 25 that the most eminent people tend to be conceived in largest numbers at temperatures at least 6° F. lower than the optimum for physical vigor among people in general. Does this have anything to do with the fact that the optimum temperature for mental activity is lower than for physical? It seems highly probable that two such peculiar and closely similar phenomena have a close relationship, but as yet we see no way of testing the matter. What we do see, however, is that many lines of evidence point toward relatively low temperature as favorable to mental vigor. This is the most important fact which has emerged in the last two chapters.

But what is the cause of this mental vigor? Can the temperature alter the child's genetic make-up, or does it merely influence his physical vigor? We see no reason for any difference in the average heredity of people born at different seasons. Unless the biologists make some new discoveries there seems to be strong reason for believing that on an average, in any large group of families, the innate or genetic capacities of people born at all seasons are the same. On the other hand, we have seen again and again that such matters as infant mortality, length of life, and the sex ratio indicate that persons born according to the basic animal rhythm possess more than the usual vigor. The fact that the births of eminent persons conform so closely to the basic rhythm is apparently explained in considerable part by the further fact that, if people are equal in all other respects, their achievements will vary in close harmony with their physical vigor.

Although the importance of physical vigor may not be evident among certain types of erratic geniuses, such as poets and artists who die young, it has been demonstrated again and again among eminent people in general. We have seen in this book that, even though all accidental deaths cannot be eliminated, the persons listed in the *Dictionary of American Biography* lived 68.9 years on an average, and those in the corresponding British dictionary, over 70.7 (Figure 40, page 174). This in itself is evidence of much more than the average degree of constitutional vigor. In addition to this a vast amount of evidence shows that men of exceptional ability work harder and longer than those of almost any other type. This, too, indicates great vigor. From all this we infer that fame depends not only upon innate endowments and upon training and opportunity, but also upon physical vigor. From the study of millions of births in this book we have seen again and again that reproductive vigor is greatest at certain seasons. We have seen that the children born as a result of conceptions at those seasons display unusual physical vigor. We have also seen that the world's great leaders show a pronounced tendency to come from among these vigorous children in greater numbers than from among those with less vigor.

It must not be supposed that vigor necessarily means great physical strength. What it really means is an harmonious adjustment of the organs of the body in such a way that they function well year after year. Thus they interfere as little as possible with the delicate mental processes which are the primary essential of genius, and with the hard, steady work which is usually essential if brilliant ideas are to be brought to full fruition. The degree to which people possess this kind of vigor appears to be greatly influenced by the health of their parents at the time of conception. In this book we have stressed the effect of the climatic factor upon the health of the parents. Other factors, however, may be equally important. By varying people's diet sufficiently throughout the year we might cause seasonal fluctuations in the birth rate and the production of geniuses as pronounced as those associated with variations in the weather. In fact, we must by no means overlook the idea that part of the fluctuations with which we are here dealing are due to seasonal changes in diet. Seasonal changes in occupations, recreations, dress, and general manner of living may also produce distinct results. The essential point is that variations in health and vigor, no matter how they are caused, are a potent factor in altering not only the number but also the quality of births.

One further fact must not be overlooked. Our data indicate that the most eminent people in many different countries were conceived in maximum numbers at a temperature some 6° or 8° F. lower than that at which the maximum number of conceptions takes place among people in general. Is it possible that in some unknown way conception at these lower temperatures exerts a favorable effect upon the nerves, the brain, the ductless glands, and the other organs that influence the amount and nature of mental activity? As yet we cannot answer this question, but the connection between relatively low temperature and mental achievement seems clear.

CHAPTER XVII

THE ABNORMAL AND THE INSANE

If the birth of genius is especially sensitive to the influence of the seasons, the same may be true of persons at the opposite extreme. Ellis in *British Genius* concludes that idiocy and genius are akin in certain ways. Lombroso, in *Men of Genius*, sets forth the hypothesis that insanity, rather than idiocy, is the mental defect most closely akin to genius. Everyone agrees that genius, idiocy, and insanity are extreme departures from the normal. But there is one great difference between genius and the others. Environmental conditions may drive a genius insane, or even convert him into an idiot, but it is impossible to change an idiot, or even an insane person, into a genius, unless the capacity for genius is present in the germ cells. Geniuses can arise only through the birth of persons with an especially favorable combination of genes; idiots and insane persons can be produced not only by defective genes, but by a multitude of environmental causes at any stage from conception onward. Any large group of insane persons or idiots presumably includes some whose deficiency is due to defects in germ plasm, and many others whose defects are the result of accidents and other unfavorable conditions of environment.

Even if the weather, diet, and other conditions that affect the health of the parents before conception do have a distinct effect upon the future vigor of offspring, any harmful effects thus produced cannot easily be distinguished from the similar effects produced during pregnancy, at birth, or during infancy. We can draw seasonal curves of births based solely upon people who were born with an unusually favorable genetic inheritance, but we cannot easily draw similar curves of persons bearing mental defects which date from the time of conception. The only seasonal curves of defectives now available are based partly, and perhaps largely, upon persons whose defects have arisen from environmental influences at unknown seasons, or perhaps at all seasons.

With this limitation in mind, let us examine three seasonal curves of birth pertaining to children who were born with malformations of body. Such malformations are often, al-

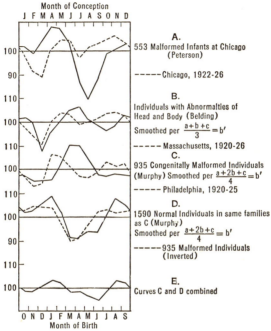

A.
553 Malformed Infants at Chicago
(Peterson)

-----Chicago, 1922-26

B.
Individuals with Abnormalties of Head and Body (Belding)

Smoothed per $\frac{a+b+c}{3} = b'$

----- Massachusetts, 1920-26

C.
935 Congenitally Malformed Individuals (Murphy) Smoothed per $\frac{a+2b+c}{4} = b'$

----- Philadelphia, 1920-25

D.
1590 Normal Individuals in same families as C (Murphy)

Smoothed per $\frac{a+2b+c}{4} = b'$

-----935 Malformed Individuals (Inverted)

E.
Curves C and D combined

FIG. 93.—Season of Conception of Congenitally Malformed Individuals.

though by no means always, accompanied by mental weakness. The first of these curves, *A* in Figure 93, is based upon data contained in an interesting and suggestive publication by Petersen (1935). On the basis of about 400 malformed children in Chicago he concludes that malformed or physically defective infants tend to be conceived in largest numbers in March and April, and that their defects are due to barometric instability at that time. In order to ascertain whether the births show a seasonal fluctuation different from the normal, he expresses the births of the malformed infants as percentages of what would be expected if their seasonal distribution varied as does that of all recent births in the United States. We have seen, however, that this method must be used very cautiously because the seasonal distribution of births varies greatly from region to region and decade to decade. Moreover, data derived from a small number of cases can be depended upon only when supported by other evidence. Therefore, having calculated and smoothed Petersen's data according to the method used in this book, we have merely plotted them according to the month of *conception* (the solid line of *A*, Figure 93). In order to enlarge the numerical basis we have included malformations of arms and legs, which Petersen omitted as of relatively small importance, but this makes no essential difference.

The second curve showing the seasonal distribution of conceptions resulting in malformed births (the solid line of *B*, Figure 93) is based upon data collected by Belding (1937) in Massachusetts. The third curve (the solid line of *C*) is based upon 935 congenitally malformed individuals studied by Murphy (1936) in Philadelphia. I have recalculated his data to allow for differences in the length of the various months, and have smoothed them by our usual method. Murphy's conclusion, with his own italics, is that there is *"no* evidence . . . to support the view that in Philadelphia there exists any significant, seasonal trend toward the conception of congenitally malformed children."

Taken as a whole the curves of the malformed in Boston (*B*) and Philadelphia (*C*) are much alike. They show a major maximum of conceptions in June or July and a major minimum in February or March. The Chicago curve, with its main maximum in April or May and its minimum in August, is quite different, but inasmuch as it is based on only 553 cases we need not attach great weight to it. Nevertheless, it is interesting to note that it bears a strong resemblance to the curve for starred American scientists (*C*,

Figure 68, page 300), but with its main maximum a month earlier and its main minimum a month later.* This resemblance may be pure accident. On the other hand, it may indicate that malformed children tend to be conceived in maximum numbers not only in hot weather, as happens in Massachusetts and Philadelphia, but at the time when geniuses are conceived in greatest number, that is, when the stimulus which leads to the spring maximum of conceptions is approaching.

The seasonal curves of malformed individuals seem to differ significantly from those for the entire population. This is seen on comparing them with the dotted lines in *A*, *B*, and *C* (Figure 93) which are based on all conceptions resulting in living births in Chicago, Massachusetts, and Philadelphia, respectively, during a recent period of 5 to 7 years. These three curves are essentially alike, as might be expected from our previous studies. Their minimum in February or March agrees with a minimum in all three of the curves for the malformed. Their maxima occur fairly uniformly in April or May, but are separated by one or two months from the corresponding maxima of the curves for the malformed. A more important disagreement is found during the summer. In Boston and Philadelphia, but not in Chicago, a summer minimum of conceptions among the population as a whole is confronted by a maximum in the curves for the malformed. Later in the season there is a similar, but less marked, contrast between a minor autumn minimum in the curves for the entire population and a minor maximum in that of the malformed.

This opposition between the malformed and the normal is strongly evident in data prepared by Murphy. The solid line of *D* in Figure 93 shows the season of birth among 1590 normal children born in the same families as the 935 malformed children of *C*. The opposition between the solid lines of *C* and *D* is obvious. Its exact nature can be still

---

* Note that Figure 68 is plotted according to month of birth, whereas Figure 93 is according to month of conception.

more clearly seen by comparing the solid line of D with the dotted line there which is the inverted curve for the malformed children. When the malformed and normal children of these families are combined, their seasonal curve of birth (E) is approximately the same as that for the entire population of Philadelphia (C, dotted) except that it is flatter. This shows that the families used by Murphy, when taken as a whole, are fairly representative of the entire population so far as season of birth is concerned. On the other hand, the normal children in Murphy's Philadelphia families show a seasonal distribution closely similar to that of Petersen's abnormal group in Chicago. This leaves the whole matter in such a state of doubt that no dependable conclusion is possible.

The seasonal distribution of births among mental defectives is puzzling for the same reason as that of the malformed. I have gathered statistics as to the month of birth of about 45,000 mental defectives in institutions for the feeble-minded. It has been possible to do this through the cordial co-operation of the responsible authorities in the institutions named in Appendix A, to all of whom I would express the deepest gratitude. Their earnest desire for exact knowledge as to the problems of mental deficiency is one of the most hopeful signs of the times. The institutions represented in our final results are scattered from Massachusetts to Minnesota, and southward as far as Baltimore. Since the seasonal distribution of births throughout this area varies comparatively little, and most of the data belong to the tier of states from southern New England westward, it seems legitimate to put them all together.

Curve A, in Figure 94, shows the seasonal distribution of births among 6500 idiots with intelligence quotients below 20; B for 15,000 imbeciles with I.Q.'s of 21 to 50; and Curve C for 23,000 morons, mainly with I.Q.'s of 51 to 70, but including a few above 70. Curve D sums up the preceding curves. As a control on which to base comparisons Curve E has been added, showing the seasonal distribution of births in Pennsylvania, Michigan, and Minnesota from 1920 to 1925. Inasmuch as Pennsylvania contains more than twice as many people as the other two states combined, this gives a fairly accurate representation of the conditions in the entire region from which the data as to mental defectives are drawn.

One of the most important facts about Figure 94 appears to be that the curve for idiots (*A*) is different from the other

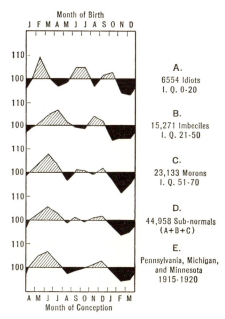

FIG. 94.—Season of Birth among Mental Defectives in the United States.

curves. Another is that the resemblance of the other curves to the general curve (*E*) increases as we go upward in the scale of mentality (downward in Figure 94). The curve for idiots shows three maxima. Those in February and October are presumably the same as those of the general population in March and September. If so, each of them has been shoved one month toward cold weather, just as have the corresponding maxima in the curves for Americans in the *Encyclopædia Britannica* and for starred American scientists (*B* and *C* in

Figure 68, page 300). The Chicago curve for malformed children shows a corresponding advance of one or two months toward cold weather in each of its two maxima.

The systematic quality of these relationships suggests that some of the idiots may owe their deficiency to an excess of the same conditions which foster genius. According to the hypothesis to which we have been led in studying men of genius, it seems probable that the genes which produce genius are able to achieve their fullest results only when the secretions of the ductless glands, the general metabolism, and other bodily functions are stimulated to just the right degree —neither too much nor too little. One of the circumstances which favor such a well-balanced stimulation appears to be certain conditions which arise in the parents before conception as the result of weather somewhat cooler than the optimum. By some process which is not yet wholly clear the weather appears to have an effect upon both parents when the reproductive cells are being formed and also, presumably, upon the mother during the earliest stages of pregnancy. This effect lasts throughout the life of the child. If this hypothesis is correct, an excessive stimulation, or one which affects only part of the cell or embryo, or perhaps only one of the two cells which meet in reproduction, might do great harm and produce idiocy. There are many examples of circumstances where a given cause produces both good and bad results according to its degree, mode of application, and time of action. The even and prolonged application of heat to a board makes it dry smoothly, but the sudden application of the same amount of heat to one side produces a severe warp. A little alcohol may make people merely merry and companionable; a larger amount makes them violently and disagreeably drunk.

The third maximum of births in the curve for idiots (A, Figure 94) comes in June and July (conceptions in September and October). This is the time when the births of eminent people are at a minimum. It is later by three months than the maximum of births among malformed infants in

Boston and Philadelphia.*   This adds to the complexity of the problem.   If we disregard the malformed infants, we may surmise that the summer maximum in the birth of idiots may be due to the same unfavorable conditions which produce a minimum of geniuses.

The exact relation between the curves of birth at the two extremes of mentality may be seen in *A* and *B*, Figure 95,

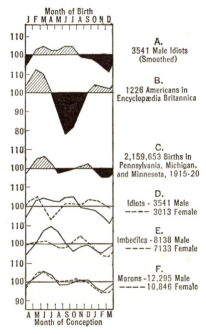

FIG. 95.—Season of Birth Among Mental Defectives by Sex, Compared with Americans in the *Encyclopædia Britannica*.

where the smoothed curves for 3541 male idiots and 1226 Americans in the *Encyclopædia Britannica* are compared. In both curves the upward bulge in February or March and the smaller bulge in October are evident, although the latter is very slight among the idiots.   In summer, however, the contrast between an upward bulge in the curve for idiots

* Bear in mind that Figure 94 is plotted according to month of birth and Figure 93 according to month of conception.

and a deep downward bending of the curve for the encyclo-pedia people is very pronounced. Section D of Figure 95 indicates that although the curves for male and female idiots do not agree very closely, presumably because of the small number of cases, they both show the three maxima. Among imbeciles (E), although there is considerable difference be-tween the two sexes, both curves show only two maxima. The June-July maximum has disappeared, a point which we shall consider in a moment. When we reach morons (F) and are able to use numbers large enough so that the curves for the two sexes are almost identical, the curves are not es-sentially different from those for people in general (C). There is no hint of the summer maximum, although those in March and September are evident.

In estimating the importance of Figures 94 and 95 we must remember that we are dealing with three possible causes of mental deficiency. The first is pure heredity, that is, the presence of genes in such combinations that normal develop-ment is impossible. The percentage of mental deficiency arising from this source presumably remains constant at all seasons, unless the weather has an hitherto unsuspected in-fluence upon heredity. The second cause of deficiency is not truly hereditary, but nevertheless dates from approxi-mately the time of conception. It is the physiological condi-tions of the spermatozoa and ova as determined by diet, weather, mental attitude, and other environmental circum-stances which influence the parents. The hypothesis which seems best to explain the facts now before us is that a certain amount of mental defect may arise from either an excess or marked deficiency of the climatic conditions which at the time of conception are normally favorable to high mentality. The third and probably most important cause of mental de-ficiency is environmental conditions which act upon the child during pregnancy, at birth, and onward throughout life. The majority of sufferers from this last type of deficiency were presumably derived from normal embryos. Therefore, an unknown, but presumably large, percentage of mental defectives must have a seasonal curve of births like that of the general population.

This leads to the idea that in Figure 94 Curve *A* represents a combination of three tendencies. First, the children derived from embryos which were normal at the earliest stages of pregnancy would give a curve like that of people in general (*E*). Second, the excessive or misplaced action of the conditions which make for eminence may shift the normal maxima a little toward cold weather both in the spring and fall. Third, the weak development of these same conditions may cause a minor maximum among the births of idiots in midsummer.

But is such an explanation in harmony with Curves *B* and *C* (Figure 94), showing the season of birth among 15,000 imbeciles and 23,000 morons? In answering this, the first point is that among imbeciles and morons the proportion whose mental defect is environmental in origin must be higher than that among idiots. The truth of this will be evident when we consider what would happen if all persons were equally endowed at birth. A few, by reason of extremely poor nutrition, very inadequate care, unusually severe accidents, or other environmental conditions, would become idiots. A much larger number, suffering in the same way but less severely, would become imbeciles or morons. On this basis a possible explanation of the curves for imbeciles and morons is that among them the number of persons with defects due to environment is so large that the proportion of what may be called "spoiled" or arrested geniuses is low. Such being the case, the spring and fall maxima of the curves for imbeciles and morons would show little tendency to occur in weather that is cooler than that in which the maximum of conceptions in general takes place. According to this interpretation Curves *B* and *C* in Figure 94 are mainly the result of the normal seasonal trend plus a slight tendency toward obliterating the minimum of births which occurs in the normal curve (*E*) during May, June, and July. Thus a tendency which causes a pronounced summer maximum in

Curve *A* of Figure 94 might simply draw the spring and fall maxima toward warmer weather and diminish the summer minimum as in Curve *B*, or leave the two main maxima in their normal position and produce a very slight maximum in summer, as in Curve *C*.

It is not easy to determine what degree of reliance should be placed upon the preceding discussion, but we can at least test the reliability of our curves and the degree to which our various types of data dovetail together to make a consistent whole. In Figure 70 (page 308), we found that 6000 cases gave a curve which seems to be practically final, but in Figure 95 we see that, with 8000 male and 7000 female imbeciles, the curves for the two sexes are still different. The reliability of the differences between the maxima and minima of the curve for idiots (*A*, Figure 94) may be tested mathematically on the basis of Table 26, which gives the actual number of cases, and the corrected number that there would have been had each month consisted of 31 days.

Using the corrected figures in the last column of Table 26,

TABLE 26

BIRTHS OF IDIOTS IN THE UNITED STATES BY MONTHS

	Actual		Corrected		Total	
	M.	F.	M.	F.	Actual	Corrected
January	292	260	292	260	552	552
February	293	254	322	279	547	601
March	306	252	306	252	558	558
April	307	218	317	225	525	542
May	297	251	297	251	548	548
June	308	256	318	264	564	582
July	326	257	326	257	583	583
August	293	249	293	249	542	542
September	281	264	290	272	545	562
October	311	259	311	259	570	570
November	254	248	262	256	502	518
December	273	245	273	245	518	518
Total	3541	3013	3607	3071	6554	6678
						556.5 Average

there is 1 chance in 54 that a maximum as high as that of
February may occur by accident, and 1 chance in 185 of a
minimum as low as that of November and December combined. The chances of accidentally getting both of these
conditions and of having them agree with other curves to
the observed extent sink to only 1 in thousands or hundreds
of thousands. The chances of accidentally getting a maximum like that of June and July, however, even when the two
are combined, rise to 1 in 22. Therefore, though that maximum is probably real, its reliability is by no means so great
as that of many other features of our curves. There seems,
then, to be a tendency for defectives in either body or mind
to be conceived in greatest numbers under the seasonal conditions which are least favorable for normal conceptions, or
else under an extreme development of the conditions which
favor genius. Nevertheless, this conclusion is tentative. It
is by no means so well grounded as the conclusion that the
development of genius is favored by conception during the
fairly cool temperatures which prevail slightly before the
maximum of the basic animal rhythm.

Let us now turn to other kinds of defects. We will begin
with one that is probably partly physical, partly mental, and
partly social, namely crime. Through the courtesy of Dr.
Emil Frankel data are available for the births of 10,000
prisoners in the New Jersey State Prison. Approximately
70 per cent of the prisoners appear to have been born between 1890 and 1909. Except for its greater amplitude and
the strong development of the September peak (conceptions
in December) the curve for prisoners (A in Figure 96) agrees
closely with our original Belgian curve as given in Figure 1
(page 30). When the prisoners' curve is compared with
Curve B for 17,502 New York school children who were
born between approximately 1915 and 1925 the two curves
are seen to be a good deal alike. The smoothed curves of
Section C at the bottom of Figure 96 bring out the resemblance very clearly. It is a curious fact that the curve for
prisoners, although based on the smaller number of persons,

is the more regular, and has much the greater amplitude. There is only 1 chance in many million that so great an amplitude will occur by chance when the number of cases is 10,000.

This looks as if births in families of the types that produce criminals tended to follow the basic animal rhythm much more perfectly than births in ordinary families. In this respect the criminals are like geniuses. The very low

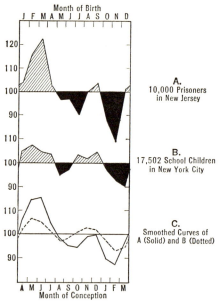

FIG. 96.—Season of Births among Prisoners and School Children.

dip of the criminal curve in November, however, is very different from anything that we have found in curves for people of eminence. Before we attempt to explain this curious condition we must learn more about several other types of people whose seasons of birth are like those of criminals.

Let us next consider insanity. Figure 97 provides interesting food for thought in respect to dementia praecox. This form of insanity is now more commonly called schizophrenia.

or splitting of the mind, according to the original Greek. It is a form of insanity which often appears in adolescence and in which heredity seems to play a marked rôle. The power of both mental and physical development seems to be lacking. A peculiar and often complete disorganization of personality appears, and with this go changes of will power and temperament of such a kind that the unconscious to a large extent replaces the conscious. This psychosis is accompanied by an extreme development of fantastic delusions and hallucinations. Its cause is highly debatable. Some authorities ascribe it to auto-intoxication, and others believe it to be related to endocrine disorders, originating in the sex glands.

Figure 97 is based on more than 10,000 cases of schizophrenics whose dates of birth were most kindly furnished by the persons and institutions listed in the Appendix. Our debt to those who gathered the statistics used in this chapter is very great. In Figure 97 the births have been divided according to the decades in which they occurred. In each case the general curve of births in Massachusetts during the same decade has been added as a dotted line. At the top, Curve A for 585 schizophrenics born from 1915 to 1924 has its maxima and minima at the same dates as those of people in general. In the general curve (the dotted

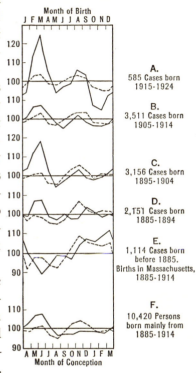

Fig. 97.—Monthly Births of Persons Suffering from Dementia Praecox Compared with Monthly Births of the Population of the Same Age in Massachusetts.

line), however, the second maximum (in August) stands at practically the same height as the first, whereas in the curve for insane persons the March maximum is much the higher. Another interesting point is that the schizophrenic curve is almost identical with that of the prisoners in Figure 96. This resemblance becomes still more extraordinary when we note that the schizophrenic curve is based on less than 600 persons and the other on 10,000, but the amplitude in the two cases is practically the same.

Among the 3511 schizophrenics who were born between 1905 and 1914 (*B* in Figure 97) the essential features of the seasonal curve of births are the same as those which we have just seen among the 585 who were born a decade later, but the amplitude is much less. Here, too, however, the maximum in March rises well above that of the curve for people in general, while the later maximum in August is lower. In fact, it is also lower than the corresponding maximum in the general curve in spite of the great difference in the number of cases. In Curves *C* and *D* for earlier decades the same conditions are repeated. Only in *E*, for 1114 persons born before 1885, does the spring maximum for the insane fall below the corresponding normal maximum. The 1114 cases of *E*, however, are mainly persons who did not suffer from insanity until late in life. Their mental breakdown was therefore much more likely to be due to environmental conditions during their lives as a whole than to anything dating from the time of their conception. Hence we should expect them to include a large majority who are normal so far as season of birth is concerned.

This calls attention to a feature of Figure 97 which may be significant. In general, although with some irregularity in Curve *C*, the difference between the curves for schizophrenics and normal people diminishes as we go from persons who became insane in early youth to those who became insane later in life, that is, from top to bottom in Figure 97. This is equivalent to saying that in early youth dementia praecox is especially likely to attack persons born at the height of the basic animal rhythm of reproduction. As life goes on, the number of people who are susceptible to insanity because of conditions prevailing at the time of their conception diminishes through death, which occurs relatively early among such people (Dayton, 1931). On the other hand, the proportion who are susceptible because of the general environment of their lives increases.

Another point worth noting is that, although both insanity and crime tend to be especially common among people who are born at the maximum of the animal rhythm, this does not happen to anything like so great a degree among people born at the later maximum in August. This later maximum, it will be remembered, depends upon conceptions at the season when people's ability to work is at a maximum. The difference between the two maxima is especially clear in F (Figure 97) where the 10,000 schizophrenics of Curves A to E have been combined. We have already seen that the August maximum which is almost missing in the curve for schizophrenics, but very clear in the dotted curve for people as a whole, is especially well developed in prosperous, well-fed regions, and among groups such as the British landed gentry where the economic standards are very high. Thus we are led again to a conclusion which we reached before on quite other grounds. At the time of the annual recrudescence of reproductive activity according to the basic animal rhythm, the maximum percentage of increase in conceptions appears to occur among the wrong type of people. It occurs among those who temperamentally or physically are not fit to have children, thereby causing a high percentage not only of children with low intelligence quotients, but of children who become criminals or develop insanity. On the other hand, the autumn increase in conceptions occurs especially among well-nourished, vigorous people who suffer relatively little from these deficiencies and disorders.

Dementia praecox is not the only kind of insanity which shows a peculiar relationship to the seasons. Figure 98 indicates that the same relationship prevails among sufferers from manic-depressive insanity. This type, it will be remembered, is characterized by alternate periods of wild mania and quiet depression. Among the manic depressives born from 1895 onward (Curve *A*) the maximum in March is much higher than for the population as a whole, while the later maximum in August is only a little higher. The manic-depressives born before 1895 (Curve *B*) show a still greater excess of births at the first maximum, and at the second their curve falls distinctly below that of people in

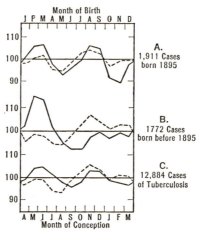

FIG. 98.—Month of Birth of Sufferers from Manic-Depressive Insanity and Tuberculosis Compared with Births in Massachusetts at Same Period, 1880–1909.

general. It seems quite clear, then, that the manic-depressive and schizophrenic types of insanity behave essentially the same as criminality so far as season of birth is concerned. The only exception is Curve *E* in Figure 97. If the 1114 cases there employed are combined with the 1772 manic-depressive cases born at the same period (*B*, Figure 98), the combined curve is much like Curve *D* in Figure 97. It conforms to the general rule.

People who are weak in health agree with the insane and criminals in showing an unusually strong tendency toward birth at the maximum of the basic animal cycle. Section *C* of Figure 98 shows this for persons suffering from tuberculosis.

Figure 99 indicates that it is also true among Negroes in comparison with whites. In Baltimore and the states of Maryland and Tennessee the relation between the whites and the colored is like that between criminals or insane persons and those who are normal. The Negroes show a higher maximum than the whites in the early part of the year and

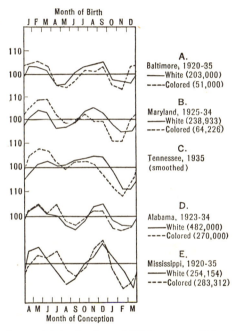

FIG. 99.—Seasonal Distribution of White versus Colored Births.

a lower maximum as well as a lower minimum in the later part of the year. The general opinion is that they differ from whites in practising less self-control. They also differ in being more poorly fed and having poorer health. In other words, they have qualities of weakness akin to those we have postulated among the parents of persons who have an especially strong tendency toward crime, insanity, and tuberculosis. In the far South the difference between the distribution of births among whites and Negroes is reduced to small proportions in Alabama and Mississippi. What this means we do not understand, unless it be that in the far South the white people are living under conditions to which they are not well adapted. Therefore, although they have a lower death rate than the colored people, their seasonal distribution of births is practically the same as that of their darker neighbors, aside from some condition, presumably cultural, which causes the bulge in Curves D and E in April.

Illegitimate births display a characteristic seasonal distribution identical with that of criminals, the insane, sufferers from tuberculosis, and Negroes. This is evident in Figures 8, 9, and 10 (pages 52, 54, and 56). In every one of the 7 sections of those figures the illegitimate maximum of births in the winter or spring is higher than the legitimate maximum. This is not because of the small number of cases, for hundreds of thousands of illegitimate births are included. Moreover, in every case the secondary later maximum in September or December, as the case may be, is lower in the illegitimate curve than in the legitimate. This accentuation of the first maximum—the one belonging to the basic animal rhythm—and the corresponding suppression of the later maximum indicate that among all these relatively weak types of people the basic animal rhythm is very highly developed.

We are now ready to inquire the reason for this curious situation. What leads to the excessive births of weak types at the height of the basic animal rhythm? And why are highly successful people also conceived in unusually large numbers at approximately the same time that criminals, insane persons, sufferers from tuberculosis, Negroes, and illegitimate children are conceived? And why do the births of eminent people rise notably in the autumn whereas those of these weaker types generally fall to a minimum in November?

The most probable explanation of these diverse and seemingly contradictory facts seems to be that weak types of people react to the basic animal rhythm of reproduction in a different way from more vigorous types. All types appear to feel the stimulus to reproduction that occurs when the temperature rises toward the physical optimum in the spring. There is, however, a great difference in the degree to which the different types yield to it. Even in the days when contraception in its modern form was unknown there was a great deal of birth control through continence, onanism, and other methods. The amount of this varied enormously from one type of family to another. It was at a maximum among the most far-sighted, self-controlled, and considerate types. It disappeared among the weak-willed, passionate, unintelligent, and shiftless. Such people yield easily to the impulse of the moment. Hence the seasonal curve of births among them not only follows the basic animal rhythm very closely, but rises unusually high at the height of the rhythm in May and June, or later in more northern countries. It falls correspondingly low in the coldest weather not only because that is the low point of the sexual urge, but because a large percentage of the possible mothers are at that time already pregnant. Such weak types of people are the ones from whom spring the majority of illegitimate children, criminals, and physical or mental weaklings who suffer from tuberculosis or become insane.

Still another weak type also swells the number of conceptions at the height of the animal rhythm. This consists of couples where one or both is physically below par, and hence unable to procreate children under normal conditions. Many older married couples must belong to this type. We have seen that the children of such couples—the later children—do not live so long or become so famous as the first children (Table 19B, page 293). The advent of the mating season must raise the reproductive powers of such people as well as of others. The result must be that a considerable number of physically weak couples who are unable to have children most of the year produce them when the rhythm reaches its height. This may be one reason why sufferers from insanity and tuberculosis show so marked a maximum of births in March.

Still another point is that none of these weaker types shows the normal tendency toward increased conceptions when the temperature falls to the physical and then to the mental optimum in the autumn. Still less do they show a tendency to throw the spring maximum back into cooler weather, as occurs among the most intellectual types. In other words, here again we have evidence that the stronger types of people physically, intellectually, and morally are at their best in weather cooler than that which forms the optimum for less vigorous types.

Still another difference between the higher and lower types of births is connected with the fact that the August maximum is very low in the weaker type. In previous chapters we have seen that a maximum of births may arise from July to September not only because of the unusual physical and mental vigor which prevails in the best climates during the late fall and early winter, but because men who have been working away from home often return to their families in the fall when outdoor work comes to an end. The majority of such men are in the prime of young manhood. They are usually physically sound, and they come home full of vigor because of their summer's work out-of-doors. Moreover, their wives are young and hence are more nearly at the ideal age for childbearing. Such couples must tend to have strong, healthy children. This would raise the August and September maxima of births in general in comparison with the births of the weaker types who become criminals, or who suffer from insanity or tuberculosis. Thus there seem to be abundant reasons why weak types of people show a great predominance of births at the height of the reproductive season.

Insanity and other evidences of unbalanced mentality show a strong seasonal relationship not only in the matter of births, but still more in the season at which they become manifest. About a century ago Esquirrol (1838) published data showing that in Paris there was a strong tendency toward a maximum of outbreaks of insanity from May to July and a minimum in December. Lombroso (1911), Ammann (1914), Kollibay (1921), Ellis (1916), Wilmanns (1920), Blum (1932), Wetzel (1920), Hoche (1910), Meier (1922), and Norbury (1924) have all confirmed this conclusion. Some of them, especially Ammann, Lombroso, and Wilmanns, have

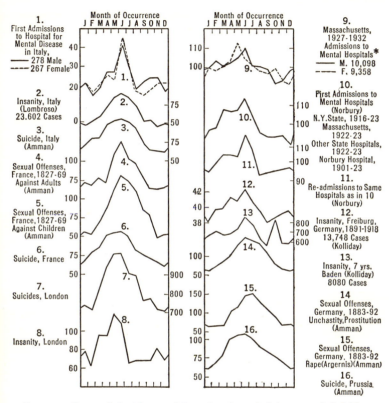

FIG. 100.—Seasonal Incidence of Insanity, Sexual Crimes, and Suicide.

shown that sexual crimes and suicide also follow the same seasonal course.

The whole matter is summed up in Figure 100, which is taken from many different sources. At the top Curve 1 shows how small a number of cases is needed to give a very pronounced seasonal curve of the outbreak of insanity. The solid line shows seasonal variations in the admission of 278

male patients suffering from insanity to a hospital in northern Italy during the years 1930 to 1934, according to Bonfiglio (1935). The dotted line shows a similar curve for 267
female patients. June had twice as many admissions as the
winter months, and men and women behaved alike. Curve 2,
from Lombroso, shows the season at which a much larger
number of patients, more than 23,000, were admitted to
Italian hospitals. June again shows a maximum, with the
winter months only a little more than half as high. In
Curve 3 we see that suicides in Italy, as reported by Ammann,
follow almost the same seasonal course as outbreaks of insanity.

Coming to France, Curve 6 indicates that suicide follows
the same seasonal course as in Italy. Curves 4 and 5 add
a new feature. They indicate that sexual offenses also follow almost the same course as insanity and suicide, except
that they rise to a maximum with special suddenness in
May and June. It has often been supposed that sexual offenses reach a summer maximum because of the opportunities offered by outdoor life at that season. Careful students
are practically a unit, however, in concluding that this cannot be the case, because if it were, there is no good reason why July and August should so systematically show a
drop. We have seen abundant evidence of this in previous
chapters where illegitimacy was discussed. In Figure 100
we note especially that Curve 5 for sexual crimes against
children has a greater amplitude and rises more steeply than
Curve 4 for similar crimes against adults. This suggests very
strongly that the increase in sexual offenses is not due to
the opportunities afforded by warm weather and outdoor life
in anything like so great a measure as to the sexual urge
which becomes strong at this season in man just as in animals.

Going on with Figure 100 we find that in London the evidences of mental instability indicated by suicide reach a
maximum in May and June (Curve 7), while admissions to
hospitals for the insane rise highest in May. Among the 18
curves of Figure 100 this and the dotted line of 9 are the only

ones with a maximum in May. One other (15) rises highest in August, but the remaining 15 all have their maxima in June. On the right of Figure 100 some American curves agree with the others. The first two (9) show the admission of both males and females to hospitals for mental diseases in Massachusetts from 1927 to 1932 according to data which were kindly furnished by Dr. Neil A. Dayton. The next two curves are based on data collected by Norbury from his own hospital and various state hospitals. They represent first admissions (10) and readmissions (11) of patients suffering from insanity.

The remaining curves are all from Germany. Curve 12 shows admissions on account of insanity to hospitals in Freiburg during 28 years, while 13 shows the same thing for the entire province of Baden during 7 years. In Curves 14 and 15 the seasonal distribution of sex offenses in Germany is illustrated. The fact that Curve 15, based on cases of rape, reaches a maximum in July rather than June may indicate the influence of the opportunities afforded by summer weather in addition to the urge of the basic animal rhythm. The slight bulge in July and August in Curve 14, showing cases of unchastity and prostitution, may be of similar origin. Then in Curve 16 we have the seasonal distribution of suicide in Prussia. Data from other regions and other periods might be added in large amounts, but all that we have been able to find agree with the situation as set forth in Figure 100. All the 18 curves there given have essentially the same form. Moreover, that form is practically the same as that of the curve of conceptions as we first found it in Belgium. In other words, the Belgian curve of births, with which we began our study of seasonal curves, is typical of the seasonal curves of sex offenses, suicide, and the outbreak of insanity, provided we shift it three months so that it becomes a curve of conceptions.

There has been much speculation as to the reason for this agreement between sex offenses, insanity, and suicide but Wilmanns (1920) appears to be the only one who has correctly interpreted it. He suggested very tentatively that all three of these departures from the normal might be manifestations of the same sexual impulse which causes births to reach a maximum in March, and which causes animals like the stag to become madly furious during the rutting season. Before reading Wilmann's brief article I had reached the same conclusion. It seems to me that the facts set forth in this book leave little room for doubt as to its reliability. The seasonal distribution of sex offenses certainly finds a full and complete explanation in the basic animal rhythm of reproduction, plus a small allowance for the effect of warm weather in allowing opportunities for clandestine meetings. As for insanity and suicide it is well known that when animals are in heat a kind of madness comes over them. The females search wildly for the males, and the males still more wildly for the females. Both sexes become oblivious to danger and will rush unheeding into situations that mean death and that they would ordinarily avoid. The males are the worse, and Kollibay thought that among human males the seasonal fluctuation in insanity is greater than among females. Curves 1 and 9 in Figure 100 do not support this view, for the amplitude of the female curves is in both cases slightly the greater. Be that as it may, the males certainly are wilder in their actions during the season of sexual activity than are the females. The males of animals fight furiously with one another. They often attack other creatures which they think are getting in their way. They even go so far as to attack inanimate objects, and kill themselves thereby. Thus the actions of animals during the mating season display a close parallel to the sexual crimes, the insanity, and the suicide which in man reach a climax at the time when the mating instinct is at its height.

This conclusion is strengthened by Kollibay's analysis of the seasonal distribution of admissions to mental hospitals according to the age of the patients. Among the four age groups which she used she found that in Freiburg the seasonal peak in late spring and early summer is clearest at ages

15 to 30; it remains clear at ages 30 to 45; it is postponed to July or August at ages 45 to 60; and above 60 it gives place to two peaks in March and December, respectively. These facts should be considered in connection with the ages at which different types of insanity are most likely to appear. Figure 101 shows the rates of admissions to hospitals for three diverse kinds of insanity in New York State from 1929 to 1931, according to Malzberg (1935). At the top we see that

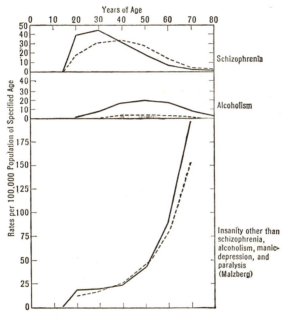

FIG. 101.—Age at Onset of Mental Derangement in New York State, 1929–1931.

schizophrenia, which is generally supposed to have an especially close connection with the sex organs, manifests itself with great suddenness immediately after puberty, especially in males. It reaches a maximum in men at not far from 30 years of age, and among women before 40. As old age approaches, the occurrence of new cases greatly diminishes. Manic-depressive insanity, the other most common type in early maturity, follows a similar course, but reaches a maximum among men at about the age of 50. The contrast between the sudden onset of schizophrenia and the gradual rise and decline of insanity due to alcoholism (*B*, Figure 101) is very impressive, as is the different kind of contrast between schizophrenia and the gradual increase of insanity due to senility (*C*).

A final evidence of the close connection between the season of maximum sexual activity and the outbreak of in-

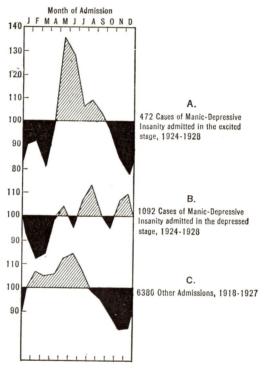

Month of Admission

A.
472 Cases of Manic-Depressive Insanity admitted in the excited stage, 1924-1928

B.
1092 Cases of Manic-Depressive Insanity admitted in the depressed stage, 1924-1928

C.
6380 Other Admissions, 1918-1927

Fig. 102.—Admissions to Mental Hospital in Florence, Italy. Smoothed curves.

sanity is seen in Figure 102. This is based on data from Amaldi (1928) as to the extent to which the mental hospitals of Florence during the years 1924 to 1928 admitted patients suffering from the manic as opposed to the depressive states of manic-depressive insanity. In this type of insanity, it will be remembered, the patients suffer from alternations between a highly excited state in which they often imagine themselves

to be of marvelous quality, and a greatly depressed or melan-
cholic state in which they suffer terrible hallucinations as to
their own debasement. Curve *A* of Figure 102 shows that admissions to mental hospitals on account of the manic or excited stage rise with extraordinary speed from an index number of about 81 in March to 136 in May. From May onward
there is an almost steady decline to a level of only 78 in December. The contrast between this curve and the one for admissions in the depressed state (*B*) is most illuminating.
Not only is Curve *B* irregular in comparison with *A*, but it
reaches a maximum three months later, as if by reason of
reaction after the violence of May. In this respect it is quite
different from the curve for admissions because of other types
of insanity (*C*). These reach a maximum in May and June,
but lack the explosive quality of the admissions due to the
excited phase of manic-depressive insanity. The explosion
certainly occurs at the very time when sexual activity is increasing most rapidly, and there is every reason to think that
the conditions of glandular activity which lead to sexual
desire also lead to a breakdown of the mind and to great excitement among persons with the hereditary constitution and
the environmental conditions which predispose them to
this form of insanity.

These conditions furnish another link in the chain which
connects the basic animal rhythm of reproduction with an
increase in the following factors: (1) normal conceptions,
(2) illegitimacy, (3) prostitution, (4) ordinary rape, (5) at-
tacks upon female children, (6) the outbreak of insanity in
general, (7) the explosive outbreak of the manic or excited
stage of manic-depressive insanity, and (9) suicide. Increased activity of the reproductive organs under the stimulus of the return of warm weather and perhaps of other seasonal conditions is apparently the primary change which sets
all the others in motion.

The chain of cause and effect can be carried further to the
time when the people who became unbalanced by reason
of the sexual urge were conceived. The people who in later

life are especially likely to become criminals, or to suffer from schizophrenia, manic-depressive insanity, or tuberculosis, are especially likely to have been conceived at this same time of heightened sexual activity. Perhaps it is the unrestrained sexual excesses of persons with an hereditary tendency toward these afflictions which causes so many people of these types to be conceived at that period, or possibly the general raising of reproductive activity causes people of less than normal vigor to produce children at that time and not at others. At any rate the conception of people who will at some future time suffer from these forms of weakness occurs with unusual frequency at the same season when outbreaks of insanity and suicide are most common.

This brings to a close our survey of facts as to the seasonal distribution of births and of related conditions. In the two following chapters we shall sum up our conclusions and show how they apply to human evolution as it manifests itself in the origin of our species, and to the measures which must now be taken to insure a favorable future both for man himself and for his civilization. The most remarkable feature of this whole study is the way in which a great many facts from highly diverse fields dovetail into a single harmonious fabric.

CHAPTER XVIII

THE EVOLUTION OF *HOMO SAPIENS*

The facts now before us have a direct bearing on the problem of human evolution. This will be more readily apparent if we first sum up our main conclusions. The first conclusion is that in man, just as in animals, an annual rhythm of reproduction is of great importance. The existence of such a rhythm has long been recognized. This book brings together a great body of data which show that the rhythm is universal, and is evident in the seasonal distribution of births all over the world. One of our chief tasks has been to detect the fluctuations in the birth rate due to cultural conditions such as seasonal migration, religious prohibitions, festivals, and other social customs. We have found this possible in most cases, and it could doubtless be done universally if our knowledge of local habits were sufficient.

When variations in season of birth arising from cultural causes are eliminated, we can compare the residual variations with the physical environment. We thus discover that the seasonal distribution of births depends largely upon the weather, and varies from region to region in almost perfect harmony with the climate. The maxima of conceptions, and to a less extent of births, show a tendency to occur as nearly as possible under the same conditions of weather in all parts of the world. Temperature appears to be the main factor in causing the seasonal fluctuations. As the weather grows warmer in the spring, reproductive activity increases. Taking some 80 regions into account, we find that conceptions which result in living births tend strongly to reach a maximum at temperatures which cluster around an average of 62° F., or 17° C., for night and day together. This temperature therefore appears to be the optimum for conception.

There is evidence of increased reproduction not only when the temperature rises toward 62° but also when it falls to that level or lower after having been higher. Rising temperature produces much the more important effect. This may mean that increasing sunlight stimulates reproduction in man, as it does in many plants and animals. Light, however, can scarcely be more than a minor factor. A temperature of about 62° is accompanied by the maximum rate of reproduction under conditions of light as various as those which prevail in India during November or February, in New Jersey during May, and in Quebec during July. In all these cases the temperature is approximately the same, but the amount of sunlight is quite different. Moreover, under certain conditions, especially in regions or social groups where prosperity and comfort attain an especially high level, the return of the temperature to 62° after it has been higher stimulates reproduction regardless of the amount of light. Thus our general conclusion is that seasonal variations in temperature are the main factor in setting in motion the basic rhythm of reproduction.

Another conclusion is that, although departures in either direction from an average of 62° F. lower the number of conceptions, high temperature has a far greater effect than low. This is especially evident when seasonal curves of birth for regions like Japan and Florida, with long, hot summers, are compared with those for regions like Manitoba and Finland, with long, cold winters.

The importance of good health among parents at or before the time of conception is surprisingly far reaching. In this book we have seen how great a part the weather plays in this matter. It seems probable that other conditions, such as the diet and general hygiene of the parents, are no less important in giving children a good start in life even before they are conceived. We have discovered in this book that one evidence of a good start is that people born at the height of the basic animal rhythm are more equally divided between the two sexes than are those born at other times.

Other evidences of this are their lower death rate during infancy and their long lives. In the eastern United States persons born in March live on an average nearly 4 years longer than those born in July. The relation of all these favorable conditions to season of birth, to weather, and to the health of the parents at the time of conception appears hitherto to have been overlooked. Going on with this catalogue of advantages we meet the problem of the season of birth among persons of eminence, a subject which has been widely debated for some time. In this book the use of a much larger body of material than has hitherto been available leaves little doubt that the births of people of unusual ability conform to the basic animal rhythm much more closely than do those of people as a whole. This advantage, like the others enjoyed by people born at the height of the basic animal rhythm, appears to arise from favorable conditions among the parents at or before the time of conception.

Abundant statistics enable us to go farther than this. They indicate that eminent persons are especially benefited by cool weather. Relatively speaking, the conception of such people falls off in hot weather much more than does that of ordinary people. The converse of this is also true. The optimum temperature for the conception of persons of unusual ability is distinctly lower than that for ordinary people. Thus cool regions, as well as cool seasons, provided they are not too cold, have a great advantage over warm regions. They may not produce any greater number of persons whose inherited capacities are of unusually high order, but from the time of conception onward they apparently endow such persons with the physical capacities which are needed to make their mental capacities productive.

Turning now to the defective or handicapped classes of society, we find them surprisingly numerous among the people conceived at the height of the reproductive season. Persons who become criminals, suffer from tuberculosis or insanity, or merely have low intelligence are especially likely to be conceived under the influence of the maximum phase of the basic animal rhythm. On the other hand, there is some indication that mentally or physically defective children show more than the usual tendency to be conceived in hot weather, but this is not very clear. There is no doubt, however, that the season of maximum sexual stimulation in May and June is characterized by certain very undesirable features, even though the children conceived at that time include many who live long and become eminent. One such feature is a marked increase not only in all kinds of sexual irregularities, but also in suicide and insanity. In view of all these varied conditions the season at which people are born is obviously a very important and practical matter.

One of the most interesting problems that has concerned us in this book is the reason why a temperature in the neighborhood of 62° is the optimum for reproduction. Why not 40° or 80°? We have come to the conclusion that the reason is found in a selective process which occurred among our primitive ancestors. In climates of an intermediate type, neither very cold nor so warm that they are monotonous, the children who are conceived when the average temperature rises to about 62° F. are born in the early spring when reasonably warm weather first arrives. That is the time when the supply of food begins to increase after the scarcity of winter. In other words, birth occurs at the season which is best for the survival of the infant, just as happens among animals. It is best for two reasons. First, the infant begins life at a time when the food available to the mother will steadily increase in amount and variety, so that she will have the maximum supply of milk with which to feed it. Second, the infant is able to gain strength through several months of life before it faces the great hazards that accompany hot weather. It will be still more mature before facing another kind of hazard in the form of the scarcity of food which among primitive people often ensues during the winter.

A major feature of this book is the discovery that the optimum temperature for reproduction is also the optimum for physical health in general. Previous studies and experiments in many countries and among diverse races have shown that the optimum temperature for our species as a whole is an average temperature of approximately 62° F., or a little higher. With an average of 62° the thermometer rises at midday to somewhere near 70°. The reason why the optimum for physical health and comfort occurs at this temperature and not at some other has been a puzzle ever since the reality of the optimum became evident. We now find a very cogent reason for this. Modern infants have the lowest early death rate and the survivors live longest when conceived at seasons during which the optimum temperature prevails. The same was probably far more true of primitive infants. We therefore conclude that our enjoyment of temperatures of 68° to 70° in the rooms where we are sitting apparently owes its origin to the time when *Homo sapiens* acquired his present physical characteristics. A drastic selective process presumably favored the survival of individuals whose health and powers of reproduction were especially stimulated when the temperature reached such a level that it ranged from perhaps 55° by night to 70° by day, and averaged somewhere near 62°. Thus a definite optimum of temperature became a primary, innate quality of our species.

Still another highly significant fact has come to our attention in connection with the temperature at the time of birth rather than conception. The optimum temperature for mental as contrasted with physical activity has received comparatively little attention. Nevertheless, a number of lines of evidence indicate a distinct mental optimum at a temperature which averages somewhere in the vicinity of 45° F., or 8° C. The reason for such an optimum has hitherto been even more elusive than the reason for the physical optimum at 62°. The explanation of the physical optimum, however, leads at once to what seems to be a full explanation of the mental optimum. If children are conceived in the late spring or early summer when the temperature rises to an average of about 62°, they will be born in the late winter or early spring when the temperature is appreciably lower, provided of course they live in a climate with at least a moderate difference between summer and winter. The parental qualities most essential to the survival of children are not quite the same at conception and at birth. At the time of conception, the most important thing is that the health of both parents should be as perfect as possible, thus giving the child the greatest vigor and the best possible start in life. At the time of birth, however, a naked, unprotected species like man stands in special need of mental alertness. No amount of brute strength or good health will keep the mother well fed and the baby well protected if the parents are stupid. During the first month or two of life, far more than at any other time, the survival of the child depends on the mental alertness of its parents. Thus the same sort of selective process which gave *Homo sapiens* a physical optimum at a temperature of 62°, thus bringing the maximum of births at the most favorable season, appears to have given him a mental optimum at about 47°, thus giving the parents the maximum ability to preserve the child's life. This solution of the perplexing problem of both a physical and a mental optimum seems to be one of the most important features of this book.

Certain minor coincidences of a wholly unexpected nature have also engaged our attention. They seem to confirm our conclusion as to the hereditary adaptation of man to a certain definite type of climate. The most conspicuous of these is a set of curious and complicated facts which emerge from old Belgian statistics. The statistics show that in the third month of life Belgian infants rather suddenly acquire an unexpected power to resist the harmful effect of seasonal fluctuations in the weather. This ability gradually diminishes during the succeeding three or four months and has practically disappeared in the eighth month. Such a condition is in itself very strange, but a far stranger fact is that in the fifteenth month, or thereabouts, the same power of resistance appears once more, only to disappear again in the course of the next few months. If we accept the view that a physical optimum near 62° and a mental optimum near 47° were the most favorable temperatures for conception and birth respectively when *Homo sapiens* acquired his present characteristics, an explanation of the peculiar conditions among Belgian infants seems ready to our hand. As soon as the mean temperature rises above the physical optimum, the death rate among young infants shoots up with extreme rapidity. Hence if primitive children were born mainly in the early spring according to the basic animal rhythm, those which inherited more than the average power to resist the effect of hot weather during the three or four warmest months would be favored in the race for survival. The recurrence of this special type of resistance a year later would be a still further favorable factor.

An equally extraordinary adaptation is shown by adults in Belgium, Denmark, and New York during the reproductive period. At that time, but not at earlier or later stages of life, the months from March to June are characterized by a curious accession of vigor which materially diminishes the death rate. The effect upon women is especially great. Thus, during the months when both birth and conception are at a maximum according to the basic animal rhythm, people who may become parents are temporarily endowed with a kind of strength denied to others. The case is analogous to that of infants, but with exactly the changes needed to adapt it to fathers and especially mothers, thus giving the children a better chance to survive. Unfortunately, we have as yet found no other data by which to test either of these peculiar adaptations. Nevertheless, the facts are so systematic, so completely unexpected, and so perfectly in accord with other evidence that they deserve considerable weight. They appear to represent a biological inheritance which mankind as a whole has preserved from some early habitat. There, through mutation and selection, as we suppose, our species apparently acquired a climatic adaptation so deep seated that it still persists, although man has now migrated to all sorts of other climates.

This brings us back to our main conclusion that the basic animal rhythm of reproduction permeates our lives in many ways that have been little suspected. The season at which people are born affects the number of births, the percentage of boys compared with girls, the rate of infant mortality, the duration of life after the dangers of infancy are passed. It also affects the percentage of criminals, tubercular patients, and persons who suffer from insanity. Later in life the on-set of the active phase of the annual reproductive cycle creates a kind of excitement which manifests itself in sexual crimes, insanity, and suicide, and probably in many other ways. The season at which people are conceived, and the temperature of the region where they are conceived, also have a good deal to do with the number who rise to the heights of fame. And finally an inherited adaptation causes us to react to the weather in different ways according to our age from infancy onward. When the indirect effects of such conditions are considered there seems to be scarcely a person or a phase of life which is not vitally influenced by the season at which people are born and the season at which the reproductive urge becomes strongest.

Let us apply all this to the problem of human evolution. We will begin by inquiring what it indicates as to the climate in which *Homo sapiens* acquired the climatic adaptations which we have been studying in these pages. It should be carefully noted that we are talking about our *species* and not about the genus *Homo*. The genus may have originated a million years ago. It has included several extinct species, among which are the ancient men of China, Java, and South Africa, as well as the Neanderthal man of Europe. Our species, on the other hand, is comparatively young, dating only from the last glacial epoch 30,000 to 60,000 years ago. In considering the climatic adaptation of this new species we must remember that the statistical data in this book pertain to people who practise modern methods of clothing and shelter. Therefore it is probable that their climatic optima, both physical and mental, are somewhat lower than those for primitive, poorly clad, and poorly sheltered savages, even though the savages and ourselves have exactly the same inherited adaptations. In order to avoid confusion, however, let us ignore this for the present and simply inquire what kind of climate is most nearly ideal according to the data now before us, together with such other data as may seem pertinent.

1. The first condition of such a climate appears to be a *mean temperature of 62° in June* at the height of the season of sexual activity, this temperature being also the optimum for physical health.

2. The next is a *temperature of 47° in March* at the season of maximum births and of maximum mental activity. Figure 103, based on daily deaths in New York City from April, 1882, to March, 1888, shows that approximately this same temperature was the best for the health of young children before the advent of modern hygiene.

3. The Belgian mortality curves of Figures 63 and 64 indicate that children suddenly acquire *a special power to resist the influence of the changing seasons* during their third month of life, and show

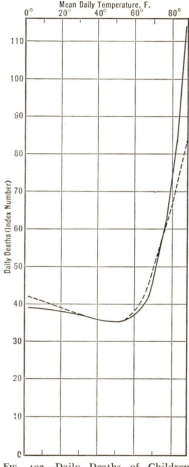

—— Day on which temperature occurred
– – – Average of 3 and 8 days after a given temperature

FIG. 103.—Daily Deaths of Children under Five Years of Age from All Causes except Pneumonia and Influenza Compared with Mean Temperature in New York City, 1882-1888.

it again approximately a year later. This would mean that children born in March when the temperature averaged 47° would acquire this power in May when the temperature would average about 58° F. Figure 103 shows that at this temperature the curve of deaths among young children begins the rapid upward sweep which carries it so high in Figures 29 (page 108) and 39 (page 168).

4. The Belgian mortality curves of Figures 63 and 64 also indicate that *the special power of children to resist the influence of the seasons lasts into the seventh month of life,* which would mean into September for children born in March. In continental climates the temperature in September generally averages a degree or two lower than in May, but in coastal regions there is a corresponding difference in the other direction. For our present purposes we may assume that September is essentially the same as May. The duration of the period when infants show special resistance to seasonal influences is important because it gives a clue to the length of the season when special danger is to be anticipated on account of the heat. Thus it also affords an indication as to the month when the height of the reproductive season should be placed.

Putting the Belgian data as to deaths of infants according to the month of life (Figure 63) with the New York data as to deaths of infants on days with specific temperatures, we see that our ideal climate appears to be one in which the following conditions are met: (1) the dangerous period begins when the mean temperature reaches 58°; (2) it lasts from the third to the seventh month of the life of the child; (3) it presumably ends when the temperature drops below 58° once more; (4) if the temperature of the month of conception is to be 62° and that of the month of birth 47°, the foregoing conditions can be met only where the temperature averages about 62° in June and births are at a maximum in March. If the maximum of births is put in February the period of hot weather becomes too long to fit the Belgian data, and if in April, too short. Of course the temperatures stated above will be higher when we make allowance for the inability of primitive man to protect himself from wind and weather, but that need not concern us just yet.

5. Although *variability of temperature* from day to day has been discussed in this book, it requires further explanation. Several lines of evidence indicate that one of the most important elements in promoting health is a fair amount of change of temperature from day to day—interdiurnal variability. This is illustrated in Figure 104, based on tables published in *Weather and Health* (Huntington, 1930). The figure is based on weighted averages in which the effect of the mean temperature has been eliminated.* Thus the upper curve in Figure 104 indicates that at temperatures of 71° to 85° F. there were 23 periods of 10 days each during which the average difference between the temperature of one day and the next was only 1° F. The deaths on the last days of these 22 periods averaged nearly 105, when the average for all days with similar temperature is taken as 100. On the last days of 144 periods in which the interdiurnal change of

* In Figure 104, the effect of mean temperature has been eliminated as follows: In Table 6 of *Weather and Health,* page 160, daily data for the years 1882 to 1888 are tabulated according to 5° intervals of *mean* temperature and 1° intervals of average interdiurnal *change* of temperature. The figures given in the table are the average number of deaths per day on the last days of 10-day periods having a given mean temperature and interdiurnal variability. In preparing Figure 104 these numbers have been expressed as percentages of the corresponding average for the last days of *all* 10-day periods having the specified mean-temperature, regardless of the interdiurnal variability. Then the percentages for 3 mean-temperature groups at each degree of interdiurnal change have been weighted, added, and averaged. For example, during the period 1883 to 1888, there were seventeen 10-day periods when the mean temperature averaged from 81° to 85°. Their average index-number of deaths per day was 58.0. Two of these periods had an average interdiurnal change of temperature of only 1°. The number of deaths in those two periods was 119, or an average of 59.5. When expressed as a percentage of 58.0, this amounts to 102.6. Therefore, the upper left-hand entry of Table VI in *Weather and Health* becomes 205.2. This is the weighted index-number of daily deaths at the end of two periods having a mean temperature of 81° to 85° and a mean interdiurnal variability of temperature of 1°. When all the other 10-day groups having temperatures of 81-85°, 76-80°, and 71-75° have been treated in the same way the index-numbers for all three mean temperatures at each degree of interdiurnal variability can be combined. Thus the effect of the mean temperature is eliminated.

temperature averaged 2°, the deaths averaged 100.5. At the end of the 189 periods with a change of 3° the deaths fell to 98.6, but with greater changes they again rose a little.

In the second line of Figure 104 we see that at temperatures of 56° to 70° the number of 10-day periods during which the average interdiurnal change of temperature was only 1° was too small to be used. It was actually 9, and these have been combined with the 74 that had an average change

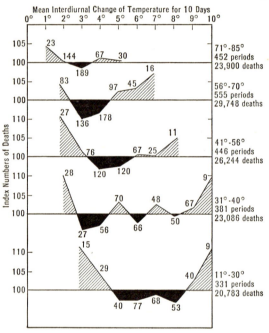

FIG. 104.—Deaths in New York City, 1883–1888, in Relation to Mean Temperature and Interdiurnal Change of Temperature.

of 2°, thus making 83 for the left-hand end of the diagram. On the last day of these 83 periods the deaths amounted to over 104. With an average interdiurnal change of 3° the deaths fell to only a little more than 95; but with greater changes they rose until finally at the end of periods with great variability (an average of 7°) the deaths amounted to 107.

So it goes at every level of temperature. Of course the average change from day to day increases as the weather becomes colder, but always the periods with the least change of temperature from day to day end with a high death rate. An intermediate degree of change is followed by a low death rate, while great changes again lead to high death rates. Thus Figure 104, when taken in conjunction with other evidence, makes it clear that our adaptation to climate is of such a kind that we are stimulated and our health is improved by a moderately high degree of variability from day to day, whereas our health is injured by great changes and still more by monotonous uniformity. The degree to which people can benefit by interdiurnal changes of temperature varies according to the climate to which they are accustomed, but the people in all parts of the world seem to be distinctly benefited by such changes provided they are not too severe. Therefore we conclude that *Homo sapiens* inherits a climate adaptation of such a kind that he benefits from a fair degree of variability, that is, a fairly frequent occurrence of the ordinary cyclonic storms which bring our "weather."

6. Another condition which plays a large part in determining the quality of a climate is *atmospheric humidity*. In spite of a widespread opinion to the contrary, fairly high humidity is desirable so long as the temperature does not rise much above the physical optimum. At high temperatures an abundance of atmospheric moisture is very undesirable, but at the optimum or lower the best condition is a relative humidity averaging about 80 or 90 per cent for night and day together. This is evident in practically every careful investigation that has yet been made. The relation of humidity to reproduction is not yet clear, but any climatic condition which has an effect on health must also have some effect on reproduction. Moreover, essentially the same relation to humidity seems to characterize all kinds of people. Therefore we may consider that the climate in which *Homo sapiens* acquired his final climatic adjustment not only had a mean temperature of 47° F. in March and 62° in June, but was fairly humid and variable, without going to great extremes. The most common reason for such characteristics

is frequent storms of the ordinary type, but mountains and seacoasts enjoy them to a certain degree.

Having set up a series of criteria by which to judge the climate in which *Homo sapiens* presumably took the final steps in his evolution as a species, let us inquire whether the climate in any part of the world now meets these criteria. That will pave the way for a similar inquiry concerning the climates which appear to have existed during the glacial epoch when the present species of man originated. For the present we shall continue to use the data for well-clothed, well-sheltered people of the modern kind.

It is astonishing to find how few places have climates which agree with the few simple criteria set up by our study of births and deaths. Only two types of climate can be considered, and one of them departs quite far from what we may for convenience call the norm, or ideal. One type consists of oceanic climates in fairly high latitudes, and mainly on west coasts or on islands. The other is found at high altitudes about 30° from the equator. The most conspicuous region of the first type centers in the peninsula of Brittany in northern France. There Nantes has a mean temperature of 45° F. in March and 62° in June. Bordeaux with 47° in March and 64° in June lies on the southern edge of the area where the norm is very closely approached. Paris (43° and 62°) and London (43° and 59°) lie on other borders, but of course there is no sharp line of demarcation. This west European area fits the requirements of our norm not only in temperature, but in its rather high humidity and its cyclonic storms which bring frequent moderate changes of temperature from day to day.

Three other regions of this same type lie in the so-called newer parts of the world. In the Willamette Valley and Puget Sound area of the northwestern United States the conditions found in Brittany are quite closely approximated except that cyclonic storms are not so regularly distributed at all seasons. Portland and Roseburg, Oregon, with temperatures of 46° in March and 62° in May come very close to the norm so far as temperature is concerned. Olympia in northern Washington, with temperatures of 44° and 59°, may be regarded as near the border of this area. A third area of the same general type lies in New Zealand. Ophir, well to the south in the interior of the southern island, has a temperature of 46° in September, corresponding to March, and of 60° in December, corresponding to June. The very small region which is thus represented enjoys good conditions of atmospheric humidity and storminess, although the degree of variability may not be quite sufficient. Finally, on the east coast of South America the coastal city of Bahia Blanca has temperatures of 53° in September and 68° in December, and the region a little farther south comes somewhat closer to having 47° and 62° in these months. The conditions of humidity and of the seasonal distribution of storms do not approach the norm so closely as in the other three regions of this high-latitude type. Like them, however, the Argentine region has an invigorating and healthful climate. The other three regions, centering in Brittany, the Willamette Valley, and the southern island of New Zealand, come close to being the best parts of the world so far as health is concerned.

There is not the slightest probability that any of these regions was the place where *Homo sapiens* took the final step which made him a distinct species. Practically all authorities agree that that step occurred during the last great advance of the ice at a time when the earth's climate was cooler than now. Keith, according to a statement at the International Symposium on Early Man in Philadelphia (1937), believes that certain cave deposits in Palestine carry *Homo sapiens* back some 60,000 years to the early part of the last or Wisconsin glacial epoch. Other authorities put the origin of *Homo sapiens* no farther back than 30,000 years, and connect it with the later of the two advances of ice in the Wisconsin epoch. In either case the present species of man originated at a time when the climate was much more severe than at present, as is generally agreed by anthropologists.

The reader may well be reminded once more that we are talking about the species *Homo sapiens,* and not about the genus *Homo.* After the genus originated, there were repeated crises during which different species of man originated. The ancient human species of China, Java, South Africa, and the Neanderthal man of Europe were much more primitive than our own species. They appear, to be sure, to have learned how to use fire, prepare skins for bedding, and use caves as shelters. But whether they built shelters and were genuinely clothed is not so clear. For our present purpose the essential point is that during the last ice age from about 30,000 to 60,000 years ago a new and more highly developed species of man came into existence. The facts in this book suggest that under the stress of a glacial climate he acquired certain climatic adaptations which are so deep-rooted that they still persist and have suffered only minor modification in the many new climates into which *Homo sapiens* has made his way.

Viewing the matter in this way it is clear that, although Paris, London, Portland, and other places may now have climates that closely approach the norm for our species, they did not have such climates when that norm was established. On the contrary, they were so cold as to be practically uninhabitable. They are important in the scheme of human evolution, but their importance lies in recent times and not in the far past.

The other type of region in which we now find temperatures of approximately 47° in March and 62° in June may have been the place where *Homo sapiens* originated as a species. All the examples of this type lie at high levels in low latitudes about 30° from the equator. The official temperature at Simla on the slope of the Himalayas is 52° in March and 67° in June at an altitude of about 7000 feet. At approximately 8500 feet the temperature comes close to our exact norm of 47° in March and 62° in June. Similar conditions are found at high altitudes in the same latitude in other parts of the world. The other, similar regions are limited to a small area in southern China, a larger area in the plateaus of Afghanistan and Persia, and a very small area in the Atlas Mountains of Morocco. South Africa and South America also have small areas of the same kind, but there is no reason to look to them for the origin of *Homo sapiens*. All these areas where the conditions of temperature agree with our norm have a fair degree of atmospheric humidity because of their altitude and coolness, but are deficient from the standpoint of variability from day to day because of their lack of cyclonic storms. They are decidedly healthful regions compared with the lowlands around them, but by no means so good as regions such as Brittany and the Willamette Valley.

Let us now go back to the glacial period when our species apparently originated. At that time the snow line on the mountains was 3000 or 4000 feet lower than now and the mean annual temperature at least 10° F. and perhaps 20° F. lower than now. Our newly evolved species was presumably so primitive that only the most rudimentary forms of clothing and shelter were available. Therefore we are probably justified in assuming that the temperature most stimulating to reproduction was perhaps 5° F. higher than the 62° which we have found most stimulating among well-clothed and well-housed moderns. This would, of course, bring the maximum of births at a correspondingly lower temperature. Let us also assume that the mean temperature at its lowest averaged 15° F. lower than now, and that the period of most extreme temperature exercised a preponderant influence in determining the biological adaptations to climate which we have been studying in this book. We must also take account of other respects in which the climate of glacial times differed from that of today. One such difference was presumably an increase in the range of temperature from summer to winter. In latitudes as low as 30° this increase must have been small, but it must have had a measurable effect in shoving the region where March and June have a difference of 15° a little toward the equator. It is not probable that the shoving amounted to more than 5° of latitude at the outside, for at the equator the contrast between the seasons can scarcely have been much greater than at present.

Taking all these conditions into account, it appears that at the height of the last glaciation a climate of approximately the type which we have called the norm, but about 5° F. warmer, prevailed at an altitude of approximately 2000 to 6000 feet between latitudes 25° and 30° in Asia and Africa. This location is determined as follows: Starting with a temperature of 62° in June today at an altitude of 8500 feet, we raise the temperature 5° on account of primitive man's lack of clothing and shelter. This would be equivalent to a descent of about 1500 feet, that is, to 7000 feet. We then descend again to allow for the lowering of temperature during the glacial period. We should have to descend nearly 5000 feet if the glacial lowering of temperature was 15° F. This gives an altitude of 2000 to 3000 feet. But we must ascend again about 1000 feet because we move 3°, let us say, toward the equator in order to allow for the increased contrast between the seasons which probably occurred during times of glaciation. This gives us an altitude of 3000 to 4000 feet above sea level. Inasmuch as our calculations are at best very rough and depend on a good many assumptions, we may enlarge these limits and say that the type of climate for which we are seeking must have prevailed between altitudes of 2000 and 6000 feet above sea level. The latitude where it occurred is open to much less question than the altitude. A difference of 15° F. between March and June corresponds to a difference of about 25° F. between January and July. There is little probability that so great a difference occurred within the tropics even at the height of glaciation. On the other hand, so small a difference certainly did not occur farther north than at present. Therefore when we say latitudes 25° to 30° we must be coming quite close to the actual facts.

In our day deserts prevail for the most part in latitudes 25° to 30°, but such was not the case when icesheets spread over much of northern Europe. Climatic principles and archeological evidence agree in showing that in those days cyclonic storms must have followed a much more southerly course than at present. Even in our day a faint band of such storms follows the Mediterranean Sea, crosses Mesopotamia and southern Persia, reaches northern India where it traverses the Indo-Gangetic plain in attenuated form, and finally struggles across the Burmese mountains and revives somewhat in southern China. During the glacial period this belt of storms was probably much intensified, and brought with it not only moisture, but the kind of interdiurnal variability which we have found to be especially good for health. Thus on mountains and plateaus at a height of somewhere between 2000 and 6000 feet, between latitudes 25° and 30°, the climate at the climax of the last glaciation appears to have closely resembled the type to which man as a species seems to be intimately adapted. The areas where such a climate presumably prevailed are as follows: (1) a plateau in southern China in the provinces of Yunnan and Kweichow; (2) very limited areas on the southern slope of the eastern Himalayas; (3) a large Iranian area of plateaus in Baluchistan and southern Persia; (4) a limited area around the northern end of the Red Sea including a part of western Arabia, together with smaller areas in the Sinai Peninsula and among the mountains east of the Nile; and (5) a small area in the northern part of the Ahaggar plateau in the central Sahara. From a purely geographical standpoint the size of the Iranian area, its location in respect to storm tracks, and its position between such early centers of civilization as Mesopotamia and northern India would lead us to choose it as more likely than any of the other four regions to be the home of the earliest man of our particular species.

The conclusion to which we have just come is especially interesting because of its relation to other, independent lines of research. When this study of man's innate climatic adaptations was begun I had no idea of attempting to locate the place where *Homo sapiens* originated. It is, therefore, especially gratifying to find that our statistical study brings us directly to the region where we should look for that origin not only on the basis of traditions such as are embodied in the Bible, but of archeological explorations and the findings of anthropologists. The method here employed is undoubtedly crude, and can be greatly improved. Nevertheless, it seems logical, and its results are certainly in harmony with a vast body of facts derived from other sources.

Chapter XIX

THE SEASONS AND HUMAN PROGRESS

When people first learn of the connection between season of birth on the one hand, and health, longevity, and eminence on the other, they are likely to react in two ways. First, they think of their own birthdays: "Was I born at a season that is good or bad?" Second, they think of children, their own or those of others: "Ought not people to plan so that their children will be born at the best possible season? Would not this give them better health, longer life, greater success, and more happiness?"

The season of our own birth is of course important, but there is nothing we can do about it. If we were born at an unfavorable season we can comfort ourselves with the thought that many great and long-lived people have been born at that same season. Moreover, heredity, diet, and mode of life, when taken together, doubtless have far more effect upon health, longevity, and achievement than has season of birth. The climate where we are born, as well as the weather, also has a great effect. Nevertheless, it may be better to be born of healthy, long-lived, well-nourished parents at the worst season in the worst climate rather than of anemic, short-lived, poorly nourished parents at the best season in the best climate. All this is worth saying only because people often think that a book like this magnifies one single factor at the expense of all others.

Let us try to estimate how important it is to be born at the right season and in the right climate. The climatic enthusiast may say that on an average the chances of permanent fame are 50 to 100 per cent greater among Americans born in February than among those born in June. In the eastern United States, the people born in March live nearly

4 years longer than those born in July. If the average expectation of life at birth is 62 years, the people born in the hot climate of Queensland die about 10 years sooner than Australians born in the cooler climates of England and the Australian state of Victoria. Their span of life is less than that of the others no matter in what part of Australia they happen to live at the time of death. Prolonged summer heat results not only in a reduction of conceptions, but in a still greater reduction in the proportion of scientists and other leaders. Birth in hot weather, or conception at the end of a long hot summer, or in a hot climate, seems to be a disadvantage from which people never recover. The climatic enthusiast may also state that in the worst climates the average span of life is 20 to 40 years less than among people born in the best climates, and the number of world leaders is negligible. He may clinch his argument by asserting that, if the weather is bad enough, potential parents may be so weakened that there will be no conceptions that give rise to living, healthy infants. Therefore he may conclude that climatic influences are of supreme importance. At one extreme they prevent conceptions or lead only to those that result in abortions and imperfect children who never have much vigor. At the other extreme they make it possible for the most perfect types of human beings to be born.

Although the preceding statement is true, its real significance can be appreciated only when it is weighed in comparison with similar statements as to other factors. The enthusiastic student of diet, for instance, may say very truly that, if the diet of potential parents is extremely scanty and lacks certain essential elements, conception may be absolutely prevented, or the embryos may be imperfect. He may insist that where the diet of the parents is most nearly perfect, the children also are most nearly perfect. Similar claims may be set up in respect to disease. Where parasitic diseases, for example, have been most nearly conquered, defective or poorly developed children are far less common than in the regions where such diseases run riot. Therefore some people may conclude that defectives will almost disappear when the diseases due to parasites and viruses are finally conquered. The same broad claim may also be set up as to occupations, social habits, hygienic practices, and other aspects of life. Any one of these may be so bad as to prevent conception, or cause the progeny to be born with defects that are never eradicated. On the other hand, where each is most nearly perfect, the children also rise to a high standard, and great achievements are common.

The over-enthusiastic believer in heredity has little patience with such claims on behalf of purely environmental factors. Do not long-lived parents tend to have long-lived children, regardless of climate, diet, and hygiene? Does not heredity play the main part in determining whether an infant is a hopeless defective or a potential genius? Does not talent run in families for generation after generation? Is not the number of relatives in encyclopedias far beyond what would happen merely by chance?

When the claims of physical environment, cultural environment, and heredity are stated in this crude fashion, it becomes clear that each starts with an important truth and ends with an egregious fallacy. It is easy to see this fallacy in others, but not so easy to recognize that much of our own thinking is equally fallacious. All too often we behave as though we really believed that if unfavorable conditions in respect to factors in which we are interested were corrected, perfect conditions would ensue. Millions of earnest teachers, clergymen, scientists, sociologists, and others are so deeply and subconsciously imbued with this fallacy that they let it guide their lives. In reasonable moments, to be sure, they know beyond question that the complete removal of disadvantages along any one line never produces ideal conditions. They also know that the attainment of the ideal, or even any reasonable approach to it, requires the co-operation of many factors. If perfect children are ever to be born in this world, their parents must be genetically perfect, but those same parents must also be perfectly nourished, they

must be engaged in occupations which permit perfect physical and mental equilibrium, and their lives must be so or-
dered that their physical and mental health suffers no disturbance from excesses of any kind. In addition to this they
must live in the ideal climate and their children must be
conceived at the ideal season. We cannot attain the ideal,
but if we are to keep our feet on the road that leads thither,
we must realize that all the conditions set forth above must
be kept in mind. Bad conditions in one field of effort may
nullify or attenuate the effect of efforts in every other field;
but no amount of improvement in one field can bring us anywhere near the ideal, or even keep us headed straight toward it, unless similar efforts are made in other fields.

We see this clearly enough in the case of a bridge. The
bridge may fail because of poor steel, bad foundations, ignor-
ance as to the maximum height and speed of the current, unduly heavy loads, the unbalanced weight of a draw, miscalcu-
lation as to the intensity of earthquakes, or any one of many
other conditions. The bridge is perfect only if every one of
these conditions is perfect. Even though they recognize this,
it is very hard for the environmentalist and the hereditarian,
the student of diet and of viruses, the climatologist and the
expert in public health to see their subjects in true relation
to all the others. We are like the dogs of an untrained
team. All of us are supposed to pull the same sledge, but
each is attached to the sledge by an independent line, and
each attempts to dash ahead at his own sweet will.

To change the metaphor a little, the branch of science
represented in this book is like a strange dog added to a team
which is only just beginning to pull together. The old dogs
snap at the new one, or pull away from him. The new
dog snaps back, or sits down on his haunches at the wrong
moment. Our task, as drivers, is to train old dogs and new
to work together. We must find out how much each dog
can draw and where he will work best without tangling the
traces, or fighting with his neighbors. This new dog that we
are trying to train can pull only a small part of the load,

but he is essential if the load is to be pulled easily and well. Otherwise the other dogs will have to pull him as well as the sledge. If he is properly harnessed and driven, however, he may be able, for example, to increase the average span of life by about two years even in a good climate like that of the United States, and by unknown amounts elsewhere.

Our new knowledge as to season of birth can be of practical use only if we use it in one of two ways. First, we can change the present seasonal distribution of births. Second, we can discover the exact conditions which make certain seasons favorable, and then take steps to create those conditions at other seasons. Both methods are practical, and both will probably be employed by future generations. A change in the season of birth could easily be brought about within a few decades if society were convinced that it is worth while. It will probably begin among a small and highly enlightened group, and gradually spread downward.

Suppose that all births occurred from the middle of January to the middle of April, and thus at the best season from the standpoint of general achievement as well as that of longevity and vigor. A few inconveniences might result. The hospitals would be crowded at one season, but they could serve as day nurseries the rest of the year. The doctors would have to sit up nights, but they would have plenty of time for sleep, recreation, and study during the rest of the year. The schools might have to close for the season of birthday parties, but the stores would rejoice in a birthday rush like that of Christmas. As a matter of fact, however, any such inconveniences, whether real or jocular, would be a small matter compared with a gain of two years in average length of life, and a corresponding increase in vigor and achievement. Moreover, any change of this sort is likely to occur so slowly that the necessary adjustments will take place almost without recognition.

An important point to note in this connection is that, if our reasoning is correct, the extra two years of life would not be added to the period of immaturity, or to the period of decay in old age. Each of those would be shortened rather than lengthened by a widespread improvement in constitutional vigor. Thus the working period of life would be increased by perhaps 5 per cent, while the percentage of people too old and infirm to work would not show any corresponding increase. Moreover, during the working years people would enjoy better health than now. Hence they would lose less time in illness, do their work better, and behave more sanely because less disturbed by the many minor ailments which do so much to warp our judgment and make us hard to get along with.

Any attempt at such a change in the season of births is bound to run into difficulties. The unforeseen difficulties are generally far worse than the ones that seem obvious at the start. One obvious difficulty at present is that the births at the height of the seasonal rhythm include a relatively large percentage not only of unusually able and vigorous children, but of those with low intelligence and with constitutional traits of the sort that render them especially likely to become criminals, or to suffer from insanity, tuberculosis, and other forms of weakness. Fortunately this difficulty is not so great as appears at first sight, provided we have rightly diagnosed its cause. We have concluded that children who are intellectually and emotionally weak are born in unusual numbers at the height of the animal rhythm of reproduction because weak parents of these same types are especially prone to yield to the reproductive stimulus of the optimum temperature. If all parents were urged to have children only at the optimum season, these weaker types would be affected least of all. In the first place, the intellectually and emotionally weak are the kind who act most on impulse and least on reason. Therefore, the idea of planning for the birth of their children at a particular time would have little effect on them. In the second place, they already yield fully to the seasonal impulse, hence even if thoughtful people began to have more children at the most favorable season, it would be impossible for the weak types to make any such increase.

If a widespread attempt were made to concentrate births at the most favorable season, the result might actually be a reduction in the number of weaklings. This would occur chiefly in the case of physically weak but intellectually sound parents who have children only when the annual recurrence of the animal rhythm raises their reproductive powers sufficiently to induce conception. If such parents knew that their children were likely to be physically weak, many of them would adopt contraceptive measures at that season, even though they did not find it necessary to do so at other seasons. Even in the larger and more dangerous group composed of emotional and intellectual weaklings, an understanding of the seasonal rhythm and its effects might diminish the number of these children, provided physicians, nurses, and social workers gave enough attention to the matter. If these leaders could recognize the weaklings, as is increasingly possible, they could make special efforts to persuade them to be careful in the practice of birth control at the season when there is the greatest temptation to unrestrained sexual activity. Efforts in this direction will be greatly simplified by the fact that on the whole the extra children born to inferior types of parents by reason of the upward swing of the reproductive rhythm are not wanted. They are the undesired result of a purely animal instinct. It must be remembered that birth control has now become a well-established part of our social customs, even among religious groups which theoretically frown upon it. Except for an outmoded prudery there is no reason why people should not be publicly as well as privately warned that the season for special precautions as to conception is at hand. We cannot predict how future generations will handle this problem, but we may feel certain that they will face it, and will follow methods quite different from those of the past. New knowledge demands new methods.

The facts presented in this book may have more importance indirectly than directly. The essential reason why the children born at some seasons have an advantage over those born at others is presumably that the glands and other organs of the parents function differently according to variations in the environment. In view of the triumphs of modern medicine we may confidently expect that a realization of the importance of the seasons in relation to reproduction will stimulate research. Thus we shall discover why the children conceived at certain times have an advantage. That in turn will enable us to create the desired conditions at other seasons, or in greater measure at the chosen seasons. Thus a large field of possible improvement opens before us.

Another very important point emerges in connection with our study of birth rank. The facts as to both longevity and eminence indicate that the children of reasonably young mothers have an advantage. Therefore, the present tendency of the more intelligent classes to postpone parenthood for some time after marriage is a decided disadvantage to the next generation. It may be necessary in a social system such as ours, but obviously such a system ought to be changed.

One of the main conclusions to be drawn from this book is that the time for beginning our efforts to benefit the next generation must be pushed steadily backward. We must begin by making it possible for the finest types of young people to marry early and have children promptly. At the same time, we must make them realize the importance of their own physical condition at the time of conception. The psychologists have shown that many dangerous or annoying psychoses arise from unnoted events in very early childhood. The facts in this book focus attention on a still earlier phase of life. It has long been recognized that the care of the mother during pregnancy has an important effect upon the health and happiness of the child. Most biologists agree that the health of both parents—father as well as mother—before and at the time of conception is also highly important. In this book we have found an unexpected wealth of evidence as to the great importance of the pre-conceptual period. The climatologist is concerned in this because the weather is a potent factor in causing variations of health from season to season, but when it comes to discovering how to gain the most from our new knowledge many other types of workers are needed. The physiologist must tell us what sort of diet, exercise, and mode of life will best fit prospective parents not only for health in general, but for the particular kind of health, if such there be, which will give their children the best start in life. To the social worker of every kind there opens up an almost unlimited field of usefulness in making known the discoveries of the scientists and persuading people to use them intelligently. Proper recreation, freedom from anxiety, certainty that if children are born they will be a pleasure and not a burden are only a few of the many conditions which influence parents before children are conceived, and which may have a profound effect upon the quality of the children. Preparation for the child should be made weeks or months before it is conceived.

It has been supposed in the past that eugenics is concerned only with hereditary qualities, and such is undoubtedly the case. Nevertheless, if eugenics means the applied science in which the objective is that children shall be well born, the prenatal and preconceptual influences of climate and weather come close to being included. This does not mean that there is any confusion between heredity and environment. What it does mean is that an unfavorable physical environment may depress a given group of people for generation after generation regardless of the people's genetic constitution. Thus the result may be closely similar to that which would ensue if the germ plasm were poor.

We may be dealing with what Martin (1937) has called "temporary inheritance." He suggests that, if a certain response to an environmental condition is repeated often enough, the capacity to respond increases, and may even be transmitted to offspring. For example, Kammerer (1924) attempted to produce acquired characteristics which would be inherited. In one experiment he repeatedly cut off the siphons of the ascidian *Chiona intestinalis,* hoping that their progeny would show reduced siphons. Each amputation of the organ, however, was followed by renewal, and the new siphons were actually longer than those that were cut off. Moreover, the offspring of the experimental ascidians had longer siphons than the normal of their species. Martin suggests that, when the siphons were cut off, other cells were subjected to a strong stimulus which resulted in the growth of a new siphon. Each cutting of the siphons strengthened this tendency, and finally the power to produce siphons was actually increased in the germ cells. We cannot enter into the matter further here, but many of our facts seem to fit such an hypothesis better than the more orthodox belief that new qualities arise only through mutation and selection.

In some ways the obvious ease with which man can be influenced by his climatic environment is very encouraging. It suggests that we may have discovered a new way not only of improving man's environment, but even of altering his inheritance. Be that as it may, it is quite clear that the way is open for the removal or amelioration of one of the environmental handicaps which are holding us back while we are engaged in the long and difficult process of improving man's biological inheritance. Perhaps Darwin was a more profound prophet than we have realized when he said that the main trouble with mankind is not lack of ability, but failure to use those gifts with which we are already endowed. In order to use those gifts we need release from all sorts of physical and social handicaps.

Among those handicaps the climatic factor holds only a small place. Its position, however, is strategically important. It is the most ubiquitous of all the factors in our physical environment. We can never get away from the air that we breathe and the weather that greets us morning, noon, and night. Climate and weather are also the most variable of all the factors of physical environment. Nowhere is the air at night the same as by day. Nowhere is every day exactly like every other. Everywhere there is some difference between one season and another. In many lands the contrasts between the weather of one season and another, or even between that of one day and another, are extreme. And in most parts of the earth it is hard to travel more than a few hundred miles without noting some difference in climate. Moreover, climate and weather also exert a profound influence upon other factors such as diet, occupations, and recreation.

It is desirable to emphasize the importance of climate for still another reason. It has been much neglected, especially in comparison with the marvelous biological discoveries which stem from Pasteur's germ theory and the genes to which Mendel introduced us. This neglect is beginning to be realized. Therefore it seems not improbable that the next few decades may see a rapid growth in our knowledge of the influence of physical environment. When we understand the effect of physical environment as well as we now understand parasitic diseases, the result may be as surprising as the conquests of modern medicine and hygiene have been.

Here we must bring this book to a close. We are tempted, indeed, to bridge the long gap between the original evolution of *Homo sapiens* under the impact of a specific type of climate, and his present life in climates to which he is not perfectly adjusted. If we did this we should find that the whole history of civilization may be interpreted as a prolonged and unconscious effort of man to readjust himself to climate. His primitive and apparently perfect adjustment was roughly shattered by the great climatic changes which accompanied the waning of the ice age. Since then he has been living in climates which depart in one way or another from the ideal. A curious conflict has taken place between the impulses arising from the two diverse optima. The feelings of comfort associated with the physical optimum, and the relaxation due to temperatures above the optimum, have made people enjoy warm countries. These same conditions, however, have caused people to relax, and to make relatively feeble efforts to overcome the forces of nature. Moreover, people's minds are not subject to the same periodical stimulus which is received where the temperature falls to the mental optimum.

In cooler lands, on the other hand, this stimulus and the fact that the unpleasant effects of low temperature can best be overcome by energetic action have fostered human progress. There, however, man's health has suffered until he learned the arts that provide good clothing, shelter, warmth, and dryness. Thus a tendency for the centers of civilization to move northward and oceanward has been one of the main facts in the history of civilization, but this has been retarded because of the slow progress of mechanical inventions.

If we should attempt a sketch of the history of civilization, we should immediately find that, although the climatic phase is much more important than is usually recognized, it is only one among many. The path of progress has been influenced not only by the air that man breathes, but by the soil beneath his feet, the waters that ebb and flow, the mountains that block his path, the minerals that lie in their depths, and the swarming plants and animals of the land, the air, and the water. This would by no means end the matter, for we should have to face the question of the innate qualities of different groups of people. Is there any such thing as racial differences in mental aptitudes? Does a process of selection lead to innate differences between such groups as nomads on the one hand, and urban laborers on the other? Have such differences influenced history? Even when we have discussed these difficult topics, we have left untouched the major part of the field usually covered in studies of civilization. Man's progress from the old stone age onward may properly be interpreted in terms of the extent and kind of tools and implements which he has invented as a substitute for the slow changes in bodily form which were the main feature in the evolution of animals. Or again, the whole course of human evolution since the great change which produced *Homo sapiens* has been toward a type of life in which purely physical activities have gradually become dominated by the intellectual, artistic, and ethical aspects of life.

In such a sketch of civilization, still other aspects would at once forge to the front, for civilization is the most complex of all the phenomena with which the scientist has to deal. It is the most complex because it depends upon everything else from chemistry to psychology. Therefore we must leave the great interval between the first development of *Homo sapiens* and his modern attempts at self-improvement for another book. The aim of the present book has been merely to set forth certain facts as to season of birth and climate. From these facts we have concluded that our species inherits a marvelous and highly delicate adjustment to climate, and that this adjustment enters into practically every human problem. It enters into all phases of life because it influences us every moment from the time when the germ cells of our parents first become entities until we finish our allotted span of life.

APPENDIX A

CONTRIBUTORS OF STATISTICAL
MATERIAL USED IN THIS BOOK

CONNECTICUT

Dr. *Charles T. La Moure*, Mansfield State Training School, Mansfield Depot, Connecticut.

INDIANA

Dr. *O. J. Breidenbaugh*, Director of Research, Indiana Boys School, Plainfield, Indiana.

Dr. *L. P. Harshman*, Fort Wayne State School, Fort Wayne, Indiana.

Dr. *J. V. Pace*, Superintendent of Indiana State Sanatorium, Rockville, Indiana.

MARYLAND

Dr. *W. Therber Fales*, Director of Bureau of Vital Statistics, Health Department, Baltimore, Maryland.

Dr. *A. W. Hedrich*, State Department of Health, 2411 North Charles Street, Baltimore, Maryland.

Dr. *G. H. Preston*, Commissioner of Mental Hygiene, State of Maryland, 330 North Charles Street, Baltimore, Maryland.

MASSACHUSETTS

Professor *David L. Belding*, Boston University School of Medicine, 80 East Concord Street, Boston, Massachusetts.

Dr. *Neil A. Dayton*, Director of Statistics and Research, Department of Mental Hygiene, State House, Boston, Massachusetts.

Dr. *Roy D. Halloran*, Superintendent, Metropolitan State Hospital, Waltham, Massachusetts.

MICHIGAN

American Legion Hospital, Battle Creek, Michigan.

Miss *Anna I. Austen*, Director of Social Service, Newberry State Hospital, Newberry, Michigan.

Dr. *R. L. Dixon*, Superintendent of Michigan Home and Training School, Lapeer, Michigan.

Dr. *George F. Inch*, Superintendent of Ypsilanti State Hospital, Ypsilanti, Michigan.

Dr. *H. M. Pollard*, University of Michigan, Ann Arbor, Michigan.

Dr. *Perry V. Wagley*, Superintendent of Pontiac State Hospital, Pontiac, Michigan.

MINNESOTA

Dr. *Herbert A. Burns*, Superintendent of Minnesota State Sanatorium, Ah-gwah-ching, Minnesota.

Dr. *M. W. Kemp*, Superintendent of Anoka State Asylum, Anoka, Minnesota.

Dr. D. E. McBroom, Superintendent of Minnesota Colony for Epileptics, Cambridge, Minnesota.

Dr. J. M. Murdoch, Superintendent of School for Feebleminded, Faribault, Minnesota.

Dr. W. L. Patterson, Superintendent of Fergus Falls State Hospital, Fergus Falls, Minnesota.

Dr. B. F. Smith, Superintendent of Rochester State Hospital, Rochester, Minnesota.

MISSISSIPPI

Dr. R. N. Whitfield, Director of Vital Statistics, State Board of Health, Jackson, Mississippi.

NEW JERSEY

Mr. William J. Ellis, Commissioner, Department of Institutions and Agencies, State of New Jersey, Trenton, New Jersey.

Dr. Emil Frankel, Director of Division of Statistics and Research, State Department of Institutions and Agencies, Trenton, New Jersey.

NEW YORK

Dr. R. E. Blaisdell, Medical Superintendent of Rockland State Hospital, Orangeburg, New York.

Dr. Louis I. Dublin, Metropolitan Life Insurance Company, New York City.

Dr. William Jansen, Board of Education, 500 Park Avenue, New York City.

Dr. C. G. McGaffin, New York City Children's Hospital, 65-30 Kissena Boulevard, Flushing, Long Island.

Dr. Benjamin Malzberg, Department of Mental Hygiene, State House, Albany, New York.

Dr. Charles S. Parker, Superintendent of Kings Park State Hospital, Kings Park, New York.

Dr. David J. Swartz, 900 Grand Concourse, New York City.

OHIO

Mrs. Margaret M. Allman, Director of Department of Public Welfare, State Office Building, Columbus, Ohio.

Dr. R. E. Bushong, Superintendent of The Lima State Hospital, Lima, Ohio.

Dr. Frank Notestein, Milbank Memorial Fund, 40 Wall Street, New York City. (Princeton University, Princeton, N. J.).

PENNSYLVANIA

Dr. Helen D. King, Wistar Institute, Philadelphia, Pennsylvania.

Dr. Henry I. Klopp, Superintendent of Allentown State Hospital, Allentown, Pennsylvania.

TENNESSEE

Dr. W. C. Williams, State Department of Public Health, Nashville, Tennessee.

VIRGINIA

Miss Estelle Marks, Bureau of Vital Statistics, State House, Richmond, Virginia.

APPENDIX B

BIBLIOGRAPHY

This bibliography does not pretend to be complete. It includes little except publications which have been referred to in the preceding text, and hence omits many others which are of much value. It also omits three types of books which have been used in large numbers: (1) standard books of the *Who's Who* or biographical type, (2) government publications containing statistics, and (3) genealogical books.

ALTER, W. VON. 1930. *Archiv für Soziale Hygiene und Demographie.* N.S. 5: 508-509. December.

ALLEN, F. J. 1922. Nature. 110: 40.

ALMQUIST, J. A. 1918. *Svenskt biografiskt lexikon.* Stockholm.

AMALDI, PAOLO. 1928. *Revista sperimentale de frenetrie e medicine legale delle alienazioni mentale.* 3: 466-467. "Steti affettivi delle psicosi manizco-depressive e ritmo stagionade."

AMMANN, R. 1914. "Untersuchungen über die Veränderung in der Häufigkeit der epiletischen Anfälle und deren Ursachen." *Zeit f. d. ger. Neurol. u. Psych.* 24: 617-663.

ARCTOWSKI, H. 1935. Publication of the Geographical Institute of the University of Lwow, Poland.

BALFOUR, A. 1923. "Sojourners in the Tropics and Problems of Acclimatization." *The Lancet.* 204: 1329-1334; 205: 84-87; 243-247.

BELDING, D. L. 1937. Personal communication.

BERLINER, B. 1914. *Der Einfluss von Klima, Wetter und Jahreszeit auf das Nerven- und Seelenleben, auf physiologischer Grundlage dargestellt.* Wiesbaden.

BESSON, M. LOUIS. 1935. *Annales des services techniques d'hygiène de la ville de Paris.* 16: Météorologie. Paris (Gauthier-Villars, Editeur). "Influence de la température et de la saison sur la mortalite à Paris." See also: Vol. 2 (1921) and 6 (1925).

BISSONNETTE, THOMAS HUME. 1936. "Sexual Photoperiodicity." *Jour. Heredity.* 27. 1936.

BIVINGS, LEE. 1933. "Preconceptual and Prenatal Influences Affecting the New Born." *Jour. Amer. Medical Assoc.* 101: No. 22. p. 1703.

——1934. "Racial Geog. Annual and Seasonal Variations in Birth Weights." *Am. Jour. Obstetrics and Gynecology.* 27: 725-728.

—— 1908. *Tropical Medicine.* London.

BLONSKY, P. P. 1929. "Früh und Spätjahrkinder." *Jahrbuch für Kinderheilkunde.* Vol. 124.

BLUM, KURT. 1932. "Über die Abhängigkeit psychischer und nervöser Störungen von atmosphärischen Einflüssen." *Archiv für Psychiatrie und Nervenkrankheiten,* 96: 171-196.

BONFIGLIO, LUIGI. 1935. "L'alienozione mentale nel Polesine nel quinquerinic 1930-34." *Note e riveste di psichiatrie.*

BRAUN, KARIAN. 1927. (Aug.) Feriska Lakareselskopetz Handlinger. Finland.

CAMPBELL, DAME JANET. 1929. *Infant Mortality Reports on Public Health and Medical Subjects No. 55.* London.

CASTLE, W. E. 1931. *Genetics and Eugenics.* 4th ed. Cambridge.

CATTELL, J. McKEEN. 1903. "1000 Most Eminent Men and Women." *Popular Science Monthly.*

CURINIER, C. E. 1899. *National des contemporains.* Paris.

CHILD, CHAS. G. 1922. *Sterility and Conception.* New York.

DAYTON, NEIL A. 1930. "Size of Family and Birth Order in Mental Disease." *Publication of the Am. Sociol. Soc.* Vol. XXIV. No. 2. May. pp. 123-137.

—— 1931. "Mortality in Mental Deficiency over a Fourteen Year Period: Analysis of 8,976 Cases and 878 Deaths in Massachusetts." *Proceedings of the Fifty-fifth Annual Session of the American Association for the Study of the Feebleminded held at New York, May 25-28.* pp. 127-212.

DONCASTER, L. 1914. *The Determination of Sex.* Cambridge.

DUNCAN, J. M. 1871. *Fecundity, Fertility, and Sterility.*

DURKHEIM. 1907. *Le Suicide.*

DUSING, C. 1884. *Die Regulierung des Geschlechtsverhältnisses bei der Vermehrung der Menschen, Thiere, und Pflanzen.* Jena. Or, *Jen. Zeitsch. f. Naturw.* XVII.

ELLIS, HAVELOCK. 1914. *Man and Woman.* New York.

—— 1916. *The Criminal.* New York.

—— 1927 and 1904. *A Study of British Genius.* London.

—— 1934. *Psychology of Sex.* New York.

ESQUIROL, E. 1845. (Trans. from the French edition of 1834 by E. K. Hunt.) *A Treatise on Insanity.* Philadelphia.

GEDDES, PATRICK, and THOMSON, J. A. 1890. *Evolution of Sex.* New York.

GINI, C. 1912. "Contributi statistici ai problem dell'eugenica." *Estratto dalla Rivista Italiana di Sociologia.* Anno XVI. Fasc. III-IV.

—— 1934. "Su la portata e gli effetti delle false denuncie di nascita per i nati denunciati al principio dell'anno." Extrait du *Bulletin de l'Institut International de Statistique.* Tome XXVII. La Haye.

GRENLICH, W. W. 1931. "The Sex Ratio among Human Stillbirths." *Science.* 74: 53-54.

HEAPE, W. 1907. "Note on the Influence of Extraneous Forces upon the Proportion of the Sexes Produced by Canaries." *Proc. Camb. Philosoph. Soc.* XIV.

—— 1907. "Notes on the Proportion of the Sexes in Dogs." *Proc. Camp. Philosoph. Soc.* XIV.

—— 1909. "The Proportion of the Sexes Produced by Whites and Colored Peoples in Cuba." *Phil. Trans. Roy. Soc. B 200. Proc. Roy. Soc. B 81.*

HELLPACH, W. *Die geopsychischen Erscheinungen. Wetter, Klima und Landschaft in ihrem Einfluss aus das Seelenleben.* Leipzig. Verlag von Wilhelm Engelmann. 1911, 1928.

HILLIS, D. S. 1924. "Experience with 1000 Cases of Abortion." *Surg. Gyn. Obs.* 38: 83-87.

HOCHE, A. 1910. *Geisteskrankheit und Kultur.* Freiburg.

HOLMES, S. J., and GOFF, J. C. 1923. "Selective Elimination of Male Infants under Different Environmental Influences in Eugenics in Race and State." Vol. II. pp. 247-48.

—— 1936. *Human Genetics and Its Social Import.* New York.

HAYCRAFT, J. B. 1895. *Darwinism and Race Progress.* London.

HUNTINGTON, ELLSWORTH. 1919. *World Power and Evolution.* New Haven.

—— 1920. "Air Control and the Reduction of the Death Rate after Operations." Parts I and II. *The Modern Hospital.* Vol. XIV. No. 1. pp. 10-16 and 111-114.

HUNTINGTON, ELLSWORTH. 1921. "The Relation of Health to Racial Capacity: The Example of Mexico." *Geographical Review*. April, pp. 243-264.

—— 1924. *Civilization and Climate*. 3rd ed. New Haven.

—— 1930. "Weather and Health." *Bulletin of the National Research Council No. 75*. Washington, D. C.

—— 1932. *The Ebb and Flow of Human Population*. Rome.

—— 1933. *Economic and Social Geography*. New York.

—— 1935. "Climatic Pulsations." *Hyllningsskrift Tillagnad Sven Hedin*. Stockholm.

—— and RAGSDALE, MARTHA. 1935. *After Three Centuries*. Baltimore.

HUBBARD, S. D. 1918. "Abortion in New York City." *Mo. Bull. Dep. Health*. New York City. pp. 207-210.

IRELAND, ALLEYNE. 1925. "The Month of Your Son's Birth." *Hearst's International*. May.

ISACHSEN, LOUISE. 1911. Orn Periodiske Svingninger i Blodets Sammensaetning. *Archiv. for Mathematik og Naturvidenskab*. Vol. XXXII.

JASTRZEBSKI, S. 1929. Article on Sex Ratios: Encyclopædia Britannica, 14th ed.

KAMMERER, P. 1924. *The Inheritance of Acquired Characteristics*.

KASSEL, CHARLES. 1929. "Birth-Months of Genius." *The Open Court*. Vol. XLIII (No. 11). November. Chicago.

KENDREW, W. G. 1922. *The Climate of the Continents*. 1st ed.

KING, HELEN DEAN. 1927. "Seasonal Variations in Fertility and in the Sex Ratio of Mammals, with Special Reference to the Rat." Sonderdruck aus Wilhelm Roux' *Archiv für Entwicklungsmechanik der Organismen*. Berlin.

—— 1937. Personal communication.

KOLLIBAY-UTER, HANNA. 1921. "Über die Jahreskurve geistiger Erkrankungen." *Ztschr. f. d. ges. Neurol. u. Psychiat.* Berlin.

KOPP, MARIE E. 1934. *Birth Control in Practice*. New York.

KRÜGER, HERMANN A. 1914. Deutsches Literatur-lexikon. München.

LEAGUE OF NATIONS HEALTH ORGANIZATION. Memorandum Relating to the "Enquiries into the Causes and Prevention of Stillbirths" and "Mortality during the First Year of Life." Geneva, 1930.

LEE, J. B. 1933. *Principles and Practice of Obstetrics*. Philadelphia.

LEHMANN, ALFRED, and PEDERSEN, R. H. 1907. *Das Wetter und unsere Arbeit*. Leipzig.

LINDHARD, J. 1912. The Seasonal Periodicity in Respiration. Skand. *Archiv. f. Physiologie*. Vol. XXVI.

LOMBROSO, CESARE. 1895. *Man of Genius*. London.

—— 1911. *Crime: Its Causes and Remedies*. Boston.

LOOFT, CARE. 1934. "Les enfants printaniers et les enfants d'automne, leur évolution d'intelligence." *Acta Pediatrica*. Upsala. 15: 381-395.

LORIMER, F., and OSBORN, F. 1934. *Dynamics of Population*. New York.

MADSEN, T. J. M. 1930. The Seasonal Variations of Infectious Diseases. *Public Health*. July.

MALINS, EDW. 1903. "Some Aspects of the Economic and of the Antenatal Waste of Life in Nature and Civilization." *Jour. Obstetrics and Gynaecology of the British Empire*. 103. 3: 307-319. Presidential address.

MALL, FRANKLIN P. 1908. *A Study of the Causes Underlying the Origin of Human Monsters*. Philadelphia.

—— 1917. "On the Frequency of Localized Anomalies in Human Embryos and Infants at Birth." *Am. Jour. Anat.* 22: 49-72. Baltimore.

MALZBERG, B. 1935. "A Statistical Study of Age in Relation to Mental Disease." *Mental Hygiene.* 19: 449-476.

MARTIN, C. P. 1937. Temporary Heredity and the Mechanism of Adaptation. *American Naturalist.* Vol. LXXI.

MAYR, G. V. 1924. *Statistik und Gesellschaftslehre Verlag Mohr.* Tübingen.

MEIER, E. 1922. "Die periodischen Jahresschwankungen der Internierung Geisteskranker." *Diss. and Z. Neur.* 76: 479.

MILLS, C. A. 1928. "Functional Insufficiency of the Suprarenal Glands." *Archives of Internal Medicine.* 42: 390-408.

—— and SENIOR, MRS. F. A. 1930. "Does Climate Affect the Human Conception Rate?" *Archives of Internal Medicine.* 46: 921-929. Chicago.

—— 1930. "Diabetes Mellitus. Is Climate a Responsible Factor in the Etiology?" *Archives of Internal Medicine.* 46: 569-581.

—— 1930. "Influence of Climate on Human Organism as Evidenced by the Death Rate from Certain Disease, and by Conception Rate." *Ohio Jour. Science.* 30: No. 4. Columbus, Ohio.

—— 1932. "Geographic Variations in the Female Sexual Functions." *Am. Jour. Hyg.* March.

—— 1933. (OGLE, CORDELIA, and ——) "Adaptation of Sexual Activity to Environmental Stimulation." *Am. Jour. Phys.* 105: 76.

—— 1934. *Living with the Weather.* Cincinnati.

—— 1934. "Suicides and Homicides in Their Relation to Weather Changes." *Am. Jour. Psych.* November.

MORGAN, T. H. 1914. *Heredity and Sex.* New York.

—— 1934. *Embryology and Genetics.* New York.

MURPHY, D. P. 1936. "The Month of Conception of 935 Congenitally Malformed Individuals." *Am. Jour. Obstetrics and Gynecology.* 31: No. 1, p. 106.

—— and MAZER, MILTON. 1935. "The Birth Order of 582 Malformed Individuals." *Jour. Am. Medical Assn.* 105: 849-851.

NINOMIYA, TSUKASA. 1934. "Is the Seasonal Fluctuation of Fecundity an Immanent Characteristic for Each Human Race?" *Jour. Chosen Medical Assn.* 24: 67-68.

NORBURY, FRANK P. 1924. "Seasonal Curves in Mental Disorders." *Medical Jour. and Record.* 119: pp. LXXXI-LXXXV.

PEARL, RAYMOND. 1930. "Requirements of Proof that Natural Selection Has Altered a Race." *Scientific.* 47: 175-186.

—— and RUTH PEARL. 1934. *The Ancestry of the Long-Lived.* Baltimore.

PETERSEN, W. F. 1934. "The Seasonal Trend in the Conception of Malformations." *Am. Jour. Obstet. and Gynecology.* 28: 443-444.

—— 1935. *The Patient and the Weather.* Vol. I. Part I and II. Michigan.

—— 1936. Personal communications.

PINTER, RUDOLPH. 1931. *Intelligence Testing.* New York.

—— and GEORGE FORLANO. 1933. "The Influence of Month of Birth on Intelligence Quotients." *Jour. Educational Psychology.* 24: 561-584.

PLOETZ, ALFRED. 1922. "Vitality of Children" (birth rank). *World Almanac.*

REYNOLDS, EDWARD. 1911. "Fertility and Sterility." *Jour. Am. Med. Assoc.* Vol. LXVII.

—— and MACOMBER, D. 1921-22. *Am. Jour. Obstetrics and Gynecology.* "Certain Dietary Factors in the Causation of Sterility in Rats." *Am. Jour. Obstet.* 11: 379-394.

ROBERTS, E. J. 1930. "Some Observations on the Secondary Sex Ratio in a Group of Dairy Shorthorn and Welsh Black Cattle." *Jour. Agric. Science.* 20: 359-363.

ROBINSON, A., and BARKER, J. R. 1929-30. "Discussion on Causes of Early Abortion and Sterility." *Proc. Med. Soc.* 23: 2-17. (Sect. Obst., gyn., and comp. med.)

ROBINSON, CAROLINE H. 1930. *Seventy Birth Control Clinics.* Baltimore.

ROESLE, E. 1930. "Seasonal Aspect of Conception and Birth." *Archiv für Soziale Hygiene und Demographie.* N.S. 5: 509-510.

ROGERS, J. F. 1926. "Genius and Health." *Sci. Mon.* 23: 509-18.

ROSSMAN, J. 1929. *Journ. of the Patent Office Society.* Vol. II. pp. 99-103.

ROWAN, WILLIAM. 1931. *The Riddle of Migration.* Baltimore.

RUDDER, B. DE. 1931. *Wetter and Jahrzeit als Krankheitfaktoren.* Berlin.

SCHULTZ, ADOLPH H. "Sex Incidence in Abortions." *Carnegie Inst. Publication.* No. 275.

SCHULER, EDGAR A. 1930. "The Relationship of Birth Order and Fraternal Position to Incidence of Insanity." *Am. Jour. Sociology.* 36: 28-40.

STANDER, H. J. *Williams' Obstetrics.* 7th ed. New York.

STEIGER, L. V. A. 1929. "Der jahreszeitliche Verlauf der Geburten in europäischen regierenden Fürstenhäusern des 19 Jahrhunderts." (Seasonal Aspect of Births in European Reigning Families). *Archiv für Soziale Hygiene und Demographie.* 4: 382-390.

STIX, R. K. 1935. "A Study of Pregnancy Wastage." *Millbank Memorial Fund Quarterly.* 13: 347-366.

STOCKARD, CHARLES R. 1921. *Development Rate and Structural Expression; An experimental study of Twins, Double Monsters and Single Deformities, etc.* Philadelphia. Or, *Am. Jour, Anat.* 1921. 28: 115-266.

SUNDSTROEM, E. S. 1926. "Contributions to Tropical Physiology." *Univ. Calif. Pub. in Physiol.* 6: 1-216.

TAUSSIG, FREDERICK J. 1936. *Abortion, Spontaneous and Induced.* St. Louis.

TITUS, PAUL. 1912. "A Statistical Study of a Series of Abortions." *Am. Jour. Obstet.* 65: 960-980.

——— 1925. "A Statistical Study of Abortions Occurring in the Obst. Dept. of the Johns Hopkins Hospital." *Am. Jour. Obstet.* 12: 960-80.

TOWER, W. L. 1906. *An Investigation of the Evolution in Chrysomelid Beetles of the Genus Leptinotarsa.* Carnegie Pub. Washington, D. C.

VON ALTER. *See* Alter.

WESTERMARCK, E. A. 1921. *History of Human Marriage.* New York.

WESTPHAL, H. 1911. *Geistenskrankheiten und Sahreszeiten.* Inaug. diss. Freiburg.

WETZEL, A. 1922. "Das Weltuntergangserlebnis in der Schizophrenie." *Ztschr. f. d. ges. Neurol. u. Psychiat.* Berlin.

——— G. 1896. "Beitrag zum Studien Kunstlichen Doppel-Missbildungen bei Rana fusca." Diss. Berlin.

——— G. 1895. "Uber die Bedeutung der Cirkularen Furche in der Entwicklung der schultzelschen Doppelbildungen von Rana fusca." *Arch. mikr. Anat.,* XLVI.

WHITNEY, LEON F. 1927. "The Mating Cycle of the Dog. *Chase Magazine.*

WILMANNS, K. 1920. "Über die Zunahme des Ausbruchs geistiger Störungen in den Frühjahrs und Sommermonaten." *Münch. med. Wschr.* 67: 175-177.

WINSTON, S. 1931. "The Influence of Social Factors upon the Sex-Ratio at Birth." *Am. Jour. Sociology,* Vol. 37.

WOODBURY, ROBERT MORSE. 1922. "Infant Mortality and Preventive Work in New Zealand." U. S. Dept. of Labor. Children's Bureau No. 105. Washington.

—— 1925. "Causal Factors in Infant Mortality." U. S. Department of Labor. Children's Bureau No. 142. Washington.

YAGI, TAKATUGU. 1933. *Studies on the Output Curve.* Kurasiki.

YAGLOGLOU, C. B., and MILLER, W. E. 1925. "Effective Temperature with Clothing." *J. Am. Soc. of Heat. Vent. Eng.* 31: 69-70.

YAGLOU, C. P. 1926. "The Thermal Index of Atmospheric Conditions and Its Application to Sedentary and to Industrial Life." *J. Indus. Hyg.* 8: 5.

—— 1927. "The Comfort Zone for Men at Rest and Stripped to the Waist." *Jour. Indus. Hyg.* 9: 251.

—— 1927. "Temperature, Humidity and Air Movement in Industries. The Effective Temperature Index." *Jour. Indus. Hyg.* 9: 297.

—— 1928. "The Summer Comfort Zone, Climate and Clothing." *Jour. Indus. Hyg.* 10: 350.

YERKES, ROBERT M. *see:* TAUSSIG, F. F. 1936. *Abortion Spontaneous and Induced.* pp. 68, 69.

INDEX

Asterisks indicate illustrations

A

Abnormal and insane, 388-416
Abortions, 47 ff., 225, 243 (table);
Negro, 220, 239; pregnancy, 203
(table); sex ratio, 193, 202, 227,
241; spontaneous, 203, 228 (table)
Actors, social level, 339
Adaptation to climate, 287; infants,
422; reproductive period, 423;
summers, 281
Afghanistan, 433
Africa: Central, 372; South, *see* South
Africa
After Three Centuries, 294
Age: and leaders, 297; mental de-
rangement, 412, 413*; of mother,
225, 231; reproductive and health,
283; and weather, 271, *see* Longevity
Agricultural labor, 79; Japanese, 85
Agriculture: and births, 138; and
migration, 79
Ahaggar plateau, 435
Akhenaton, 297
Alabama, 405*
Alicante, 147 ff., 148*
Allen, F. J., 453
Allman, Mrs. Margaret M., 452
Almquist, J. A., 453
Alter, W. von, 337, 453
Amaldi, Paolo, 414, 453
American Astrological Society, 358
American families, longevity and
death rate, 233*
American leaders, source of, 319
American Legion Hospital, 451
American Men of Science, 5, 313 f.
American scientists, 313, 314*
American stock, birth, 299, 300*
*American Women, the Official Who's
Who*, 319
Americans, genius and season, 346

Ammann, R., 409, 410, 453
Animal rhythm, *see* Basic animal
rhythm
Annapolis, 379
Annual rhythm, *see* Basic animal
rhythm
Arabia, 435
Arctowski, H., 8, 453
Argentina, 431; births, 154*
Aristocracy, births, 332
Artists, 320, 329; in Britain, 353; sea-
son of birth, 317; social level, 339;
in Sweden, 364
Astrakan, 63
Astrology, 26
Athletes, 322 f.
Atlas Mountains, 433
Atmosphere and man, 373
Atmospheric electricity, 375
Atmospheric humidity, 375, 429
Atmospheric pressure, 274; and con-
ceptions, 39 f.
Austen, Miss Anna I., 451
Australia, 438; births, 154*; first
births, 47*, 48, 221; longevity, 187;
sex ratio, 211; white, 190
Austria: births, 99*, 140; Jews, 215;
sex ratio, 215, 250*, 253
Authors, season of birth, 359*
Automobiles and births, 132
Autumn stimulus, 93, 117, 127, 143, 340

B

Baden, 409*, 411
Bahia Blanca, 431
Bakersfield, 125
Balfour, A., 23, 453
Baltimore, 405, 405*
Bankers, season of birth, 359*
Barcelona, 147 ff., 148*, 366
Barker, J. R., 457
Barometric pressure, 381, 389

459